# ATLAS OF Living and Surface Anatomy for Sports Medicine

*Senior Commissioning Editor:* Sarena Wolfaard
*Associate Editor:* Claire Bonnett/Claire Wilson
*Project Manager:* Frances Affleck
*Designer:* Charles Gray
*Illustrator:* Ethan Danielson
*Illustration Manager:* Gillian Richards

# ATLAS OF Living and Surface Anatomy for Sports Medicine

**Philip F Harris** MD, MSc, MBChB
Visiting Professor, Centre for Sports Medicine, Queen's Medical Centre, University of Nottingham Medical School, Nottingham, UK

**Craig Ranson** BSc, PGDip
England and Wales Cricket Board Lead Physiotherapist
Special Lecturer in Sports and Exercise Medicine, Centre for Sports Medicine, Queen's Medical Centre, University of Nottingham Medical School, Nottingham, UK

CHURCHILL LIVINGSTONE
ELSEVIER

Edinburgh London New York Oxford Philadelphia St Louis Sydney Toronto 2008

CHURCHILL
LIVINGSTONE
ELSEVIER

CHURCHILL LIVINGSTONE
An imprint of Elsevier Limited



First published 2008

ISBN-13: 978-0-443-10316-2

**British Library Cataloguing in Publication Data**
A catalogue record for this book is available from the British Library

**Library of Congress Cataloging in Publication Data**
A catalog record for this book is available from the Library of Congress

**Note**
Neither the Publisher nor the Authors assume any responsibility for any loss or injury and/or damage to persons or property arising out of or related to any use of the material contained in this book. It is the responsibility of the treating practitioner, relying on independent expertise and knowledge of the patient, to determine the best treatment and method of application for the patient.

*The Publisher*



Printed in China

# Contents

The DVD-Rom accompanying this text includes video sequences indicated in the text by the DVD icon. To look at the videos, click on the relevant icon in the contents list on the DVD-Rom. The disc is designed to be used in conjunction with the text and not as a stand-alone product.

# Foreword

The publication of this book is timely as Sport and Exercise Medicine now emerges as a fully recognized and discrete specialty of medicine. This book will appeal not only to trainees in Sport and Exercise Medicine (both those with a special interest and those pursuing full-time training) but additionally to practitioners in many other specialties including Orthopedics, Rheumatology and General Practice. It will be of value to a wide variety of others, including medical students, physiotherapists, osteopaths, and other allied healthcare professionals.

The authors have cleverly spliced together marked prosections with living anatomy and cross-sectional imaging to produce an extremely readable and useful text focusing on living anatomy and physical examination. It will have particular use for those involved in clinical practice, and indeed each chapter finishes with some clinical problems.

Sport and Exercise Medicine and Physiotherapy and many other specialties of medicine are founded upon a good grasp of human anatomy. Linked to this knowledge is competency in physical examination and I believe this text will be of value to those wishing to improve their anatomy and physical examination skills. As such, this book will provide a valuable and important reference source.

Professor Mark E Batt
Consultant in Sport and Exercise Medicine
Centre for Sports Medicine
Nottingham University Hospitals
Nottingham, UK

# Preface

The production of this Atlas was prompted by experience of teaching the anatomy module for a Masters of Science in Sports and Exercise Medicine. All parts of the body are vulnerable to injury from the wide spectrum of sporting activities. A sound knowledge of the relevant anatomy is essential for effective clinical examination, accurate diagnosis, and appropriate treatment of sports injuries.

Whilst lectures highlighting significant structures, prosection and skeletal demonstrations, radiological images, and problem-solving all contribute to learning, sports medicine practice remains a very practical and "hands-on" discipline. Therefore a thorough working knowledge of relevant living and surface anatomy is of paramount importance.

In this Atlas we describe and illustrate techniques for the identification and palpation of important structures and landmarks in sports medicine, the testing of muscle actions, and the evaluation of joint movements. Also included are techniques commonly used in testing for particular injuries, together with a DVD to help the reader perfect the practice of these maneuvers. To assist interpretation of the living and surface features we thought it would be helpful to include a selection of relevant illustrations of parts of the skeleton, photographs of prosections, and pertinent radiological images. At the end of each chapter clinical problems are presented. These can be solved using knowledge gained from material in the chapter. Also included in each chapter is a short list of further reading presenting clinical reports relevant to the structures considered.

We hope the Atlas will be useful for all those involved in managing sports injuries.

PFH
CR
Nottingham
2008

# Acknowledgements

We would like to record our sincere thanks to the athletes and colleagues who volunteered to act as models for this Atlas: Sarah Jamieson, Dr. Elizabeth Ojelade, Dr. Cheow Peng Ooi, Jana Pittman, Helen Richardson, Brenton Rowe, William Sharman, Richard Smith, Christine Sturgess, Fiona Westwood, Philip Wilson. We thank them all.

We are most grateful to Dr. Peter Gregory for helpful comments and for reviewing Chapters 1 and 2, and to Mr. Jeffery Boyle for reviewing Chapter 8.

Dr. Rob Kerslake, Dr. Nick Peirce, and Professor Richard Harris kindly provided a number of radiographic images which have enhanced the content of the Atlas.

Special thanks are due to the staff of Loughborough University Media Services. The photographs of the models, the radiographic images, and the DVD testify to the high standard of their professional skills. In particular we thank Peter Allison, Chris Conway, Steve Ashurst, Jagjit Samra, and Philip Wilson.

Dr. Margaret Pratten and Professor Terry Mayhew generously allowed access to facilities in the Department of Human Anatomy, School of Biomedical Sciences, University of Nottingham Medical School.

We are very grateful for the guidance, advice, and quiet efficiency of our publishers Elsevier Limited enabling publication of this Atlas to progress smoothly to fruition. In particular we thank Sarena Wolfaard, Claire Bonnett, and Frances Affleck with whom it has been a pleasure to work.

CHAPTER 1

# Head and neck

## INTRODUCTION

The head and neck contain the brain and cervical cord, and therefore constitute one of the most vital and vulnerable regions of the body. The region consists of three parts: the upper neurocranium covered by the scalp and enclosing the brain, an anterior part comprising the face and jaws, and the neck linking the head with the thorax and root of the upper limb. The brain, with its covering of meninges together with the organs of special senses, is intimately related to the skull. Sports injuries to this part of the head may be catastrophic. Anteriorly, the face includes the prominence of the nose, the lips surrounding the mouth and gums, the mobile lower jaw and the fixed upper maxilla together with their associated teeth, the eyes partially protected within the orbits, and the soft tissues of the face and external ear. All are vulnerable to sports injuries.

The neck can be divided into two parts. Posteriorly, the spine encloses the cervical part of the spinal cord (see Ch. 2). Depending on the level of damage, quadriplegia or paraplegia may result from cord injury here. Anteriorly are soft tissue structures including the sterno-mastoid muscles, the pharynx (behind the nasal and buccal cavities, and the larynx), and the vital airway formed by the larynx and trachea. On each side of these midline structures are the carotid sheaths extending the whole length of the neck under cover of the sterno-mastoids and containing the main blood supply to the neck, mouth, face, scalp, and brain.

## INSPECTION OF NORMAL CONTOURS

- Malar
- Nasal
- Oral
- Mandible
- Sterno-mastoid
- Larynx

There are common basic contours but these are considerably influenced by racial and hereditary factors, and also by the amount of subcutaneous fat, particularly in the face and neck.

### HEAD CONTOURS

Viewed from **anteriorly** (Fig. 1.1a), the general contour of the head may be round, oval, or more gaunt and elongated. The overall **symmetry** should be noted. Asymmetry may result from trauma but minor degrees of asymmetry are normal. From the highest point (vertex), the contour curves downward and laterally, where it is interrupted by the auricles which protrude on each side of the head. Continuing downward from below the ears, the contours converge smoothly to the point of the chin. In front of the ear, the **malar eminence** produced by the underlying zygoma contributes to the contour. The frontal regions of the vault overhang the oval contours of the **orbits,** which are separated by the root of the nose. The **nasal contour** changes, increasing in prominence at the nostrils and nasal apertures. Irrespective of the general shape of the nose, the **nasal bridge** is straight and in the midline. Deviations may indicate trauma, present or past. Below the nose the philtrum of the upper lip separates it from the **oral (buccal) fissure** between the two lips. The angles of the mouth where the lips converge are symmetrical. Asymmetry in level may indicate facial paralysis.

Viewed from **laterally** (Fig. 1.1b), the profile curves downward and forward from the vertex to reach the prominence of the **glabella** between the two superciliary ridges above the orbits. Below this point the profile recedes slightly to the root of the nose **(nasion),** but then passes downward and forward along the bridge of the nose to its tip. From the lower lip the profile passes on to the prominence of the chin, which overlies the **mental protuberance** of the mandible. The mandibular profile varies. It can be excessively protruding (prognathus) or unduly recessive (epignathus). From the chin the **base of the mandible** forms a distinct contour separating the face from the neck and continues as far as the well-defined **angle of the mandible.** From the angle the **posterior border** of the ramus continues upward toward the lobule of the ear. In front of the ear the **zygomatic arch** produces a transverse contour extending forward into the fullness of the **malar eminence** of the cheek. Behind the ear the prominence of the **mastoid process** is visible. With the superior nuchal line it forms an arching contour leading backward to the nape of the neck. From the vertex the contour curves backward and downward to the external occipital protuberance at the nape.

### NECK CONTOURS

Body type significantly influences the contours of the neck. In the short, stocky, hypersthenic subject, especially if obese, the neck is short, merging abruptly into the upper thorax and shoulders. In the tall, asthenic subject the neck is long, in which case structures are more easily defined.

Viewed from **anteriorly** (Fig. 1.1a, and see Figs 4.2 and 4.18), the head contour descends vertically from the ear, but then inclines laterally to continue with the curvature of the shoulder. Passing medially from the shoulder toward the manubrium, the **clavicle** forms a distinct contour. Above it and limited by the lateral contour of the neck is the depression of the **supraclavicular fossa.** On each side of the neck, descending from the ear and converging toward the **manubrium,** are oblique contours produced by the underlying **sterno-mastoid muscles.** A midline depression immediately above the manubrium marks the **suprasternal notch,** and about 5 cm above this is the **laryngeal prominence** (Adam's apple).

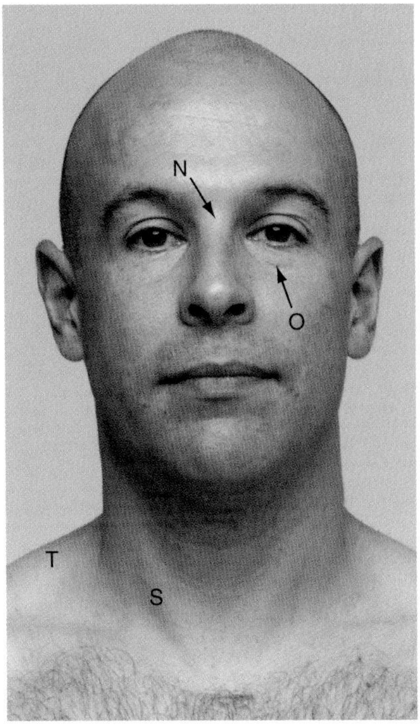


**Fig. 1.1a** Anterior contours of head and neck
Observe for symmetry or evidence of deformity and scars, especially the nose, ears, eyes, and mouth. N = nasion, O = inferior orbital margin, S = sterno-mastoid, T = trapezius

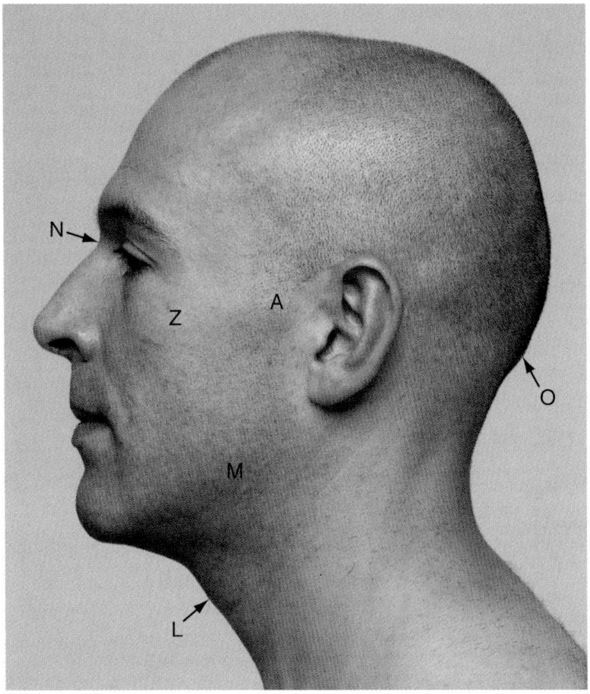


**Fig. 1.1b** Lateral contours of the head and neck
A = zygomatic arch, L = laryngeal prominence, M = body of mandible, N = nasion, O = external occipital protuberance, Z = zygoma

# LOCATING BONY LANDMARKS

- Nasal bones and aperture
- Orbital margin
- Infra-orbital foramen
- Mandible
- Zygomatic arch and zygoma
- Mastoid process
- External occipital protuberance
- Clavicle

Bony features of the skull are shown in Figure 1.2 and in radiographs in Figure 1.3.

## NOSE

With the subject seated and facing forward, the examiner locates the **root of the nose** (nasion, the junction of nasal bones with frontal) using the index finger tip. Then, opposing the pads of the thumb and index finger across the bridge of the subject's nose, the examiner draws them downward, feeling the **nasal bones,** until reaching the sharp, bony edges of the **anterior nasal aperture.** The thumb and index finger are then used to define the lateral margins (fronto-nasal process of maxilla) on each side of the aperture, diverging as they descend. Nasal fractures are the most common facial fracture, the nasal bones often being deviated and palpably displaced. These fractures are usually contact-related and can occur concurrently with fractures to the nasal process of the maxilla and frontal bone. Maxillary fractures (LeFort's) may be indicated by malocclusion of the teeth, and by maxillary mobility and deformity. The extent of the fracture line in LeFort's type 1, 2 and 3 fractures is shown in Figure 1.2b.

## ORBITAL MARGIN AND INFRA-ORBITAL FORAMEN

With the pad of the index finger, the sharp margins of the **orbital aperture** can be traced around its circumference, the mobile skin being easily moved across its bony edge. The **infra-orbital foramen** lies in a shallow depression

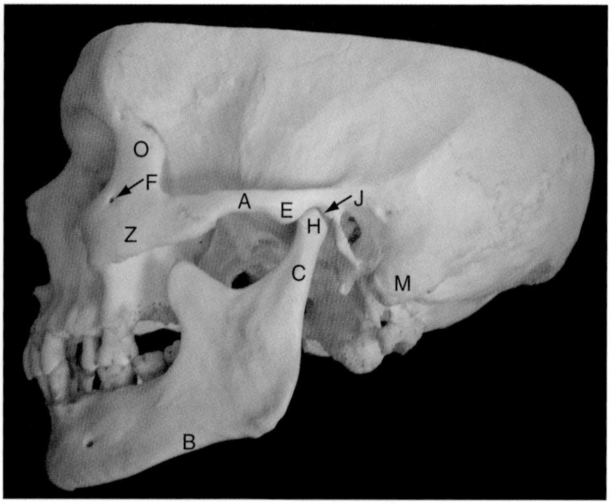


**Fig. 1.2a** Bony landmarks on the skull: lateral view
A = zygomatic arch, B = base of mandible, C = mandibular condyle, E = articular eminence (tuberosity), F = foramen for zygomatico-facial nerve, H = mandibular head, J = temporo-mandibular joint, M = mastoid process, O = frontal process of zygoma, Z = zygoma

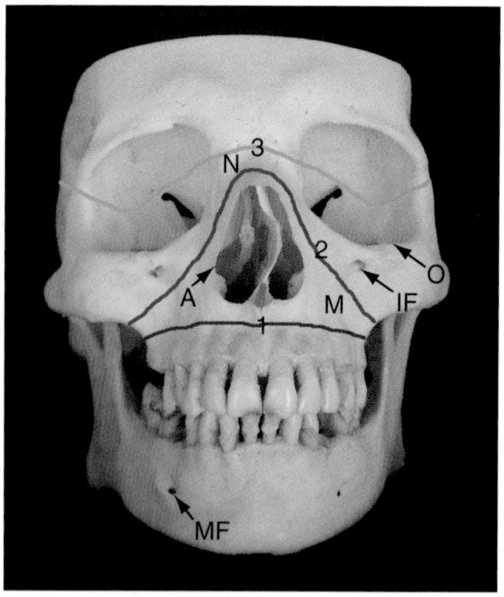


**Fig. 1.2b** Bony landmarks on the skull: frontal view and LeFort's classification of mid-facial fractures
A = anterior nasal aperture, IF = infra-orbital foramen, M = maxilla, MF = mental foramen, N = nasal bone, O = inferior orbital margin; 1 = grade 1 — LeFort fracture; 2 = grade 2; 3 = grade 3

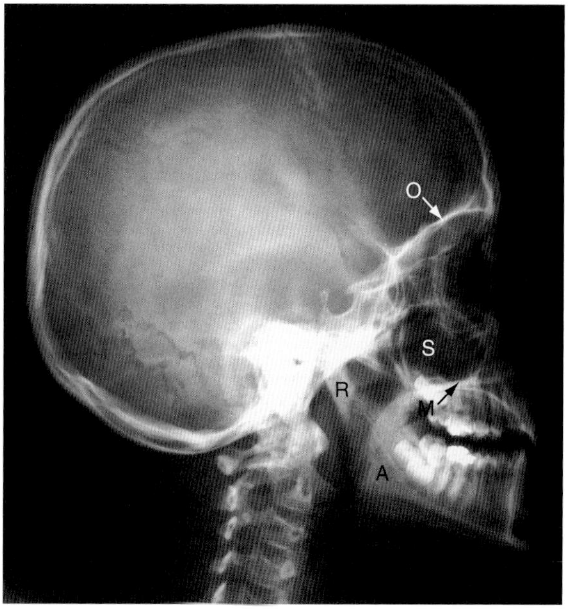


**Fig. 1.3a** Lateral X-radiograph of head
A = angle of mandible, M = hard palate (palatine process of maxilla), O = orbital roof (orbital plate of frontal), R = ramus of mandible, S = maxillary sinus

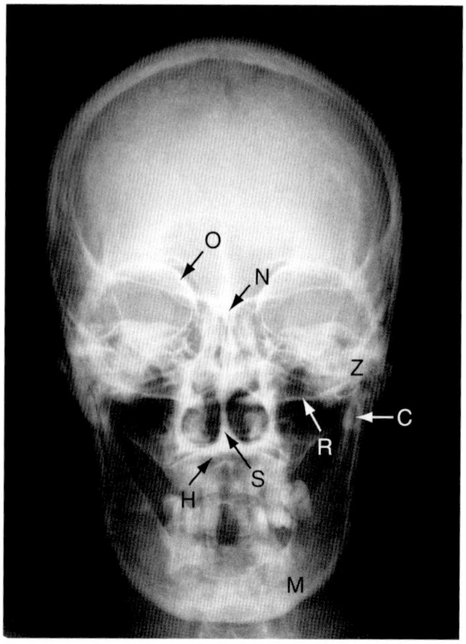


**Fig. 1.3b** Frontal X-radiograph of head
C = condyle of mandible, H = hard palate, M = body of mandible, N = nasion, O = superior orbital margin, R = roof of maxillary sinus (orbital floor), S = nasal septum, Z = zygoma

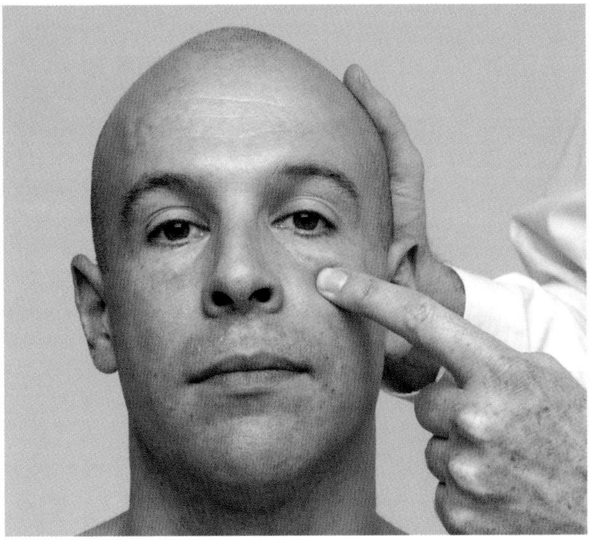

**Fig. 1.4** Locating the infra-orbital foramen

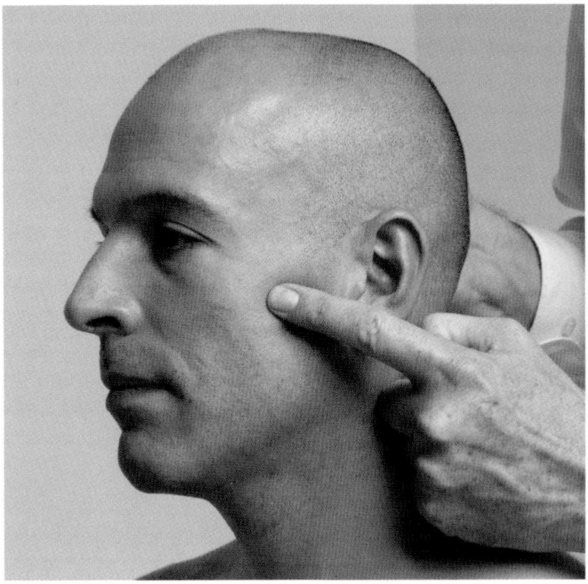

**Fig. 1.5** Palpating the zygoma and zygomatic arch

about a thumb's breadth below the midpoint of the lower orbital margin (Fig. 1.4). Deep pressure here is painful as the infra-orbital nerve is compressed. Certain ball sizes, especially squash, fit closely into the orbit and are renowned for causing orbit injuries.

## MANDIBLE

The prominent **angle** is easily located on the side of the face by rolling the tip of the index finger over it. From here the **base of the mandible** can be traced forward using firm pressure as far as the midline mental protuberance. Palpating upward from the angle, the finger can be rolled around the posterior edge of the **ramus.** Continuing upward toward the external ear, firm pressure against the back of the ramus may detect broadening into the **condylar process.** Mandibular fractures are most common at the angle and the condyle.

## ZYGOMATIC ARCH AND ZYGOMA

With the external auditory meatus as a guide, the examiner uses the pads of the middle and ring fingers to locate the **zygomatic arch,** sliding the fingers forward and rolling them across the arch to define the upper and lower borders. As the examiner continues forward, the arch is felt to expand into the prominence of the **zygoma** in the cheek. Its extent can be explored using the fingers in a massaging motion over it (Fig. 1.5). Edema over the zygoma, along with flattening or step deformities, may indicate fracture.

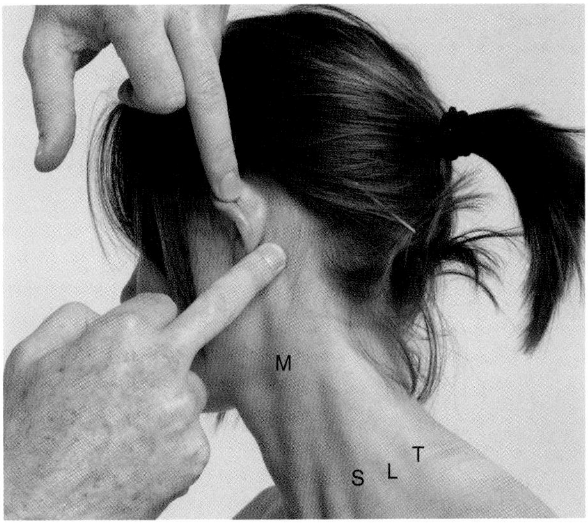


**Fig. 1.6** Locating the mastoid process
L = levator scapulae, M = sterno-mastoid, S = scalenes, T = trapezius

## MASTOID PROCESS AND EXTERNAL OCCIPITAL PROTUBERANCE

The examiner feels immediately behind the lobule of the ear with the finger tip to locate the mastoid process (Fig. 1.6), rolling it over its prominence. Keeping the finger applied firmly against the skull, the examiner guides it backward along an ill-defined, curved edge, the superior nuchal line, to reach the bony midline prominence of the **external occipital protuberance.**

## CLAVICLE

This marks the boundary between the root of the neck and the thorax. Its features are described in Chapter 4. Reconfirm that it can be palpated along its entire length from its lateral expanded end to its blunt medial end bordering the suprasternal notch.

# LOCATING SOFT TISSUES

- Parotid duct
- Laryngeal cartilages
- Scalp
- Eyelid and eye
- Ear
- Nose
- Teeth

In the living subject the soft tissues are examined by direct inspection and palpation. The subject sits or stands facing the examiner. Prosections of some relevant structures in the face are shown in Figure 1.7.

## PAROTID DUCT

A fullness, the parotid gland, may be visible below the zygomatic arch extending in front of the ear over the masseter muscle and covering the ramus of the mandible. Passing forward from the gland is the parotid duct. It is palpable where it winds round the anterior border of masseter to pass deeply into the mouth through the buccinator muscle. To define the duct the subject clenches the teeth to tense the masseter whilst the examiner draws the pad of a finger down the anterior border of the muscle to locate the duct about the midpoint between the zygomatic arch and the base of the mandible (Fig. 1.8). Facial lacerations below the level of the zygomatic arch may sever the duct.

## LARYNGEAL CARTILAGES AND TRACHEA

Two cartilages are palpable. The subject is seated or lies supine. Using the index finger, the examiner palpates in the midline from the chin downward to reach the prominent **thyroid angle (Adam's apple),** where the two laminae of the cartilage join. Continuing inferiorly, a **transverse groove** can be felt immediately below the thyroid cartilage into which the finger tip just fits. Below this is the narrow prominence of the **cricoid arch,** across which the finger can be rolled. In the depths of the groove the resistance of the **median crico-thyroid ligament** can

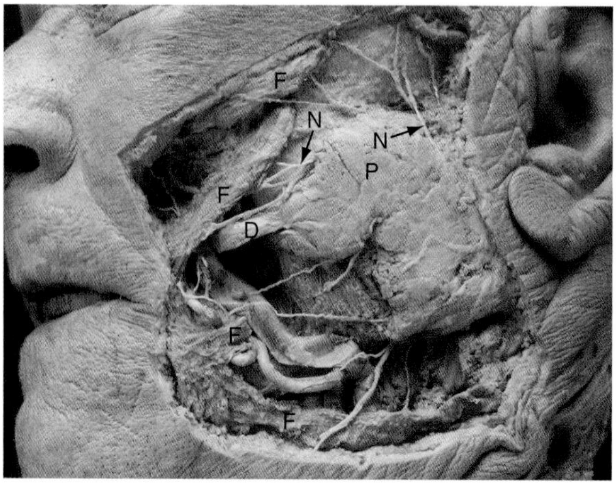


**Fig. 1.7a** Prosection showing the parotid gland, duct, and facial nerve branches
D = parotid duct, F = facial muscles, N = facial nerve branches, P = parotid gland

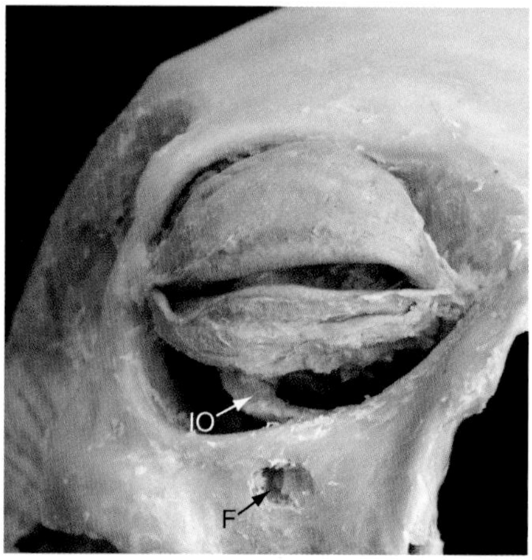


**Fig. 1.7b** Prosection of the orbit showing the inferior oblique muscle
F = infra-orbital foramen, IO = inferior oblique

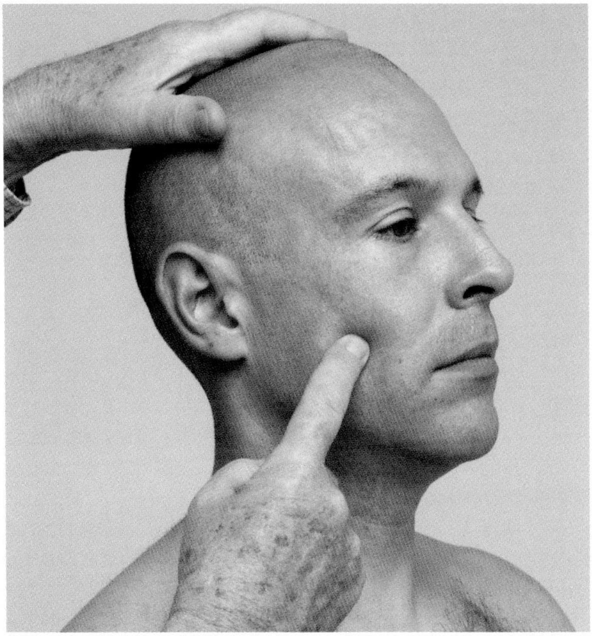

Fig. 1.8 Palpating the parotid duct

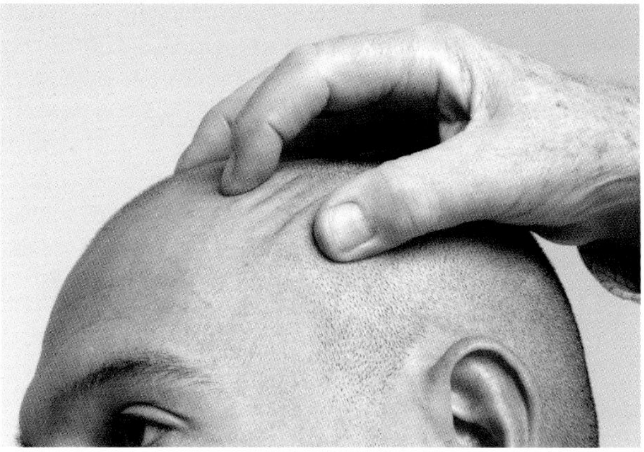

Fig. 1.10 Testing mobility of the scalp

be felt (Fig. 1.9). In an emergency, when a patent airway cannot be obtained by other methods, piercing this ligament with a sharp instrument, e.g. needle crico-thyroidotomy, provides immediate access to the airway below the level of the glottis. Below the cricoid the cartilage rings of the **trachea** are palpable in the midline down to the suprasternal notch.

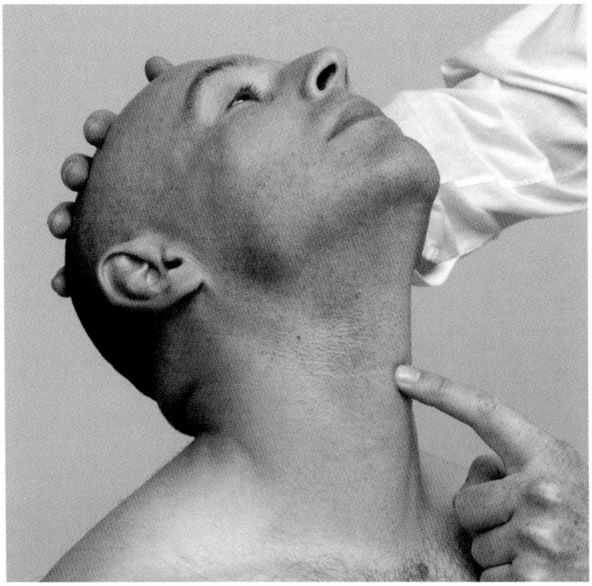

Fig. 1.9 Locating the median crico-thyroid ligament

## SCALP

The SCALP has five layers: (1) **S**kin, (2) dense **C**onnective tissue, (3) epicranial **A**poneurosis, (4) **L**oose connective tissue, and (5) **P**ericranium. It is mobile on the skull, movement occurring at layer four, which is significant in scalp injuries. Mobility can be tested if the examiner spreads the thumb and fingers of one hand across the dome of the head and massages the scalp by alternating between gripping it firmly and then relaxing the grip (Fig. 1.10).

## EYELID AND EYE

The eyelids protect the globe, which is supported within the orbit. The lids converge at the outer and inner canthi. Each lid can be gently everted to reveal a small punctum close to the medial canthus. This provides drainage for tear fluid to enter the lacrimal canaliculus leading to the lacrimal sac. The skin over the eyelids, being thin and loose, can be easily pinched up between the examiner's finger and thumb. Blood readily accumulates here ("black eye") following trauma to the head. The inside of the lids and the corneal surface of the eyeball are lined by thin conjunctiva. Subconjunctival hemorrhages are painful and visibly bright red over the sclera. On direct inspection of the front of the globe, a central dark circle marks the pupil aperture, behind which is the transparent lens; behind this is the transparent vitreous humor. Pupil sizes should be compared and are normally equal. Their size varies with light intensity and state of accommodation. Pupil inequalities and changes in size are important in severe head injuries. The iris, variable in color, surrounds the pupil aperture and separates the anterior and posterior chambers, each containing aqueous humor. It is virtually in contact with the lens.

### EAR

Whilst it has a basic morphology, the external ear varies in its size, shape, and the extent to which it protrudes. Its location and prominence on the side of the head make it susceptible to lacerations and hematomas. Undrained hematomas may fibrose, resulting in thickened "cauliflower" ears seen in wrestlers and rugby forwards. The ear's framework of elastic cartilage allows it to recover shape and position in response to displacement. The ear is examined from frontal and lateral aspects, noting symmetry, shape, and position. Skin on the back of the auricle is thin and only loosely attached to the underlying cartilage, so it can be easily pinched up.

### EXTERNAL NOSE

The tip of the nose and the nasal orifices are formed by skin covering underlying nasal cartilages. They are mobile and easily palpated with the index finger tip. The nostrils provide access into the nasal passages. By inserting a finger tip into one nostril and a thumb into the other the **cartilaginous nasal septum** can be tightly squeezed between them and its mobility tested by moving it from side to side.

### TEETH

The more anteriorly placed teeth, the **incisors** and **canines,** are the most vulnerable in facial trauma. They are easily inspected with the subject seated and facing the examiner. The subject opens the mouth whilst the examiner displaces the lips from the gums with a spatula. The white enamel of the crown covers the pain-sensitive dentine, deep to which is the pulp cavity leading down into the root embedded in the gums and bony socket of the alveolar margin. Examination of the teeth is completed by asking the subject to close the jaws firmly, at the same time baring the teeth to allow inspection for symmetrical and effective occlusion (Fig. 1.17).

## LOCATING ARTERIES AND PULSES

- Carotid
- Superficial temporal
- Facial
- Occipital
- Middle meningeal

### CAROTID

The common carotid artery ascends in the neck on the side of the trachea and larynx, and under cover of the sterno-mastoid muscle. It is an important pulse. The subject is examined sitting or lying supine. At the anterior border of the sterno-mastoid and the level of the cricoid cartilage, the fingers are pressed gently but firmly backward on the side of the larynx to compress the artery against the **carotid tubercle** (C6 vertebra) (Fig. 1.11).

### SUPERFICIAL TEMPORAL

The middle finger is used to compress the artery lightly, just in front of the tragus of the auricle where it crosses over the posterior root of the zygomatic arch.

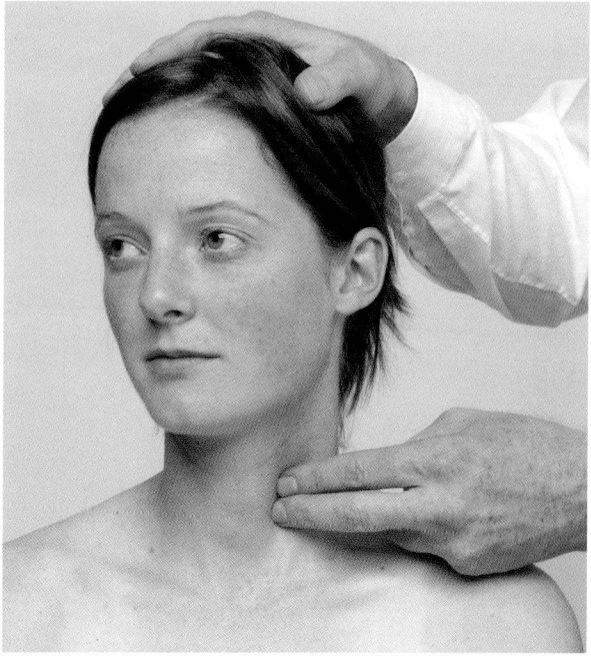

**Fig. 1.11** Locating the carotid pulse

## FACIAL

The artery is not easily felt but is located by placing the pads of the middle and ring fingers obliquely across the point where the anterior border of the masseter crosses the base of the mandible, often marked by a notch in the bone.

## OCCIPITAL

This pulse may be difficult to locate but the artery is important in the blood supply to the scalp. The examiner palpates behind and above the mastoid process, in the depression at the apex of the posterior triangle where the trapezius and sterno-mastoid muscles meet on the superior nuchal line.

## MIDDLE MENINGEAL ARTERY AND VEIN

These vessels are most vulnerable following trauma to the side of the head over the squamous temporal. They are extra-dural and in contact with the skull and endocranium. The anterior branch is located using two landmarks. With the subject seated, the examiner palpates the upper border of the zygomatic arch, then, working forward, reaches the angle where the frontal process of the zygoma can be felt passing upward behind the lateral margin of the orbit. The vessels are located at a point lying a thumb's breadth behind the frontal process and two finger-breadths above the arch (Fig. 1.12).

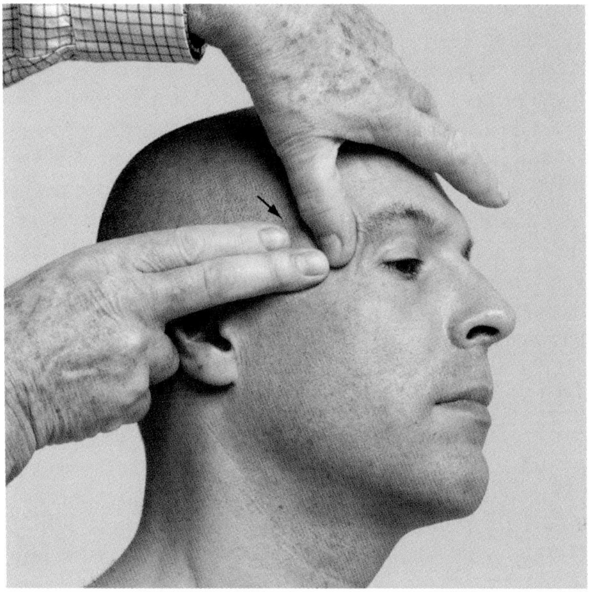

**Fig. 1.12** Locating the middle meningeal artery, marked by small arrow where borders of thumb and index finger meet.

# TESTING MUSCLES

- Sterno-mastoid
- Trapezius
- Splenius and semispinalis capitis
- Mylohyoid

## STERNO-MASTOID

These conspicuous muscles descend the whole length of the neck from the mastoid process to the sternal end of the clavicle and manubrium. Each muscle is tested by asking the subject to turn the head to the opposite side whilst the examiner resists the movement by placing the palm of a hand against the side of the head to resist the movement (Fig. 1.13). They can be tested together if the subject attempts to bend the head forward whilst the examiner applies firm pressure against the forehead to resist the movement.

## TRAPEZIUS, SPLENIUS AND SEMISPINALIS CAPITIS

The upper fibers of the trapezius contribute to the neck contour. Together with the splenius and semispinalis

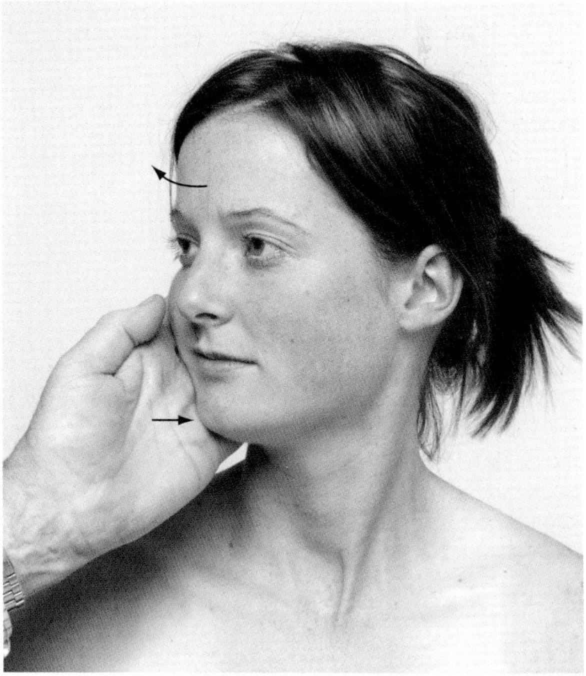

**Fig. 1.13** Testing the sterno-mastoid muscle

capitis, they are powerful anti-gravity muscles keeping the head upright. As a group they can be defined by gripping them between the thumb and fingers of one hand on the postero-lateral side of the neck on either side of the midline. They are tested by asking the subject to extend the head from a flexed position which is resisted by the examiner applying forward pressure against the occiput (see Fig. 2.9). These muscles also produce lateral flexion of the head, which is tested by the subject bending the head toward the shoulder whilst the examiner resists by pushing it in the opposite direction. Muscles in this group can be damaged during sudden uncontrolled head and neck movements ("whiplash injuries"), such as those that sometimes occur following collisions in, for example, motor sports, rugby tackles, and blows to the head during combat sports.

## MYLOHYOID

These two muscles form the floor of the mouth. Each is attached to the mylohyoid line on the inside of the body of the mandible and they interdigitate in a midline raphe which extends on to the body of the hyoid bone. They are easily tested if the subject is asked to swallow whilst the examiner applies the pad of a finger firmly upward behind the chin with the mouth closed. On swallowing, the mylohyoids can be felt to tense (Fig. 1.14). A fractured mandible may result in blood tracking along the line of the mylohyoid.

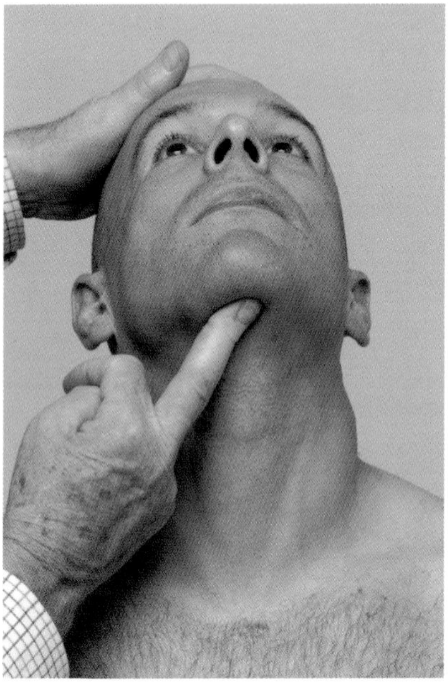

**Fig. 1.14** Testing the mylohyoid muscles

# JOINT LINES AND MOVEMENTS

- Temporo-mandibular
- Atlanto-occipital

## TEMPORO-MANDIBULAR JOINT (TMJ)

A prosection of the joint and muscles of mastication is shown in Figure 1.15a and a 3-D reconstruction in Figure 1.15b. This clinically important synovial hinge joint is between the head of the mandible and the glenoid fossa of the temporal bone. An intra-articular disc facilitates two types of movement: hinging (rotation), particularly during initial mouth opening, and gliding with wide opening. These movements can become dysfunctional and painful with derangement of the intra-articular disc. To examine function of the TMJ during mouth opening, the subject stands or sits facing the examiner who palpates both left and right TMJ using the tip of each index finger pressed firmly into the depression just behind the condyle and in front of the external auditory meatus. To assess normal mouth opening, subjects are asked to rest the tip of their tongue on the roof of the mouth whilst opening and closing the mouth (Fig. 1.16a). The examiner feels for any asymmetrical hinging of the TMJs, which can be accompanied by an uncomfortable clicking of the joint(s). Asymmetrical lateral movement of the mandible during mouth opening can be assessed by observation of the gap between the upper and lower front teeth, which should remain in line as the mouth opens (Fig. 1.16b). A toothpick wedged between the teeth can facilitate both assessment and rehabilitative exercises. Forward gliding of the mandible from the glenoid fossa is assessed in a similar manner, except that the subject is asked to rest the tongue on the floor of the mouth and open the jaw widely (Fig. 1.16c).

**Movements** at the TMJ include opening of the mouth (depression of the mandible) by the mylohyoid and digastric muscles, closing (elevation of the mandible) by the temporalis and masseter muscles, protrusion by the pterygoids, and retraction by the temporalis. Side-to-side movements are produced by a combination of muscle actions. Further consideration will be given when testing cranial nerve V. Excessive opening may lead to dislocation, especially if there is a previous history.

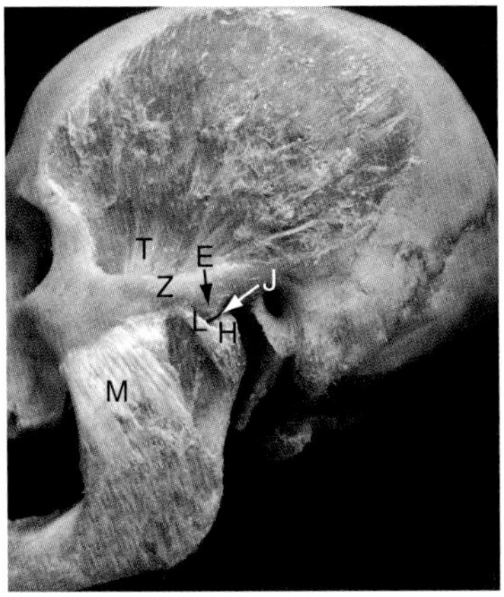


**Fig. 1.15a** Prosection showing the temporo-mandibular joint
E = articular eminence, H = head of mandible, J = joint cavity, L = lateral ligament, M = masseter, T = temporalis, Z = zygomatic arch

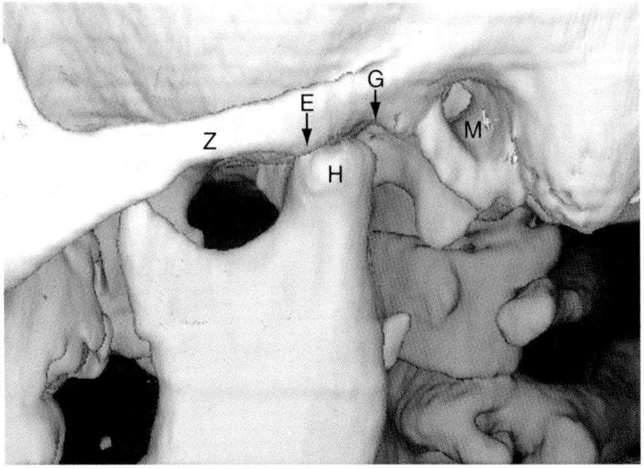


**Fig. 1.15b** CT 3-D reconstruction of the temporo-mandibular joint
E = articular eminence, G = glenoid fossa, H = head of mandible, M = external auditory meatus, Z = zygomatic arch

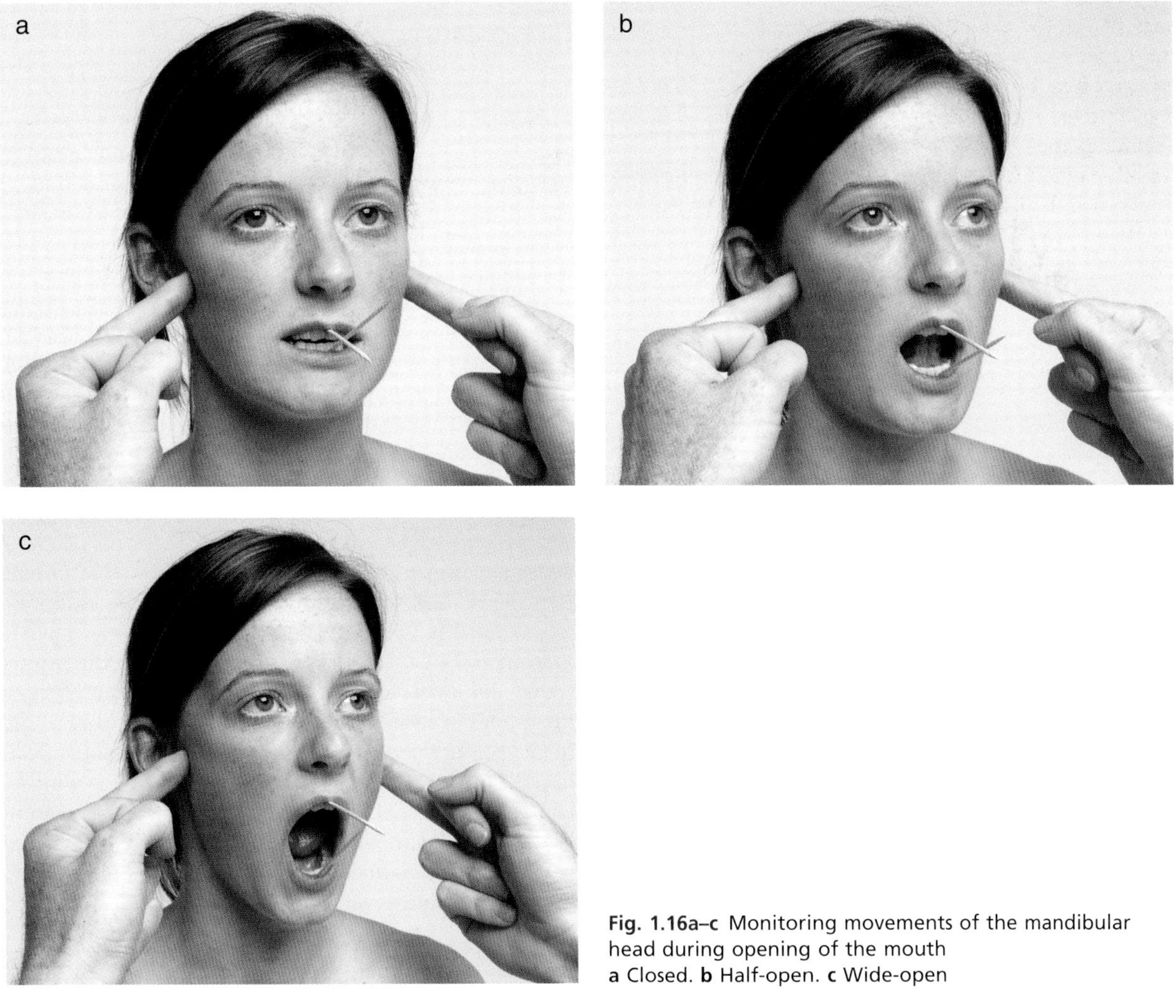


**Fig. 1.16a–c** Monitoring movements of the mandibular head during opening of the mouth
**a** Closed. **b** Half-open. **c** Wide-open

## ATLANTO-OCCIPITAL JOINT

This synovial joint lies deeply between the occipital condyles and superior facets on the atlas, and allows flexion and extension. It can be isolated from movements in the rest of the cervical spine if the examiner holds each side of the subject's upper neck firmly between the hands whilst asking the subject to bend the head forward or tilt it backward. Movement averages 30° in either direction.

# TESTING CRANIAL NERVES

- VII
- V
- III, IV and VI

Head injuries may involve any cranial nerve but consideration will be restricted to those more likely to be damaged in facial or frontal injuries, i.e. innervation of the face and eye.

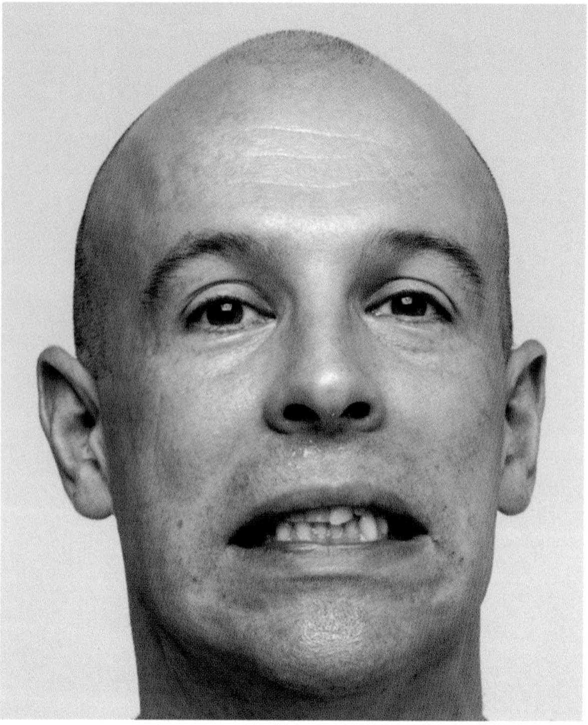

**Fig. 1.17** Testing the integrity of the facial nerve and teeth occlusion

## FACIAL NERVE (VII)

The subject faces the examiner who notes any facial asymmetry, especially at the angles of the mouth. The subject is instructed to wrinkle the forehead by looking upward, to close the eyelids tightly (the examiner can try to open them), and to show the teeth (Fig. 1.17).

## TRIGEMINAL NERVE (V)

Two components are tested: sensory and motor. Sensory testing involves light touch (cotton wool or paper tissue) and pin-prick for pain. Facing the examiner, the subject closes the eyes and responds when the face is stimulated. The three divisions of the nerve are tested in order: first by touching the forehead and tip of the nose for the ophthalmic division; then the face below the eye for the maxillary division; and finally over the body of the mandible lateral to the chin for the mandibular division. Specific branches can be tested in the areas they supply: below the inferior orbital margin for the infra-orbital nerve, over the prominence of the cheek for the zygomatico-facial, and on the medial part of the lower lip for the mental branch of the inferior alveolar nerve (Fig. 1.18). To test the motor component, the examiner places a hand over each temple above the zygomatic arch and asks the subject to clench the teeth tightly. The temporalis muscles can be felt to contract. The examiner then places a hand below each zygomatic arch over the masseter muscles, which can be felt contracting when the teeth are clenched (Fig. 1.19). During testing of the facial nerve, with the subject baring and gritting the teeth, the opportunity can be taken to check for any evidence of malocclusion.

## OCULOMOTOR (III), TROCHLEAR (IV) AND ABDUCENS (VI) CRANIAL NERVES

These nerves control eye movements and pupil responses (III). The subject is seated or stands facing the examiner, who holds the tip of a pencil or pen at eye level directly in front of the subject and about a meter away. The subject covers one eye and follows the object with the other as the examiner moves it methodically upward, downward, medially, laterally, and in correspondingly oblique positions (Fig. 1.20). The movements should be deliberate and slow, always returning to a neutral frontal position before the next movement is started. Lateral movement is exclusive to cranial nerve VI, whilst cranial nerve IV controls movement upward and outward. Pupil reaction

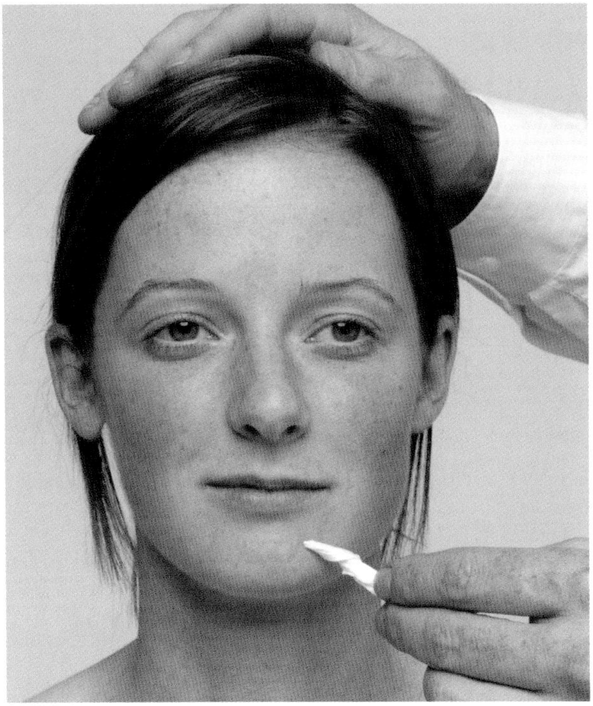

Fig. 1.18 Testing a peripheral branch of the trigeminal nerve on the face (mental branch of inferior alveolar nerve)

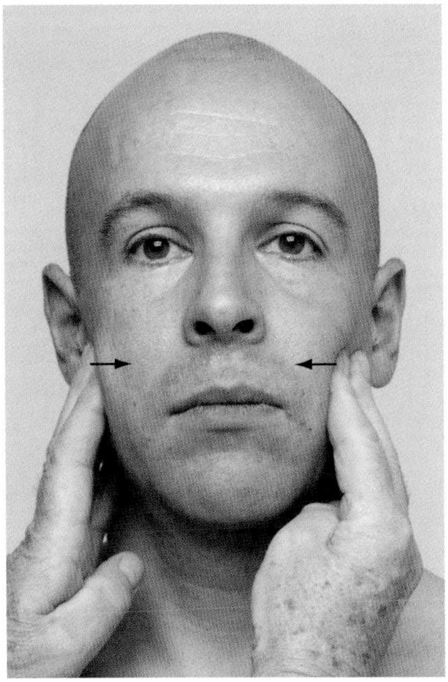



Fig. 1.19 Testing the motor component of the trigeminal nerve (masseter)

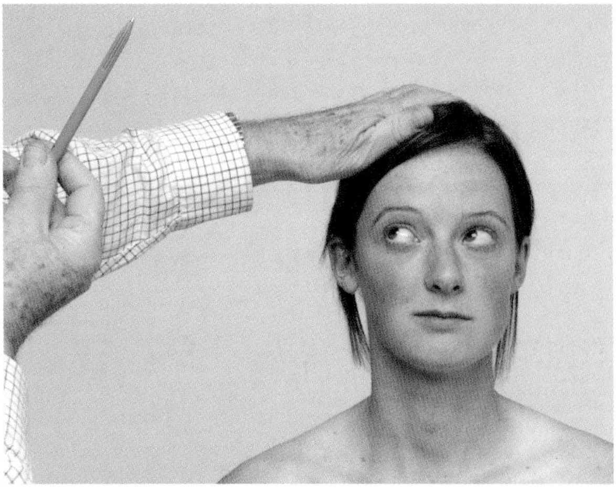

Fig. 1.20 Testing oculomotor III cranial nerve and inferior oblique muscle

is tested by covering one eye with the subject facing away from excessive light, then quickly removing the cover and noting pupil constriction in both eyes. Accommodation reflex is tested by asking the subject to stare into the distance and then focus on to a pencil held about 15 cm in front of the face, noting pupil constriction.

## SPECIAL TESTS

- Concussion
- Maxilla fracture
- Sharp–Purser test
- Alar ligament
- Facet joint
- Upper limb neural tension
- Brachial plexus compression

### SPORTS CONCUSSION

This results in a sudden, short-lived neurological impairment and is usually due to a direct blow to the head or neck. The extent of neurological impairment varies, but is generally thought to be functional rather than structural. Signs and symptoms of simple concussion generally resolve within 2 weeks, whilst complex concussion can result in persistent neurological impairment. A sports-specific SCAT (Sports Concussion Assessment Tool) may

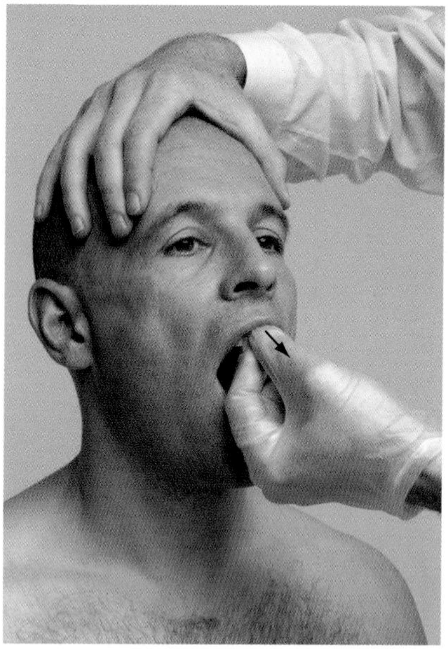

Fig. 1.21 Testing for mobility of the maxilla (Le Fort's fracture)

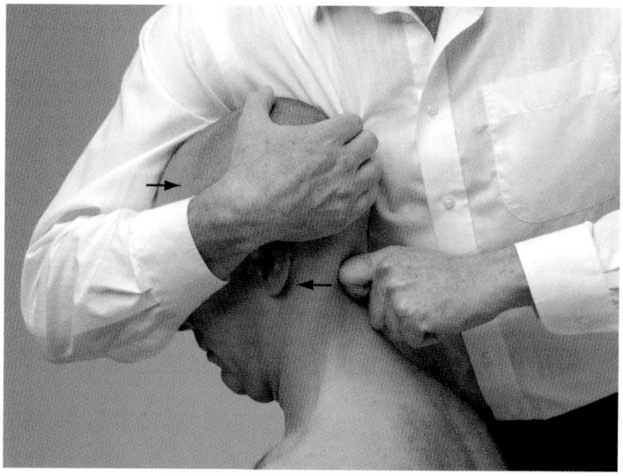

Fig. 1.22 Sharp–Purser test for the transverse atlanto-axial ligament

guide evaluation of concussion and guide the return to sport (McCrory et al, 2005).

## MAXILLA (LEFORT'S) FRACTURE

Mobility of the maxilla is tested by gripping the upper front teeth between a gloved thumb and forefinger whilst the other hand stabilizes the forehead (Fig. 1.21). The maxilla is then gently pulled forward. Movement of the maxilla without nose movement may indicate a LeFort's type 1 fracture. Movement of the entire mid-face may indicate a LeFort's type 2 or 3 fracture.

## CRANIO-VERTEBRAL HYPERMOBILITY SYNDROME: SHARP–PURSER TEST FOR THE TRANSVERSE LIGAMENT OF THE ATLAS

The subject is seated, with the neck relaxed and slightly flexed. The examiner stands at the side of the subject and stabilizes C2 with a thumb and forefinger. The crook of examiner's other arm is used to cradle the head, with the hand gripping the occiput (Fig. 1.22). The head is then glided posteriorly. A large amplitude of movement and/or a clunk may indicate laxity or disruption of the transverse ligament. This is considered a relatively safe test, as any movement will replace the anterior arch of the atlas on to the dens, increasing space for cord.

## ALAR LIGAMENT TEST

The spinous process of C2 is again stabilized between the examiner's thumb and forefinger. The other hand is used to try to flex the head laterally on the neck, ensuring no rotation occurs (Fig. 1.23). No movement represents a negative test, i.e. intact ligament on the opposite side to the direction of lateral flexion of the head.

## FACET (ZYGAPOPHYSEAL) JOINT PALPATION

In the cervical spine these joints are located opposite the spaces between the spinous processes, approximately 1.5 cm from the midline. With the subject lying prone, the adjacent superior and inferior articular processes can be palpated using the tips of the thumbs. Pressure is applied between the spinous processes and against the paraspinal muscle bulk to displace the muscles laterally, allowing palpation of the bony articular elements of the spine (Fig. 1.24). Tenderness to palpation may indicate facet joint irritation or bony pathology.

## UPPER LIMB TENSION TESTS (ULTTs)

ULTTs, or brachial plexus tension tests, can be used to assess tension and mobility of the brachial plexus and the associated upper limb nerves. Three specific tests have been described. These consist of a series of maneuvers that

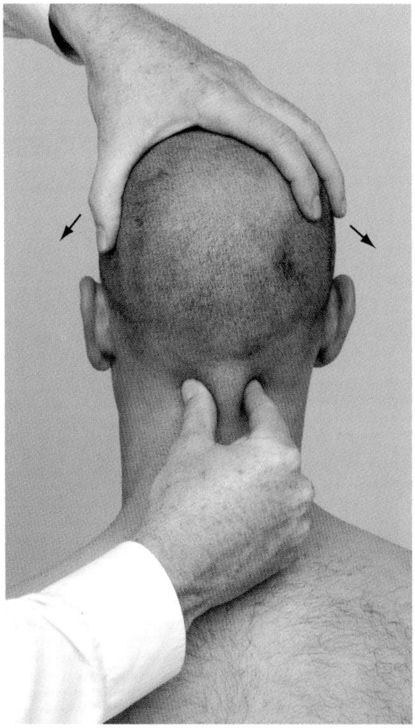

Fig. 1.23 Test for alar (check) ligament

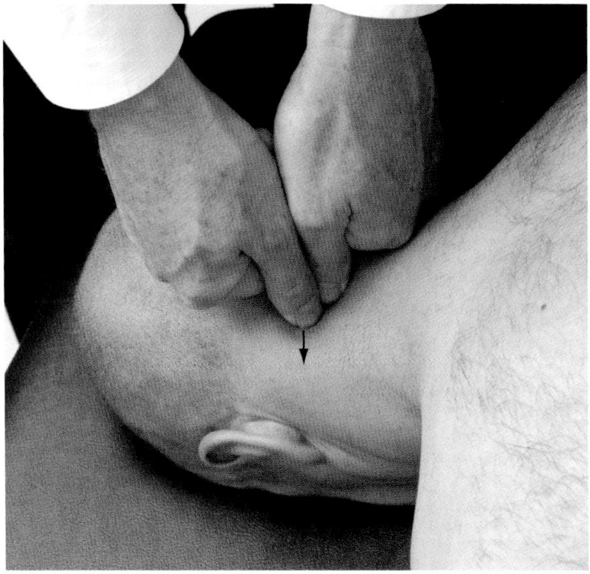

Fig. 1.24 Facet (zygapophyseal) joint palpation

place sequentially greater tension and compression on the median, ulnar, and radial nerves respectively. The ULTT1 (median nerve bias) will be described here. For descriptions of ULTT2 and 3, see Butler (1989).

### ULTT1

In the **starting position,** the subject lies supine on a couch with the head and neck in the midline. Standing facing the subject on the side to be tested, the examiner places the fingers over the subject's palm and thumb on to the dorsum of the hand to grip the distal upper limb. The subject's elbow is rested on the examiner's knee such that the shoulder is abducted approximately 45° and held in slight internal rotation. The humerus should be horizontal and the elbow flexed approximately 45°, with the wrist and fingers in neutral. Tension is placed on the proximal brachial plexus (nerve roots) when the examiner places the hand closest to the subject over the shoulder and gently induces **shoulder girdle depression** (Fig. 1.25a). If any symptoms of pain or paresthesia (tingling, numbness) are produced in the neck or upper limb, the degree of shoulder girdle depression should be reduced until the symptoms are completely alleviated. Similarly, if symptoms are produced (or resistance to movement felt by the examiner) with any of the following maneuvers, the range of movement (ROM) should be recorded and magnitude of the movement reduced so that symptoms are alleviated before moving to the next movement in the sequence. The examiner then gently adds up to 90° of **shoulder abduction** (Fig. 1.25b), which should move the brachial plexus under the pectoralis minor and coracoid. Next, further tension is placed on the brachial plexus by **externally rotating** the shoulder up to 90° (Fig. 1.25c). This is followed by **elbow extension** (Fig. 1.25d), **forearm supination**, **wrist extension,** and then lastly **finger extension** (Fig. 1.25e), movements thought to tension the median nerve progressively. Repeating the test with the subject's head and neck side-flexed (or rotated) to both (1) the opposite side (Fig. 1.25f) and (2) the same side as the arm being tested will increase and decrease brachial plexus tension respectively, and may aid differentiation of symptoms caused by adverse neural tension and other musculoskeletal causes.

## BRACHIAL PLEXUS COMPRESSION TESTS

Tests for Thoracic Outlet Syndrome (Adso's Test), Claviculo-Costal, and Pectoralis Minor Compression Syndromes are demonstrated on the accompanying DVD.

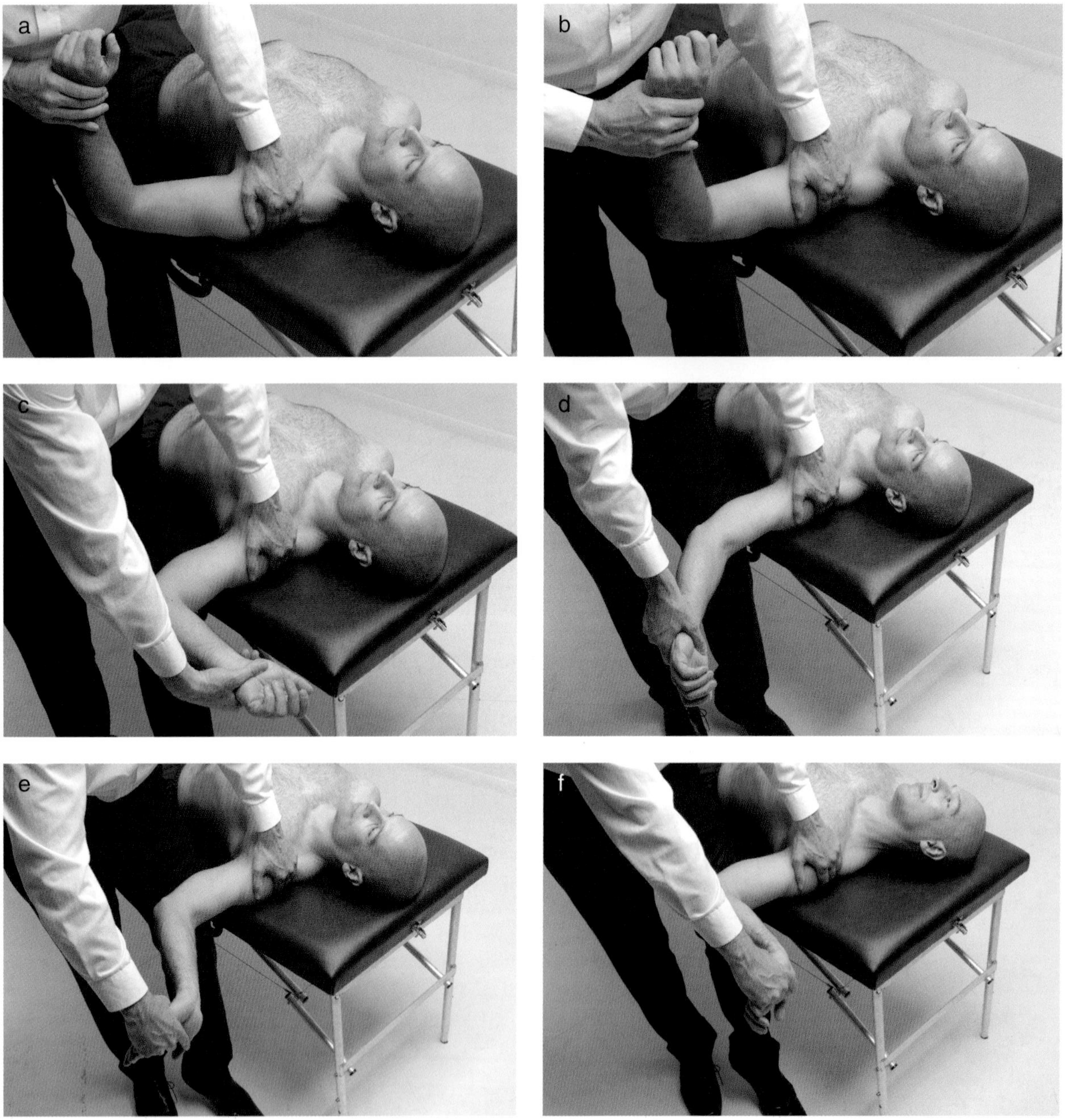


**Fig. 1.25a–f** Upper limb (brachial plexus) tension tests


## FURTHER READING

Butler DS. Adverse mechanical tension in the nervous system: a model for assessment and treatment. Australian Journal of Physiotherapy 1989; 35:227–237.

Dearing J. Soft tissue neck lumps in rugby union players. British Journal of Sports Medicine 2006; 40:317–319.

Delaney JS, Frankovich R. Head injuries and concussions in soccer. Clinical Journal of Sport Medicine 2005; 15:214–217.

Furtner M, Werner P, Felber S et al. Bilateral carotid artery dissection caused by springboard diving. Clinical Journal of Sport Medicine 2006; 16:76–78.

Gatzonis S, Charakidas A, Polychronopoulou Z et al. Unilateral visual loss following bodybuilding training. Clinical Journal of Sport Medicine 2004; 14:317–318.

Koob A, Ohlmann B, Gabbert O et al. Temporomandibular disorders associated with scuba diving. Clinical Journal of Sport Medicine 2005; 15:359–363.

McCrory P, Johnston K, Meeuwisse W et al. Summary and agreement statement of the 2nd International Conference on Concussion in Sport, Prague 2004. British Journal of Sports Medicine 2005; 39:196–204.

Nakagawa Y, Miki T, Nakamura T. Atlantoaxial dislocation in a sumo wrestler. Clinical Journal of Sport Medicine 1998; 8:237–240.

Nassar L, Albano J, Padron D. Exertional headache in a collegiate gymnast. Clinical Journal of Sport Medicine 1999; 9:182–183.

Waicus KM, Smith BW. Eye injuries in women's lacrosse players. Clinical Journal of Sport Medicine 2002; 12:24–29.

## CASE STUDY 1 • CLINICAL PROBLEMS

**Problem 1.** *During an international women's field hockey match a player receives a blow on the side of the face from an opponent's stick. There is severe bruising and a laceration requiring suturing. The team physician orders a radiograph of the head. A small hair-line fracture is noted in one of the facial bones. The wound heals and the bruising resolves. About 3 weeks later the player notices numbness over the prominence of the cheek and also complains that food seems to stick in one side of the mouth.*

a) Which bone is most likely to have been fractured?
b) What could cause numbness over the prominence of the cheek?
c) What could cause food to stick in one side of the mouth?
d) What test should be performed?

**Problem 2.** *A batsman in a cricket match is struck directly in the eye by a ball bowled at high velocity. A frontal radiograph shows disruption of the orbital floor and blood in the maxillary sinus (Fig. 1.26). Fortunately, the eye is saved. When the swelling and bruising have diminished, the subject complains of numbness on the front of the face and also double vision (diplopia) when looking in one particular direction.*

a) Which bone is particularly at risk?
b) What type of fracture is likely to have been caused?
c) What is the explanation for the numbness?
d) In which direction of gaze does double vision occur and why?

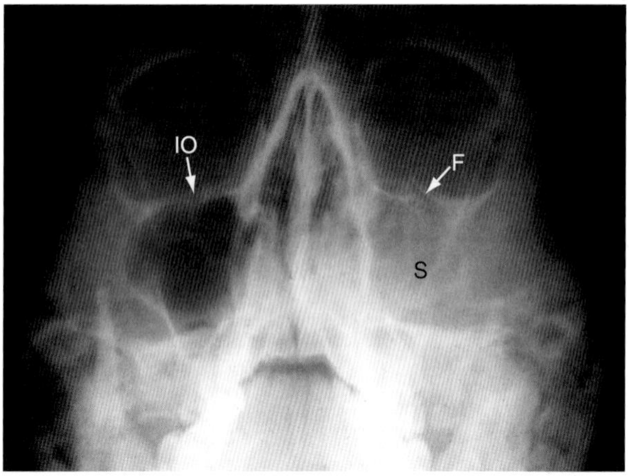


**Fig. 1.26** X-radiograph of facial skeleton: orbital fracture F = fracture, IO = infra-orbital foramen, S = maxillary sinus (opacity is due to blood in the sinus)

**Problem 3.** *During a cross country event a rider falls from her horse and receives a kick full in the face, causing avulsion of an upper front tooth. She complains of her teeth being out of line when she closes her mouth.*

a) Which facial bone is most likely to have been fractured? What other bones are at risk?
b) Which classification is used for facial fractures and in which group is this injury likely to be?
c) How can the fracture be detected?
d) What radiological investigation is indicated if the avulsed tooth cannot be found?

**Problem 4.** *A rugby winger is bending forward to gather the ball with his arm outstretched when an opponent's tackle forcibly depresses his shoulder girdle and side-flexes the neck to the opposite side. He now complains of aching pain radiating from the neck to the crook of the elbow and tingling into the thumb.*

a) What might be causing the symptoms?
b) Which tests could be used to assess adverse neural tension and which of these is likely to be positive?
c) Which dermatome is in the area of the symptoms?
d) What other (i) muscles and (ii) articulations could have been injured with this particular form of trauma?

**Problem 5.** *An ice hockey player falls to the ground and the side of his face is accidentally lacerated by an opponent's skate. The laceration is deep and located just antero-superior to the angle of the mandible.*

a) What muscle attaching to the mandible may have been injured?
b) What is the action of the muscle? How can it be tested?
c) What other structure(s) are vulnerable in this area?
d) Three months after the injury he begins to experience a painful clicking when he opens his mouth wide. What joint might be implicated and how is its movement assessed?

**Problem 6.** *During a martial arts display a karate fighter receives a blow over the front of the neck. Shortly afterwards he complains of pain in his throat and develops a hoarse voice. On local examination it is difficult to palpate any landmarks.*

a) What structure could have been injured?
b) What landmarks should be palpated?
c) What is the significance of the hoarseness?

CHAPTER 2

# Back and spine

## INTRODUCTION

Whilst the spine forms the major component of the back, other structures contribute to this region. They include the posterior parts of the ribs, which articulate with the thoracic vertebrae (considered in Ch. 3), and also the scapula and associated muscles mooring it to the trunk and arm (Ch. 4) and covering the deeper intrinsic muscles. The posterior parts of the iliac crests separate the lower part of the back from the buttock (Ch. 7).

The spine extends from the base of the skull to the coccyx and is located dorsally in the neck and trunk. Its core is the bony, segmented vertebral column terminating in the sacrum and coccyx. The column has two curvatures: a primary curve developed before birth and a secondary curve developed after birth in response to man's unique upright posture. This posture imposes particular stresses on the column, which is constructed to resist torsion and compressive forces including weight bearing, the vertebrae increasing in size caudally. Anterior and posterior longitudinal ligaments attaching to vertebral bodies span the whole length of the spine. Individual vertebrae are linked by several types of joint, including fibrous joints between spinous and transverse processes, elastic ligamenta flava between the laminae, intervertebral discs which function as shock-absorbers between vertebral bodies, and synovial joints between articular facets. These different types of joint allow small amounts of movement between adjacent vertebrae but, when summated for the whole spine, allow forward flexion, backward extension, rotation, and lateral flexion. Range and type of movement vary in different regions. The cervical spine is the most mobile and least protected part, and is therefore more vulnerable to injury. The thoracic spine is least mobile due to the attachment of ribs. The lumbar spine is substantial and adapted for bearing much of the body weight. Intrinsic muscles function as active stabilizers. They are particularly developed dorsally as anti-gravity muscles to produce and maintain the upright posture. Ligaments uniting the vertebrae are passive stabilizers of the bony column. The vertebrae, joints, muscles, and ligaments are all vulnerable to a variety of sports injuries. The spinal cord and roots of the spinal nerves are deeply placed within the spinal column, and are surrounded and protected by the meninges and cerebro-spinal fluid (CSF). These vital structures are also vulnerable to sports injuries.

## INSPECTION OF NORMAL CONTOURS

- Symmetry
- Spinous processes
- Spinal groove
- Dimples

A general inspection is made for the normal median **alignment of the whole spine,** with the subject facing away from the examiner, sitting upright on the edge of a couch, then standing and finally walking away from the examiner. The levels of the two shoulders are compared for symmetry. The subject is next asked to bend forward whilst the examiner takes a skyline view of the posterior thoracic wall on each side of the midline depression of the spine. Normally there is equal protrusion on each side of the spine. In scoliosis unequal protrusion on one side may be evident. The subject then stands upright and is viewed sideways, the examiner taking note of the normal "S"-shaped curve and any excessive curvature, especially kyphosis in the thoracic spine or lordosis in the lumbar spine (greater in the female).

Whilst the subject is standing upright, more detailed midline inspection is made from the back of the neck down to the upper end of the gluteal cleft. The detail visible varies with the amount of subcutaneous fat and musculature. A midline furrow of varying depth overlies the spinous processes of the vertebrae (Fig. 2.1a), some being more conspicuous at certain levels. When the subject bends the head and trunk forward, spinous processes in all regions are more prominent (Fig. 2.1b). In the upper part of the neck, a shallow depression may lie between the well-developed nuchal extensor muscles. Lower down the neck, the spines form a median ridge, and at the junction of the neck with the trunk, two discrete midline prominences, accentuated when the subject flexes the head, are usually clearly visible and mark the **tip of the C7 and T1 spinous processes** (Fig. 2.2). In the upper thorax, the median ridge persists but soon gives way to a groove which is accentuated by the nearby vertebral borders of the scapulae and associated muscles (see Ch. 4). The **groove** is deepest and well defined in the lower thoracic and upper lumbar regions, being further outlined by the prominent erector spinae (sacro-spinalis) muscles on each side. In the lower part of the groove, alternating elevations and depressions may outline the spines of the lumbar vertebrae in thin subjects. In the lower lumbar region, the groove is replaced by a broad, flat area over the sacrum which tapers distally into the gluteal cleft. On each side of this area, even in the moderately obese, there are distinct **skin dimples** (Venus's dimples, Fig. 2.3), which overlie the posterior superior iliac spines.

## LOCATING BONY LANDMARKS

- Skull: posterior
- Spine
- Sacrum and coccyx
- Sacro-iliac joint

### SKULL

Salient features of lateral and posterior views of the bony vertebral column, sacrum and coccyx are shown in Figure 2.4, and radiographs of the spine are shown in Figure 2.5. Whilst the subject stands, or sits on a couch, with the head

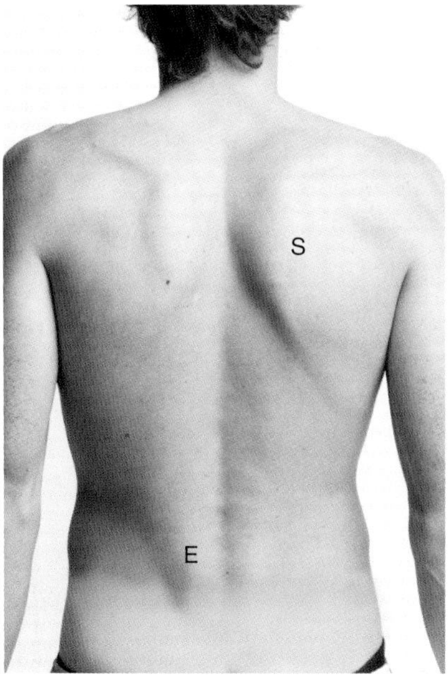


Fig. 2.1a Surface features of the back and spine
A midline furrow separates the erector spinae. E = erector spinae, S = scapula

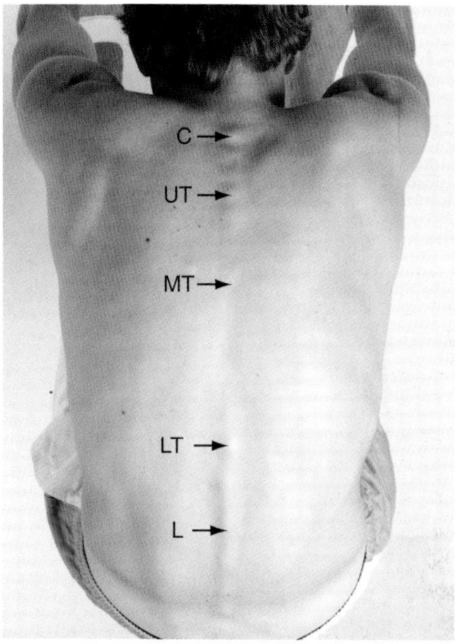


Fig. 2.1b Flexed spine demonstrating spinous processes (Compare with Fig. 2.4c) C = cervical spine, L = lumbar, LT = lower thoracic, MT = mid-thoracic, UT = upper thoracic

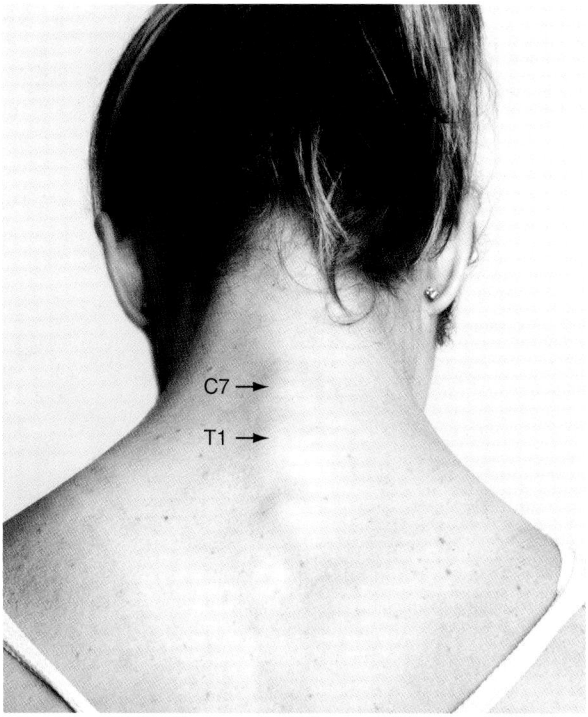


Fig. 2.2 Locating the spine of C7 (vertebra prominens)

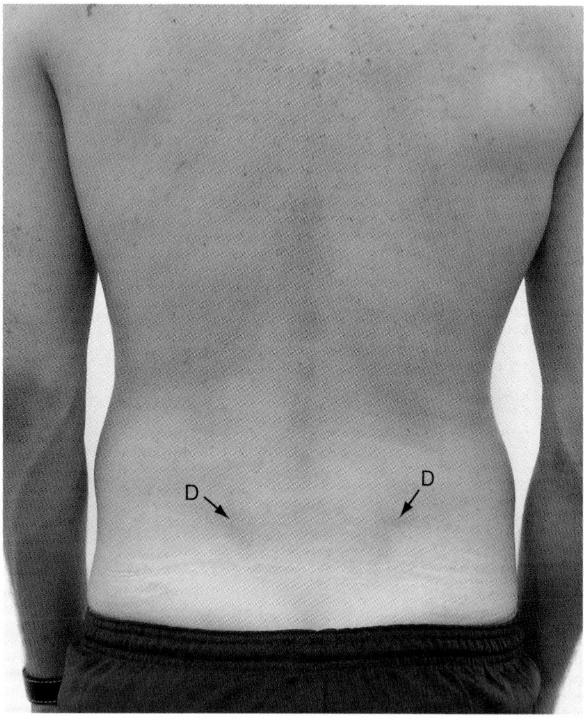


Fig. 2.3 Locating Venus's dimples (D)

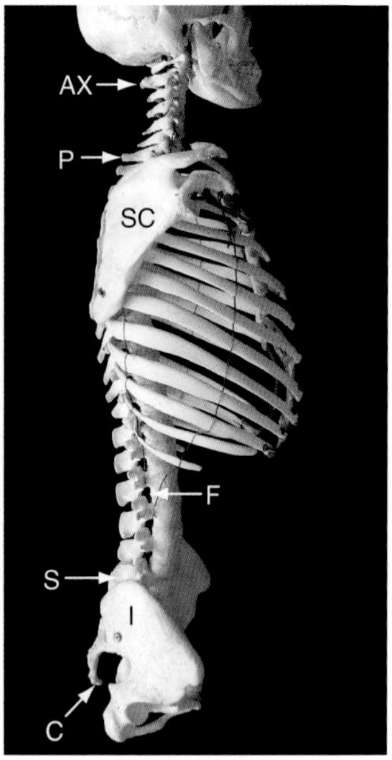


Fig. 2.4a–d Skeleton of spinal column
a Lateral view showing curvatures. Note location of ribs, scapula and ilium. AX = axis (C2), C = coccyx, F = intervertebral foramen, I = ilium, P = vertebra prominens (C7), S = sacrum, SC = scapula

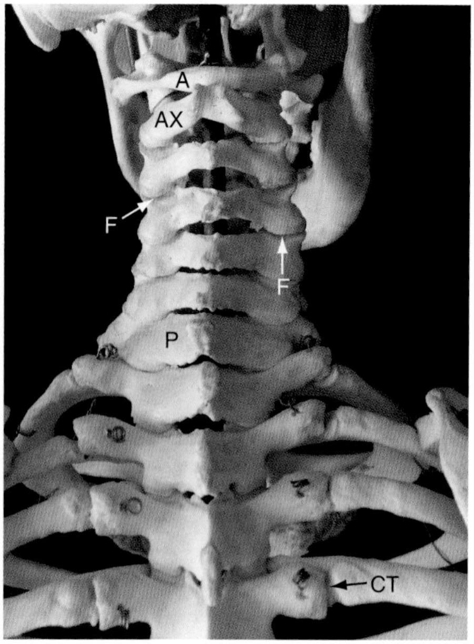


Fig. 2.4b Dorsal cervical spine
A = atlas (C1), AX = axis (C2), F = facet (zygapophyseal) joint, P = vertebra prominens (C7), CT = costotransverse joint

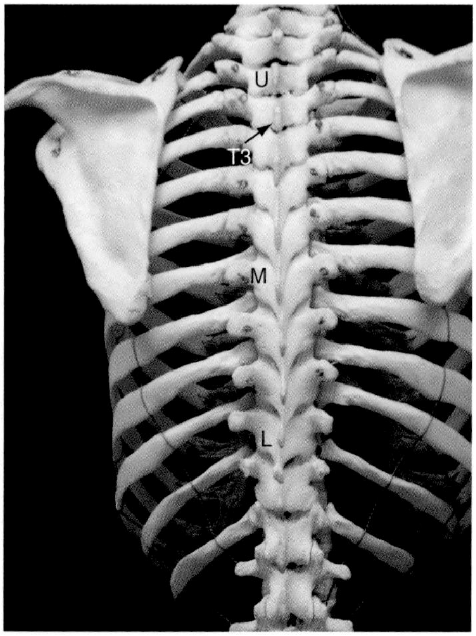


Fig. 2.4c Dorsal thoracic spine
L = lower thoracic, M = mid-thoracic, T3 = spinous process of T3, U = upper thoracic

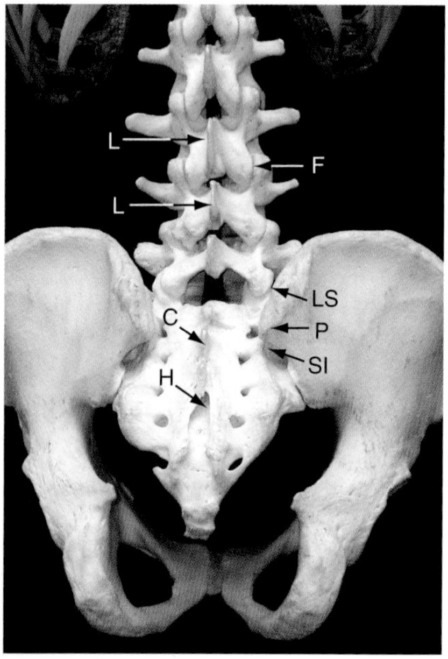


Fig. 2.4d Dorsal lumbo-sacral spine
C = median sacral crest, F = facet joint, H = sacral hiatus, L = lumbar spinous processes, LS = lumbo-sacral joint, P = posterior superior iliac spine, SI = sacro-iliac joint

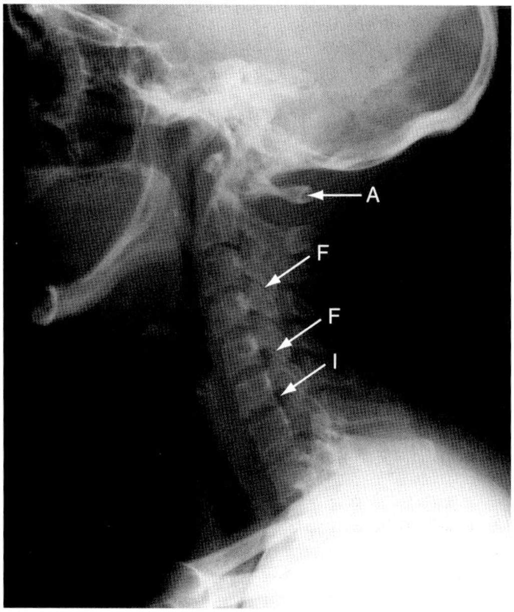


Fig. 2.5a Lateral radiograph of cervical spine
A = atlas, F = articular facet joints, I = intervertebral foramen

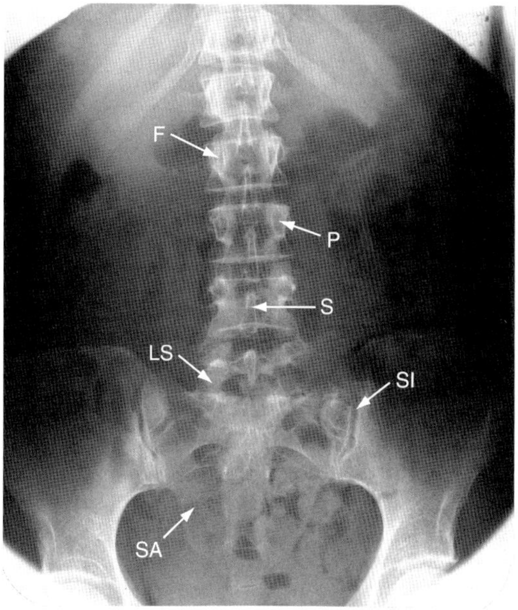


Fig. 2.5b Frontal radiograph of lumbo-sacral spine
F = facet joint, LS = lumbo-sacral joint, P = pedicle, S = spine, SA = sacrum, SI = sacro-iliac joint

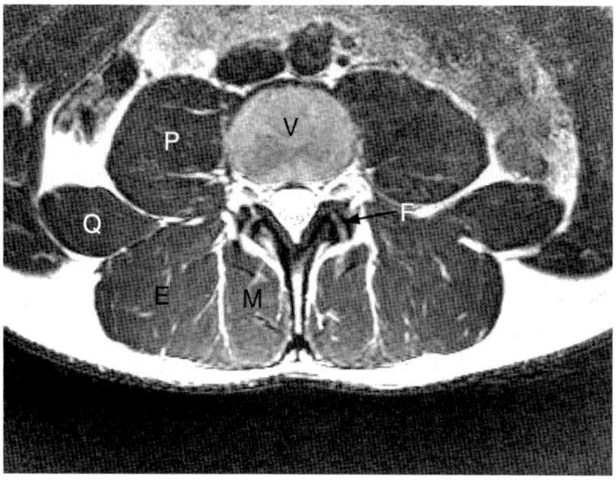


Fig. 2.5c Axial magnetic resonance image (MRI) of lumbar spine
E = erector spinae, F = facet joint, M = multifidus, P = psoas major, Q = quadratus lumborum, V = vertebral body

fully flexed, the examiner glides the tips of the index and middle fingers up the back of the subject's neck in the midline to reach a bony prominence on the back of the skull, the **external occipital protuberance,** over which the finger tips can be rolled. This marks the upper limit of the ligamentum nuchae. Ridges can be felt extending laterally from each side of the protuberance. These are the **superior nuchal lines,** which give upper attachment to the trapezius muscles.

## SPINE

Palpation of the spinous processes is facilitated by flexing the spine. The subject bends forward and downward from a standing position. This widens the interspinous spaces and emphasizes the spines. The examiner uses the tips of the index and middle fingers, drawing them firmly downward over the spines or rolling them over individual spinous processes. Except for C7, since the cervical spines are short and deeply placed beneath the ligamentum nuchae, they are impalpable. The spinous process of C7 is conspicuous and easily palpable as the **vertebra prominens** at the root of the neck (Fig. 2.2). From T1 (which may replace C7 as the most conspicuous spine) down to L5, spinous processes are palpable, although to a variable extent. In the upper and lower thoracic regions individual spines can be distinguished with care but not in the mid-thoracic region, where the long spinous processes project downward and overlap extensively (Fig. 2.4c). If the scapula is used as a landmark and the subject stands with arms dependent, the root of the scapular spine lies at level T3 and the inferior angle at level T7/8. Due to their large size and wide interspinous spaces, spinous processes are

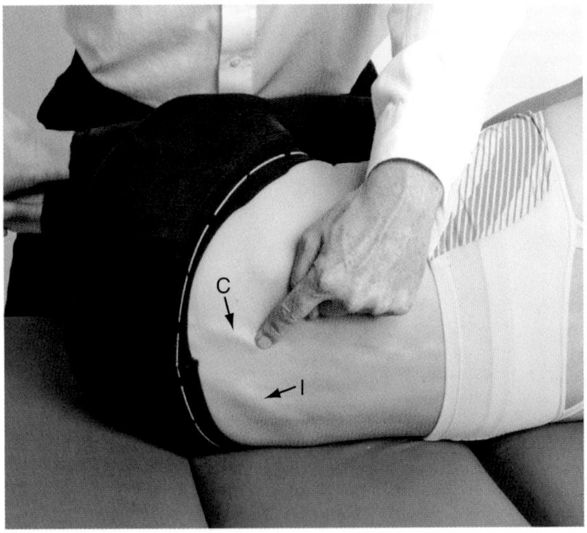


**Fig. 2.6** Locating the lumbo-sacral joint
The finger tip palpates the gap between the upper end of the sacral crest and L5 spine. C = sacral crest, I = iliac crest

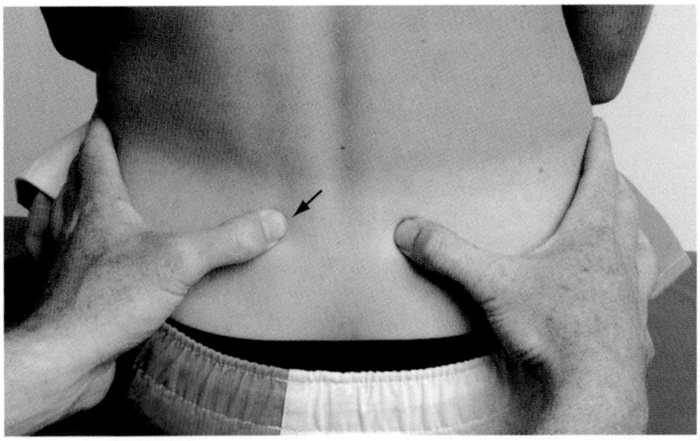

**Fig. 2.7** Palpating the sacro-iliac joints
The thumbs press into the dimples (arrow) overlying the sacroiliac joints

most easily palpable in the **lumbar region.** The **supracristal plane,** joining the tops of the iliac crests, **crosses the L4 spine.** The **intertubercular plane** joins the **iliac crest tubercles** at the level of **L5.** Individual spines can be identified by counting from L4 or from T1. With the subject increasing flexion of the lower lumbar spine to a maximum, palpation reveals a deeper depression between L5 spine and the upper border of the sacrum (Fig. 2.6). This marks the **lumbo-sacral joint.** It lies at the apex of a triangle whose lower angles are formed by the sacral dimples. Palpation can be facilitated by increasing passive flexion of the lower lumbar spine to a maximum, with the subject lying on one side on a couch (Fig. 2.6).

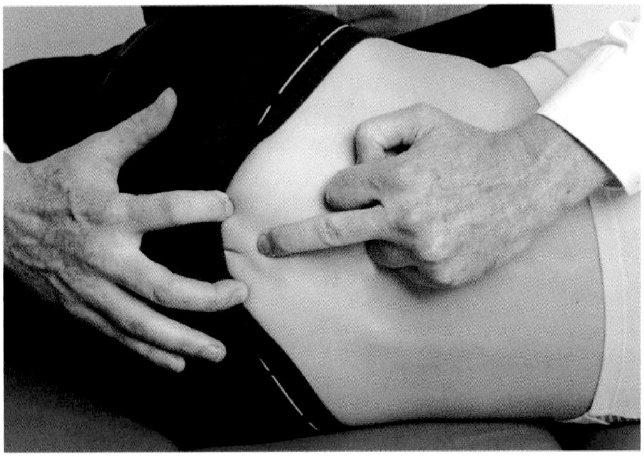

**Fig. 2.8** Locating the sacral hiatus
The middle finger tip finds the depression distal to the sacral crest and at the top of the natal cleft

## SACRUM AND COCCYX

The subject is examined standing or sitting on a couch. Using firm palpation, the pad of the middle finger is drawn across the **sacral dimple** on either side. A distinct edge in the floor of the dimple marks the posterior superior iliac spine overlying the sacrum in the posterior part of the **sacro-iliac joint.** The dimples can be examined simultaneously with the subject facing forward, whilst the examiner's hands are placed over the subject's hips with the thumbs extended medially and the pads pressing firmly into the dimples (Fig. 2.7). Palpation over the back of the sacrum, by rolling the pads of three fingers to and fro across the midline, may define the less conspicuous irregular **median sacral crest** (Fig. 2.6). Continuing palpation distally down the sacrum into the gluteal cleft, the finger passes over a bony edge into a depression. This is the **sacral hiatus** (Fig. 2.8). Below this, the finger moves across a small gap on to the **coccyx.** Alternatively, the finger tip can be moved upward from the lower part of the gluteal cleft until the bony prominence of the coccyx is reached.

# TESTING MUSCLES

- Nuchal
- Erector spinae

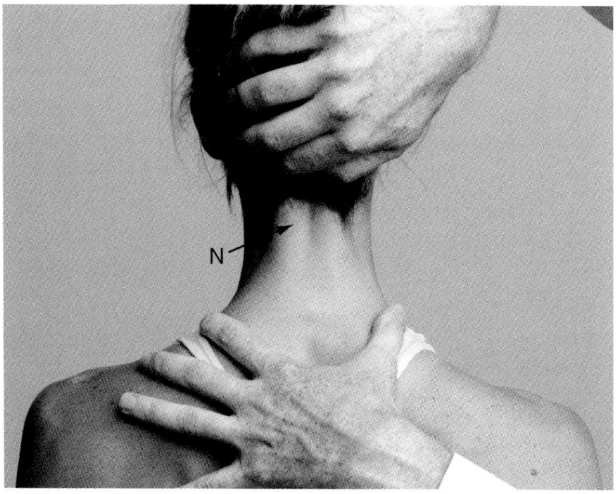


**Fig. 2.9** Demonstrating the nuchal extensor muscles
The muscles (N) contract as head extension is resisted

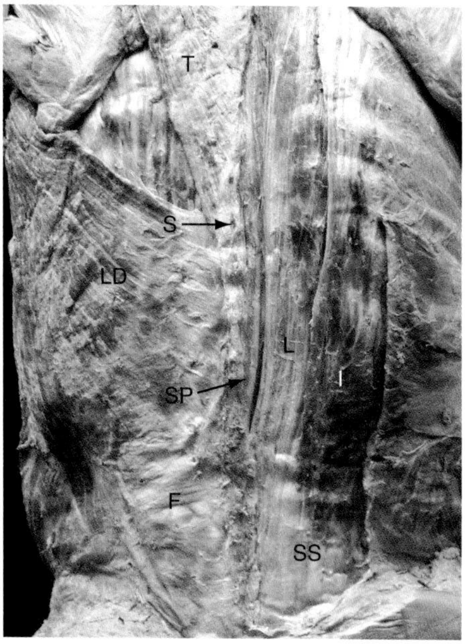


**Fig. 2.10** Prosection showing erector spinae muscles
F = thoraco-lumbar fascia, I = ilio-costalis, L = longissimus, LD = latissimus dorsi, S = spinous process, SP = spinalis, SS = sacro-spinalis, T = trapezius

Consideration in this chapter is restricted to anti-gravity muscles. Two groups of muscles are tested. Active resistance is applied whilst the subject is attempting movement and the underlying muscles are palpated as they contract.

## NUCHAL GROUP

The subject is seated or stands, and faces away from the examiner. With the head initially flexed forward, the subject attempts to extend it but is resisted by the examiner applying firm pressure over the occiput with the flat of the hand. The powerful semispinalis cervicis and splenius muscles become conspicuous on each side of the nuchal furrow and the neck–shoulder contour becomes prominent due to contraction of the underlying upper fibers of the trapezius (Fig. 2.9). Their contraction is confirmed by gripping the muscles between fingers and thumb and by palpating with the fingers flat across the dorsum of the neck–shoulder region.

## ERECTOR SPINAE GROUP

The erector spinae (sacro-spinalis) muscle group is shown in the prosection in Figure 2.10. The subject lies face down on the couch, and then lifts the head and shoulders off the couch, keeping the arms to the side of the trunk. Resistance applied by the examiner pushing downward with the palm of hand placed between the scapulae increases the profile of the erector muscles, which form well-defined ridges on each side of the spine and are particularly developed in the lower region (Fig. 2.11). Here they can be palpated as firm masses extending on to the dorsum of the sacrum.

Spinal movements are also produced by more remote muscle groups, including muscles on the posterior, lateral, and anterior abdominal walls, and these are considered in Chapter 3.

# JOINT LINES AND MOVEMENTS

- Facet
- Lumbo-sacral
- Sacro-iliac
- Range of movement

The gaps between the spinous processes contain supraspinous and interspinous ligaments, and as such are fibrous joints. They can be palpated when defining individual spinous processes (see above). The **facet (zygapophyseal) joints** are located opposite the spaces between the spinous processes about 2.5 cm from the

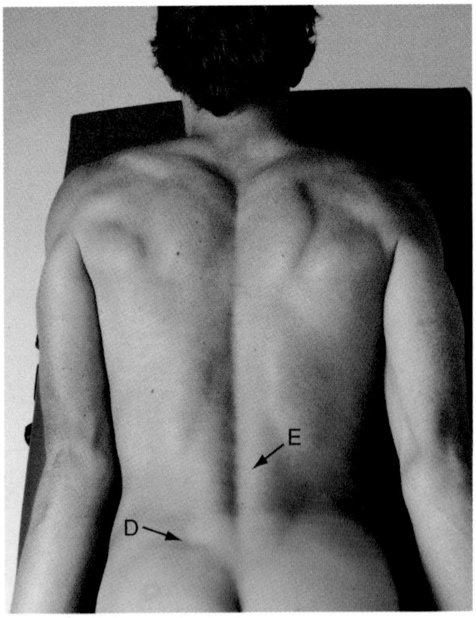


**Fig. 2.11** Demonstrating the erector spinae muscles
D = Venus's dimple, E = erector spinae

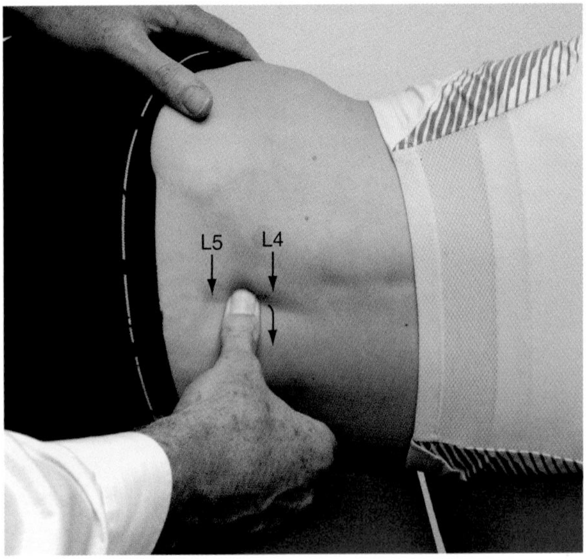


**Fig. 2.12** Locating the position of the facet joints
The thumb lies midway between the spines of L4 and L5. Deep palpation is applied whilst displacing the medial edge of erector spinae laterally

midline (Fig. 2.12). With the subject lying on their side, the adjacent superior and inferior articular processes can be palpated using the tip of the thumb. Deep pressure is applied between the spinous processes and against the erector spinae bulk to move the muscles laterally, allowing palpation of the bony articular elements of the spine. Tenderness to palpation may indicate facet joint irritation or bony pathology such as pars interarticularis stress fracture.

Intervertebral discs are symphysis-type joints and, being very deeply placed between vertebral bodies, are impalpable. Locating the **lumbo-sacral joint** and the posterior part of the **sacro-iliac joint** has been previously described.

## TESTING RANGE OF MOVEMENT

- Cervical
- Thoraco-lumbar

Spinal movements and their ranges are shown in Figure 2.13. It is practical to examine the spine as two parts: cervical and thoraco-lumbar.

### CERVICAL SPINE

Assessment of the active ROM of the cervical spine includes movements of the head at the atlanto-occipital joint, and is best performed with the subject sitting upright. The cervical spine is the most mobile region with the ability to flex, extend, rotate, and laterally flex. The subject should be asked to move through each of these movements, which can be gently guided by the examiner placing one hand on each side of the head with the fingers pointing posteriorly.

**Extension and flexion** are limited to approximately 40°. In practice, the ROM of flexion may be estimated by measuring the distance between the chin and the chest wall with the head bowed. **Rotation** is on average 45° whilst **lateral flexion** is 40–45°, and may be gauged by measuring the distance between the ear and the shoulder with the head inclined to that side.

### THORACO-LUMBAR SPINE

The subject stands upright. Since movement at the hips may mask spinal movement, especially flexion/extension, the examiner must steady the subject's pelvis firmly, grasping it from behind on both sides. **Flexion** averages 85° and can be estimated by measuring the distance between the subject's finger tips from the floor when the subject bends down and tries to touch the toes. The subject then stands upright and, with the examiner again stabilizing the

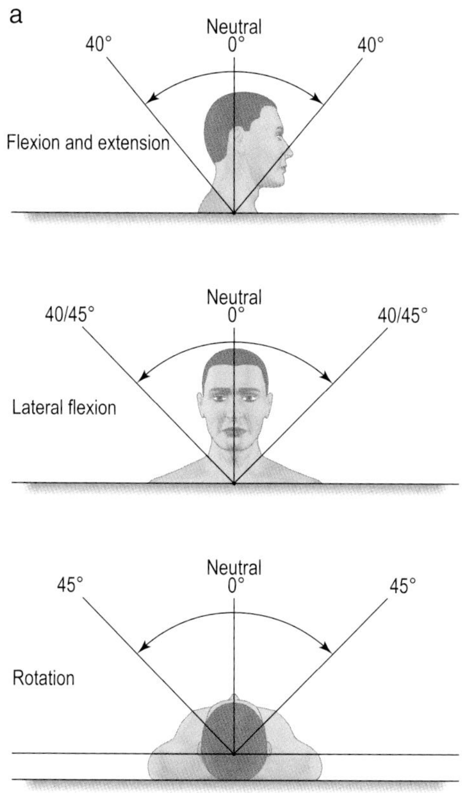


**Fig. 2.13a–d** Diagrams showing the range of spinal movements **a** Cervical spine
Redrawn from *Joint motion: method of measuring and recording.* Edinburgh: E&S Livingstone, 1965 (with the permission of the American Academy of Orthopedic Surgeons, reprinted with their permission by the British Orthopaedic Association)

pelvis, bends backward. Average **extension** is **30°**. The most accurate method to assess flexion is to use a **metal tape-measure** to record changes between two fixed points, with the subject standing upright and then bending forward (Fig. 2.14). The spine of C7 or T1 is used as the upper marker and L5 as the lower. A difference of 10 cm may be recorded in the ratio of 3 : 1 for lumbar versus thoracic spine. The tape can also be used to record **lateral flexion.** The subject stands upright facing away from the examiner, and then bends sideways. Keeping the measure joining the two bony reference points, the angle of this line with the horizontal supracristal plane is noted. Up to 35° may be achieved, and as a further guide, the examiner notes how far down the side of the leg the subject's finger tips can reach whilst bending laterally, with the knee joint as a reference point. To record **rotation,** with the subject sitting with the hands crossed over the chest, the examiner grips the shoulders firmly from behind and guides the subject in turning maximally to the left and then to the right. The movement is confined to the thoracic spine and may reach **45°**.

# SPECIAL TESTS

- Lumbo-sacral plexus tension:
  Straight leg raise
  Slump
- Detecting stress injury in the posterior elements of the lumbar spine:
  Stork test
- Sacro-iliac joint:
  Active straight leg raise
  Faber test

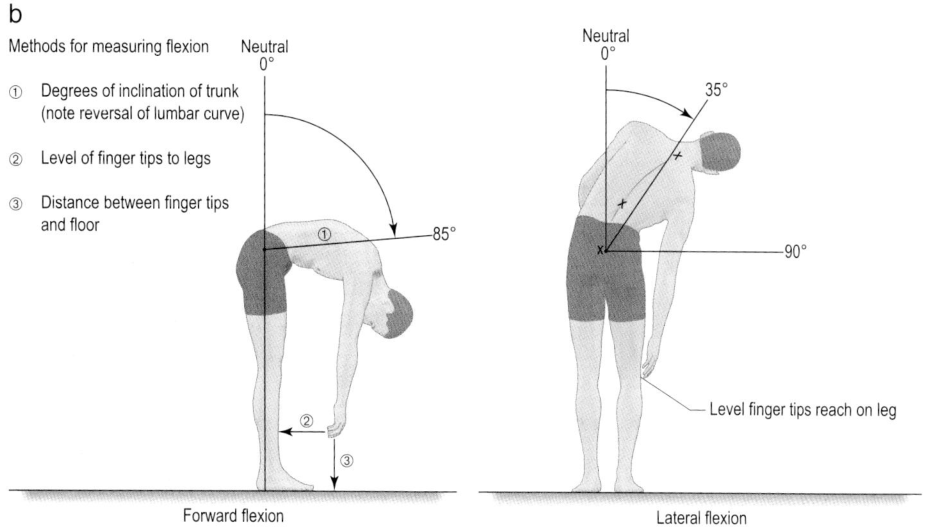


**Fig. 2.13a–d, Cont'd**
**b** Thoracic and lumbar spine

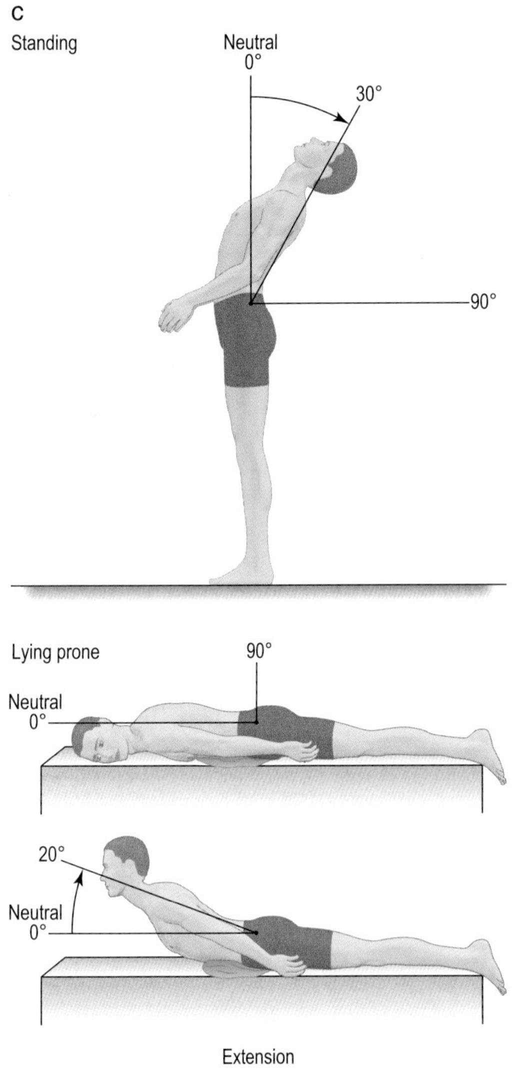


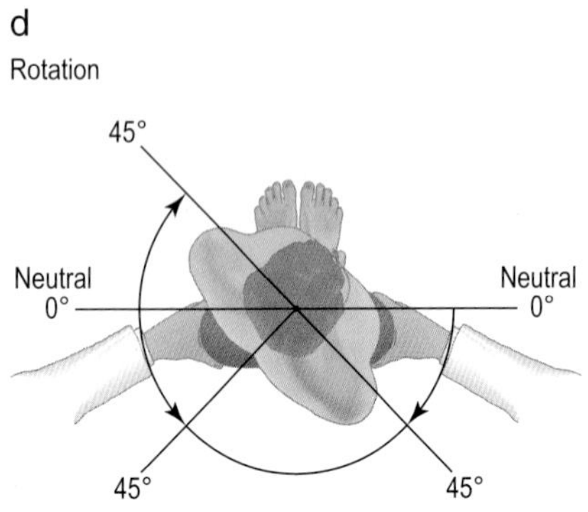


**Fig. 2.13a–d, Cont'd c** Extension
**Fig. 2.13a–d, Cont'd d** Rotation

## LUMBO-SACRAL PLEXUS NEURAL TENSION TESTS

These are used to detect adverse neural tension, which may be due to conditions such as intervertebral disc prolapse, dural or nerve root adhesions to intervertebral foramina, or also to paravertebral muscle attachments.

### STRAIGHT LEG RAISE (SLR) TEST

The subject lies supine on the couch, without a pillow and with legs extended. The examiner supports the lower leg with one hand. The subject is asked to relax the limb and report any symptoms as the limb is gradually raised by the examiner (Fig. 2.15a). The location of any symptoms, i.e. pain and paresthesia, should be noted, along with the ROM of hip flexion at which they occur. Adverse neural tension can be differentiated from musculo-skeletal origins by repeating the SLR test with the foot held in dorsiflexion (Fig. 2.15b) and with the neck positioned in flexion (Fig. 2.15c). Intensification of symptoms or a greater limitation of hip flexion ROM indicates a positive neural tension test.

### SLUMP TEST

Subjects sit at the end of the couch, with their legs dependent over the edge and their hands placed behind their back. They are then instructed to allow the head and shoulders to slump forward (Fig. 2.16a). The examiner gently maintains the subject's "slumped" position by placing one hand over the base of the neck. With the other hand, the examiner passively raises one of the subject's legs (Fig. 2.16b). The angle at which the limit of knee extension is reached, either through pain or stiffness, is noted. The subject is then asked to lift the head. If the symptoms are alleviated or a further range of knee extension can be gained, a positive test is recorded (Fig. 2.16c). Subtle signs of adverse neural tension can be detected by repeating the test with the foot held in dorsiflexion (Fig. 2.16d), increasing the stress on the lumbo-sacral plexus neural tissue.

## STRESS INJURY IN THE POSTERIOR ELEMENTS OF THE LUMBAR SPINE (PARTES INTERARTICULARES OR PEDICLES)

### STORK TEST

The examiner is positioned behind the standing subject, supporting the shoulders with both hands. The subject is asked to stand on one leg. Keeping the standing knee straight, the subject is guided into lumbar extension (Fig.

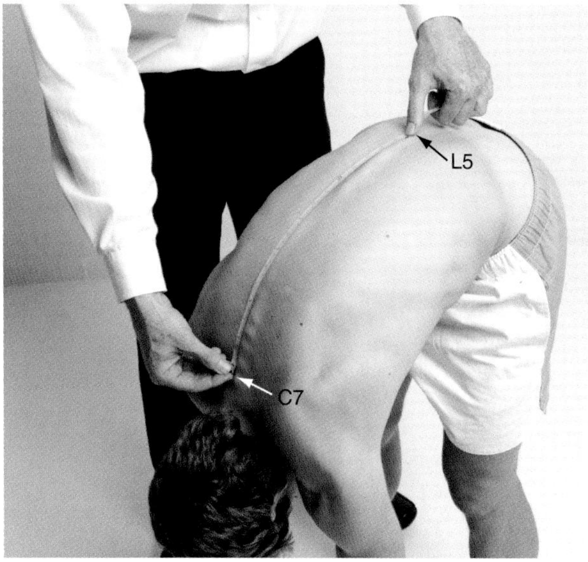


Fig. 2.14 Tape-measure method for assessing flexion of the thoraco-lumbar spine

2.17a). Pain (often unilateral) localized to a particular segment of the lower lumbar spine may indicate pars interarticularis or pedicle stress fracture. If stress injury is suspected but no discomfort is elicited with pure extension, the subject can be guided into thoraco-lumbar rotation (Fig. 2.17b) or side-flexion (Fig. 2.17c) whilst maintaining the extended position.

## TESTS FOR STRESSING THE SACRO-ILIAC JOINT (SIJ)

### ACTIVE SLR FOR SIJ INSTABILITY

Lying supine on the couch with legs fully extended, the subject raises the symptomatic limb, keeping the knee straight (Fig. 2.18a). Pain is often provoked in the presence of SIJ instability. The test is then repeated, with the examiner providing a compressive force by pressing the palms of the hands inward very firmly against the ilia (Fig. 2.18b). A reduction in symptoms or an increase in active SLR ROM with compression represents a positive test.

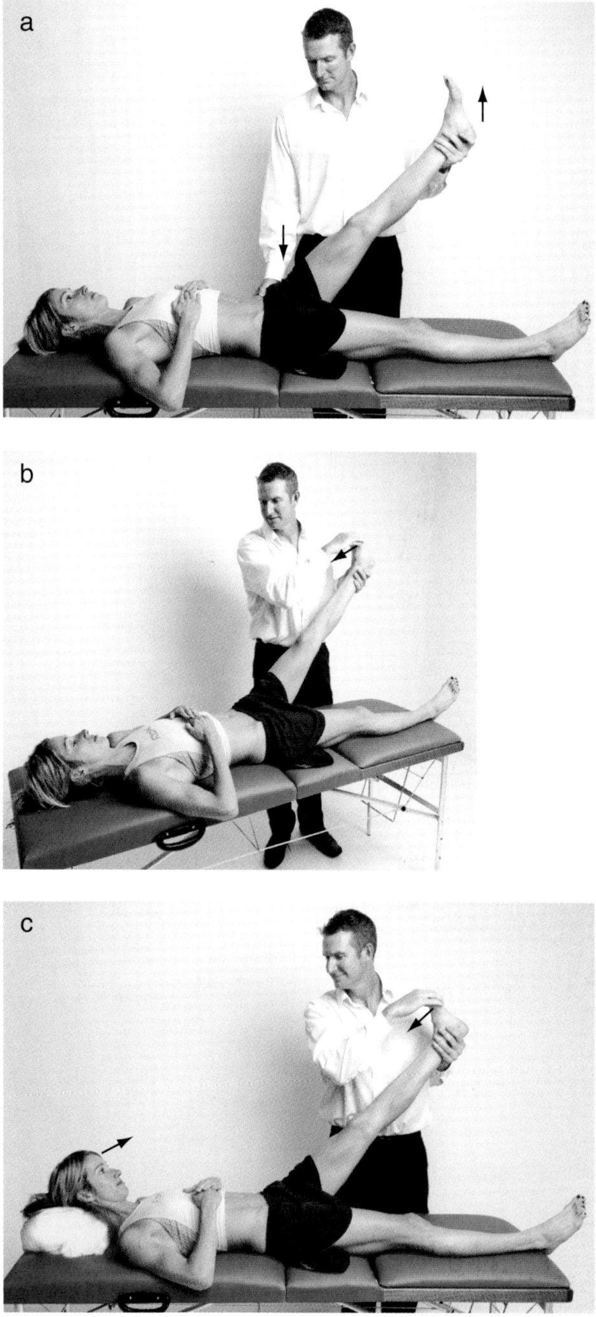


Fig. 2.15a–c Straight leg raise (SLR) test
a Straight leg raise. b SLR plus ankle dorsiflexion. c SLR plus ankle dorsiflexion plus neck flexion

### FABER (HIP FLEXION, ABDUCTION, EXTERNAL ROTATION) TEST

The subject lies supine. The limb on the unaffected side is kept fully extended. On the affected side the flexed hip is abducted and externally rotated, and the knee flexed so that the ankle rests across the other limb just below the knee (Fig. 2.19a). This test is positive if SIJ symptoms are reproduced. Further stress can be placed on the SIJ by the examiner pushing down gently with the palm of a hand over the flexed knee on the affected side (Fig. 2.19b).

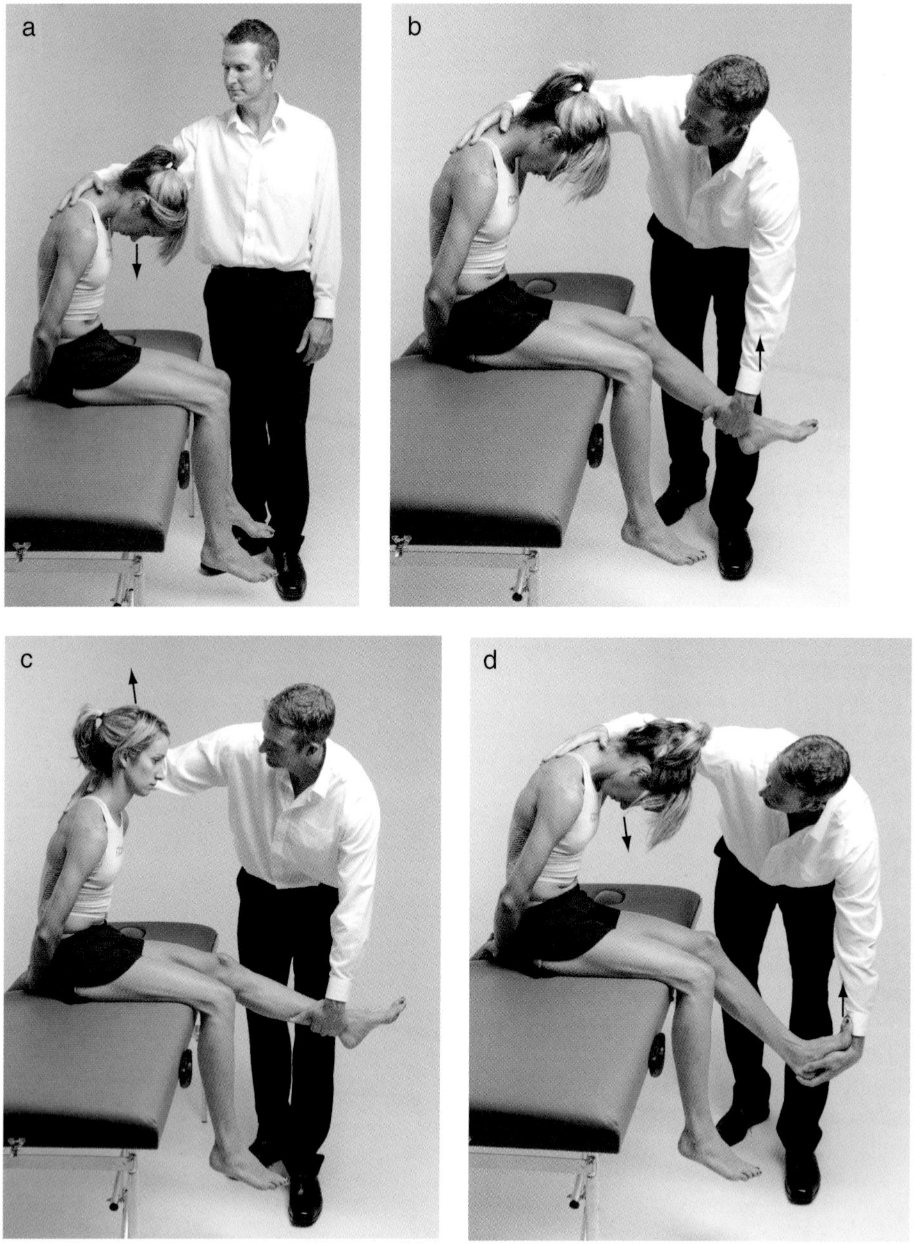


**Fig. 2.16a–d** Slump test
**a** Neck flexion. **b** Neck flexion plus knee extension. **c** Neck extension plus knee extension. **d** Neck flexion, knee extension plus ankle dorsiflexion

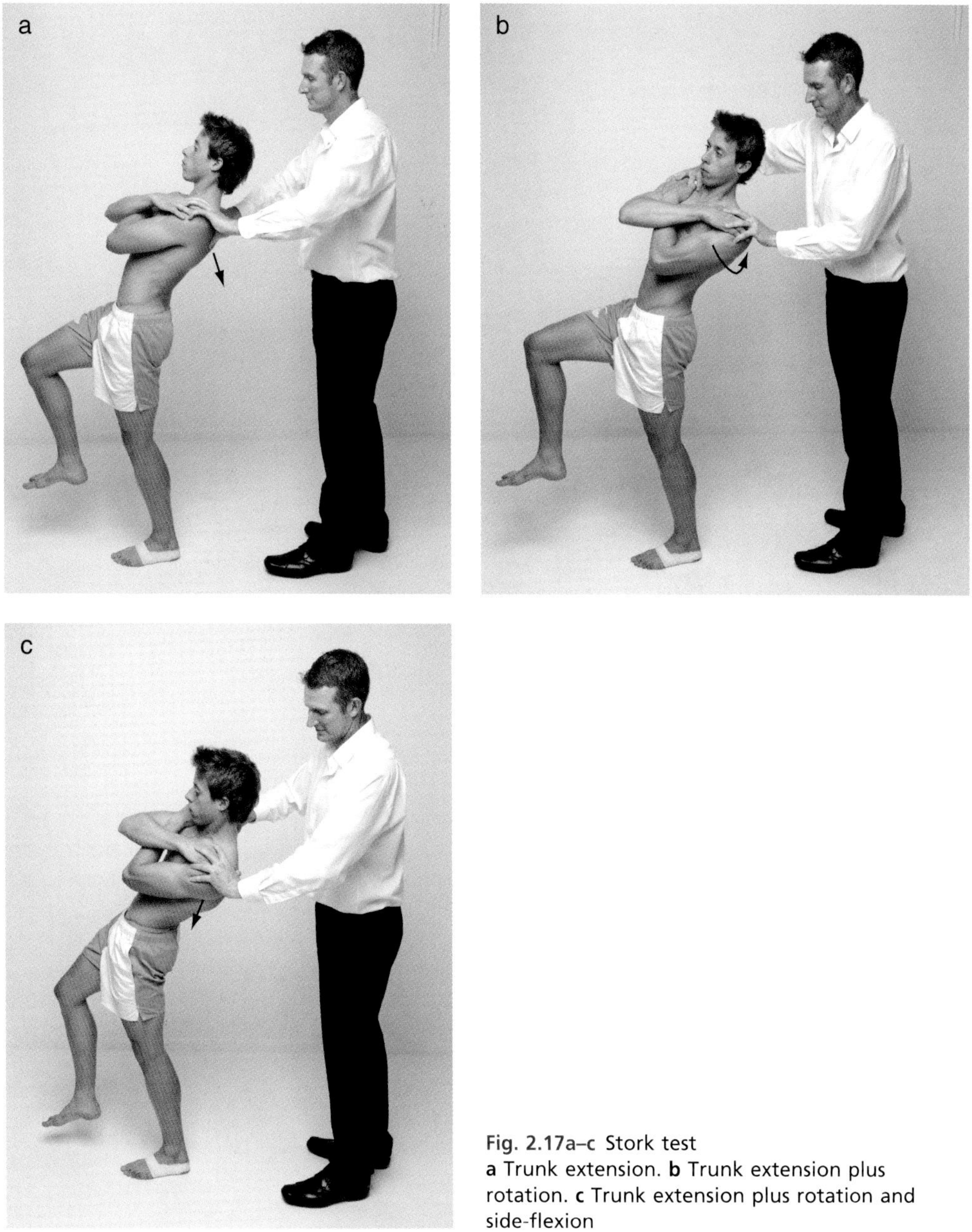

Fig. 2.17a–c Stork test
**a** Trunk extension. **b** Trunk extension plus rotation. **c** Trunk extension plus rotation and side-flexion

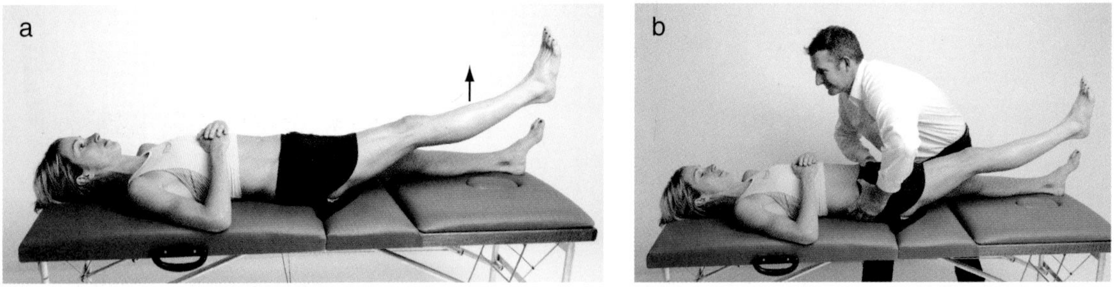


**Fig. 2.18a and b** **a** Active straight leg raise (SLR). **b** Active SLR plus ilial compression

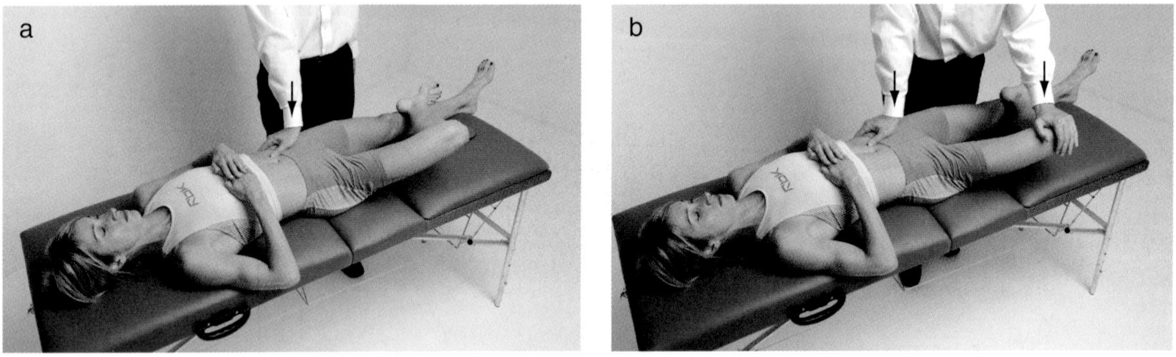


**Fig. 2.19a and b** Faber test

## FURTHER READING


Apsingi S, Dussa CU, Soni BM. Acute cervical spine injuries in mountain biking: a report of three cases. American Journal of Sports Medicine 2006; 34:487–489.

Eller DJ, Katz DS, Bergman AG et al. Sacral stress fractures in long distance runners. Clinical Journal of Sport Medicine 1997; 7:220–221.

Gerrard DF, Doyle TCA. Lumbo-sacral pain in an athlete: an unusual site for stress fracture. Clinical Journal of Sport Medicine 1998; 8:59–61.

McCormack RG, McLean N, Dasilva J et al. Thoraco-lumbar flexion–distraction injury in a competitive gymnast: a case report. Clinical Journal of Sport Medicine 2006; 16:369–371.

Miller SF, Congeni J, Swanson K. Long-term functional and anatomical follow-up of early detected spondylolysis in young athletes. American Journal of Sports Medicine 2004; 32:928–933.

Ranson C, Kerslake R, Burnett A et al. Magnetic resonance imaging of the lumbar spine of asymptomatic professional fast bowlers in cricket. Journal of Bone and Joint Surgery 2005; 87-B:1111–1116.

Sairo K, Katoh S, Sakamaki T, Komatsubara SE et al. Three successive stress fractures at the same vertebral level in an adolescent baseball player. American Journal of Sports Medicine 2003; 31:606–610.

Schmitt H, Gerner HJ. Paralysis from sport and diving accidents. Clinical Journal of Sport Medicine 2001; 11:17–22.

Standaert CJ. Spondylolysis in the adolescent athlete. Clinical Journal of Sport Medicine 2002; 12:119–122.

## CASE STUDY 2 • CLINICAL PROBLEMS

**Problem 1.** *A 16-year-old right-arm baseball pitcher complains of gradually worsening left-sided low back pain. He is now unable to pitch and reports that the pain is reproduced when he bends backward.*

a) What is the most likely diagnosis?
b) What are two possible differential diagnoses?
c) Which clinical test might be employed to diagnose bony injury?
d) What is the most appropriate initial radiological investigation?
e) What is the usual management for acute stress fracture of the pars interarticularis in adolescent athletes?

**Problem 2.** *A 60-year-old female skydiver misjudges a landing and contacts the ground with her feet flat and knees extended. She walks away from the incident but 3 weeks later she is continuing to experience severe mid-spinal pain, which is aggravated when she bends forward, coughs or sneezes.*

a) What is the likely cause of her symptoms?
b) What are at least two possible differential diagnoses?
c) What risk factors for bony injury might this athlete have?
d) How is a stable vertebral fracture likely to be managed?

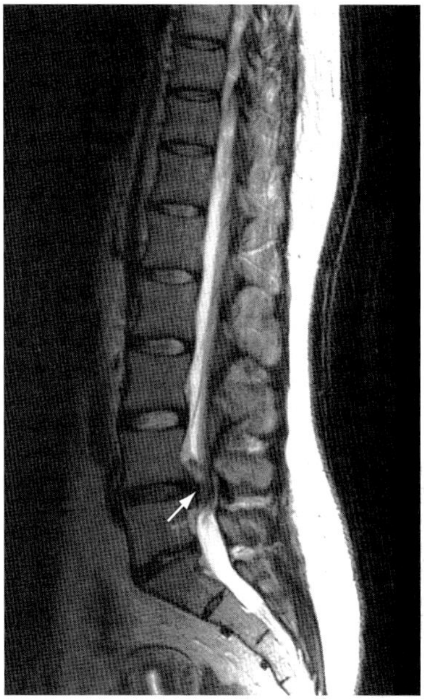

Fig. 2.20 MRI scan of lumbar spine

**Problem 3.** *A 35-year-old male triathlete experiences left lower back pain, together with pain in the buttock, back of thigh and lower leg that comes on after approximately 1 hour of cycling. He also complains of a feeling of weakness in the hamstrings when the pain starts and a reduction in foot dorsiflexion power when pedaling. There is impaired sensation on the lateral side of the leg, which extends on to the medial side of the foot. An MRI scan of the lumbar spine (Fig. 2.20) is performed.*

a) What might be causing these symptoms?
b) Name two sites or structures where the cauda equina, lumbar plexus nerve roots or sciatic nerve may be compromised in this situation.
c) Which dermatome(s) is (are) affected?
d) Would the plantar reflex be affected?
e) What is indicated by the arrow (↓) in the MRI scan in Figure 2.20?

**Problem 4.** *A 29-year-old female long jumper who is returning to training 9 months post-partum reports intermittent lumbo-sacral pain on the side of her take-off leg. She describes an occasional "clunking sensation" in this region when jumping.*

a) What joint is likely to be causing these symptoms?
b) Where can this joint be palpated?
c) What test can be used to stress this joint?
d) How might a recent pregnancy have contributed to instability of the lumbo-pelvic region in this athlete?

**Problem 5.** *When contesting possession of the ball, an Australian Rules footballer is kneed in the lower back just to the left of the spinous processes. The following morning he complains of severe, deep, left low back pain and stiffness.*

a) What damage may have been caused to the bony and soft tissue structures in that area?
b) Are lumbar transverse processes palpable?
c) The following day he reports a rusty discoloration of his urine. What might this indicate?

**Problem 6.** *A veteran race walker experiences worsening bilateral calf pain when walking more than 100 meters. It is worse walking uphill and eases as soon as he stops or if he leans forward when walking.*

a) What is the likely diagnosis and how might it develop?
b) Would the "slump test" be positive in this patient?
c) What treatment might be required?

CHAPTER 3

# Trunk and groin

## INTRODUCTION

The trunk extends from the root of the neck to the groin. It consists of the thorax proximally and the abdomen distally, separated internally by the diaphragm. The thoracic cage, formed by the sternum and ribs, encloses the lungs covered by pleura. The pleural cavities are separated by the mediastinum containing the heart and great vessels. Trauma to the thoracic wall may fracture ribs and tear the underlying lung, leading to pneumothorax. Penetrating injuries may pierce the pericardium and heart. Occasionally, flail chest results from destabilization of a segment of the chest wall. Sudden deceleration may tear the roots of the great vessels, resulting in catastrophic hemorrhage. Lying below the diaphragm and under cover of the lower thoracic wall are the upper abdominal organs, including the liver and spleen (both very vascular and easily torn), the stomach, and the kidneys in each flank on the posterior abdominal wall. The duodenum and pancreas arch across the prominence of the aorta and vertebral bodies on the posterior abdominal wall, making them particularly vulnerable. All of these organs are susceptible to tearing or perforation by blunt upper abdominal trauma.

The particular arrangement of the muscle layers in the lateral and anterior abdominal wall is structured to produce a range of movements of the trunk and spine and to control intra-abdominal pressure, important in lifting and in supporting the spine.

The lower abdomen connects with the root of the lower limb at the groin. Two anatomical features make the groin particularly susceptible to stresses and strains: first, the special arrangement of the muscles of the anterior abdominal wall in this region and the presence of points of potential weakness as a consequence of the inguinal canal, and second, the proximal attachment of muscles of the medial (adductor) group of the thigh to the nearby bony pubis.

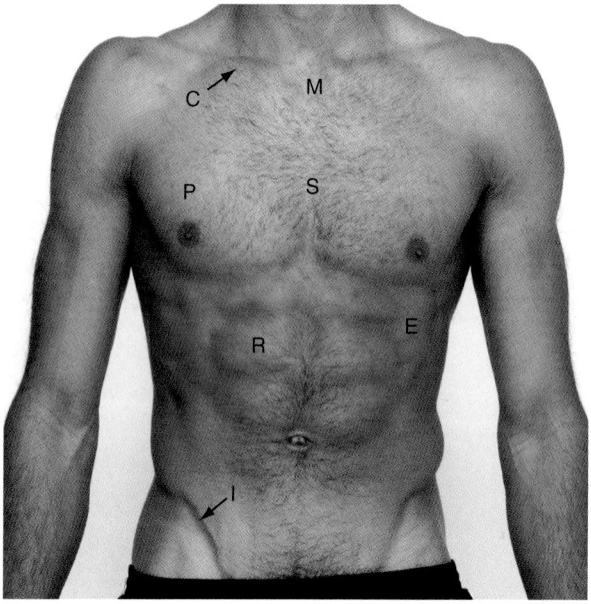


Fig. 3.1 Frontal view showing trunk contours
C = clavicle, E = external oblique, I = inguinal ligament, M = manubrium, P = pectoralis major, R = rectus abdominis, S = body of sternum

## INSPECTION OF NORMAL CONTOURS

- Clavicles
- Suprasternal notch
- Pectorals
- Sterno-manubrial angle
- Costal margin
- Rectus abdominis
- Groin

Viewed from anteriorly, the trunk varies considerably in shape, depending on body type, gender, body fat and muscular development. A frontal view of body contours is shown in Figure 3.1. From the anterior axillary folds, the lateral contour descends almost vertically but with a slight medial inclination down to the level of the waist, more marked in the female. Below the waist the contour continues to descend but with a distinct lateral curvature to the level of the hips below, which continues smoothly into the contour of the thigh. On the anterior thoracic wall the contours of the **clavicles** converge toward the midline **suprasternal notch** above the manubrium. Below the clavicles, on each side of the chest wall, is the **pectoral prominence** of the underlying pectoralis major. In the female these are obscured by the breasts. Between the pectoral prominences, across the midline, the chest wall is flat, marking the underlying manubrium and body of the sternum. In thin subjects a transverse ridge marks the **sterno-manubrial junction.** Ribs 7–10 on each side form an inverted "V" shape, the **costal margin,** converging at the lower end of the sternum at the subcostal angle. From here, in muscular or thin subjects, a shallow **midline groove** descends the anterior abdominal wall, through the umbilicus and continuing down to the pubis. This marks the underlying linea alba. On each side, parallel to the groove, **strap-like ridges** extend from the costal margin down to the pubis. In muscular subjects the upper parts may show segmentation. They are due to the underlying **rectus abdominis muscles.** The **groin** is marked by an **oblique crease** in the skin, extending from the prominent anterior end of the iliac crest downward and medially toward the midline pubes. The **inguinal ligament** lies beneath this crease.

## LOCATING BONY LANDMARKS

- Suprasternal notch, manubrium, sternal body, xiphoid process
- Ribs, costal margin, costo-chondral junction

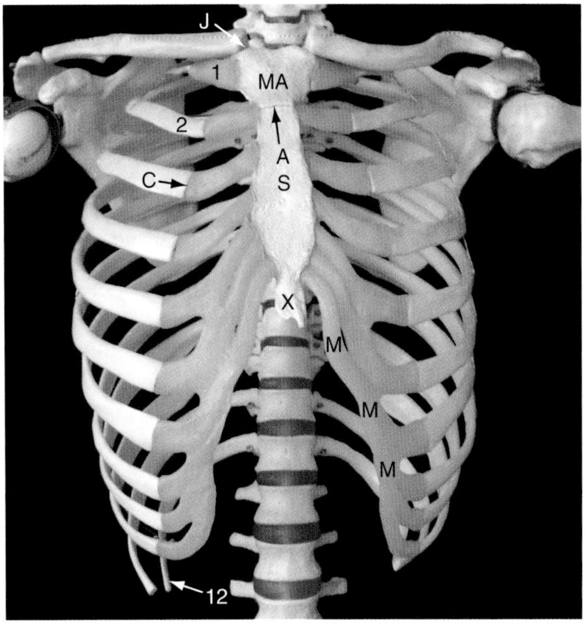


Fig. 3.2a Features of the bony skeleton of the upper trunk (thorax)
A = sterno-manubrial angle, C = costo-chondral junction, J = sterno-clavicular joint, M = costal margin, MA = manubrium, S = body of sternum, X = xiphisternum, 1 = 1st costal cartilage, 2 = 2nd rib, 12 = floating rib

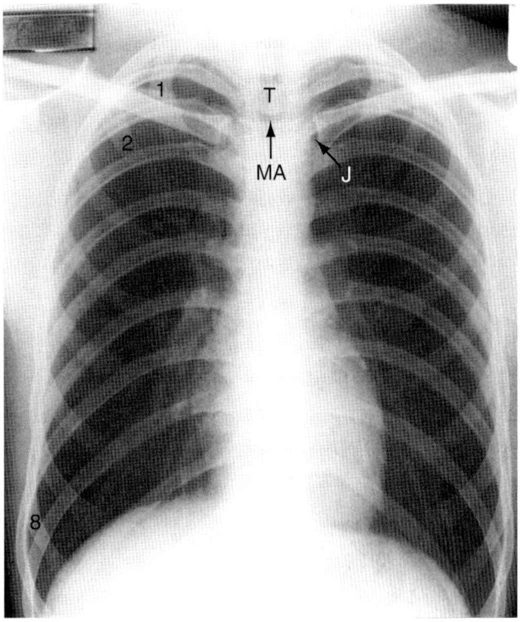


Fig. 3.2b Frontal radiograph of the chest
J = sterno-clavicular joint, MA = upper border of manubrium, T = trachea, 1, 2, 8 = ribs

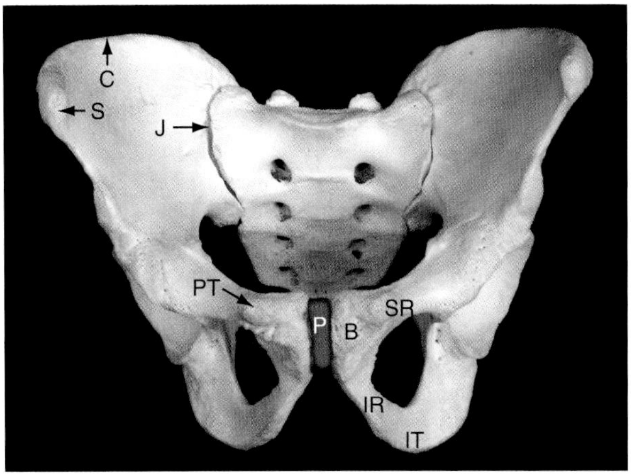


Fig. 3.3a Features of the bony skeleton of the lower trunk (pelvis)
B = body of pubis, C = iliac crest, IR = inferior ramus, IT = ischial tuberosity, J = sacro-iliac joint, P = pubic symphysis, PT = pubic tubercle, S = anterior superior iliac spine, SR = superior ramus

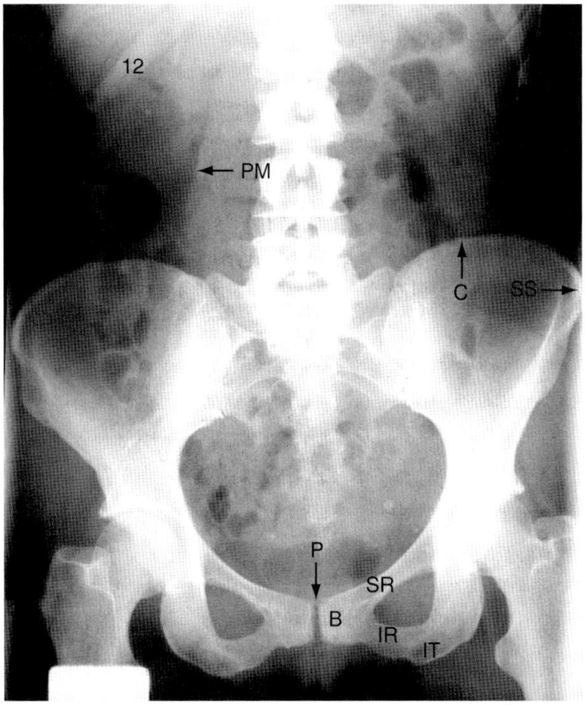


Fig. 3.3b Frontal radiograph of the pelvis
B = body of pubis, C = iliac crest, IR = inferior ramus, IT = ischial tuberosity, P = pubic symphysis, PM = psoas major, SR = superior ramus, SS = anterior superior iliac spine, 12 = floating rib

- Iliac crest and tubercle, anterior superior spine, pubic tubercle
- Symphysis pubis

## SUPRASTERNAL NOTCH, MANUBRIUM, STERNAL BODY AND XIPHOID PROCESS

Bony features of the skeleton of the upper and lower trunk are shown in Figures 3.2a and 3.3a, and radiographs of the chest and lower trunk are shown in Figures 3.2b and 3.3b. The subject lies supine on the couch. Using the index finger, the examiner feels for the upper border of the **manubrium** in the suprasternal notch. The pads of the index and middle fingers are drawn firmly down the front of the manubrium to locate a ridge, the **sternal angle,** marking the sterno-manubrial joint. Firm palpation laterally from this ridge leads to the prominence of the **2nd costal cartilage.** The fingers moving upward from here and crossing the 1st intercostal space, the medial end of the **1st rib** and its costal cartilage can be defined. This is aided by the subject reaching upward, elevating the clavicle and exposing more of the rib. Returning to the front of the sternum and palpating distally into the subcostal angle, a distinct depression marks the xiphisternal junction and leads on to the **xiphoid process,** which can be felt lying on a deeper plane and extending into the subcostal angle. It varies considerably in length and ease of palpation.

## RIBS, COSTAL MARGIN AND COSTO-CHONDRAL JUNCTION

The **costal margin** is located if the examiner draws the pads of the fingers firmly downward and laterally along the edges of the ribs, working from the subcostal angle (Fig. 3.4). To improve definition, the finger tips can be inclined upward as they move along the margin. From the lowest point of the margin, palpating in the flank with the finger tips pointing posteriorly, the free anterior ends of **floating ribs** 11 and 12 can be felt projecting forward into the anterior abdominal wall. Palpation of the ribs is completed by locating the costo-chondral junctions. This requires deep and careful palpation using the pads of the middle and index fingers, and is practicable only in thin subjects. Having defined the edge of the sternum, the examiner locates a rib and slides the fingers laterally along it, moving them firmly forward and backward over the rib, feeling for a slight ridge which marks the **costo-chondral junction** (Fig. 3.5a). This palpation may cause some discomfort. Typical junctions are shown in the prosection in

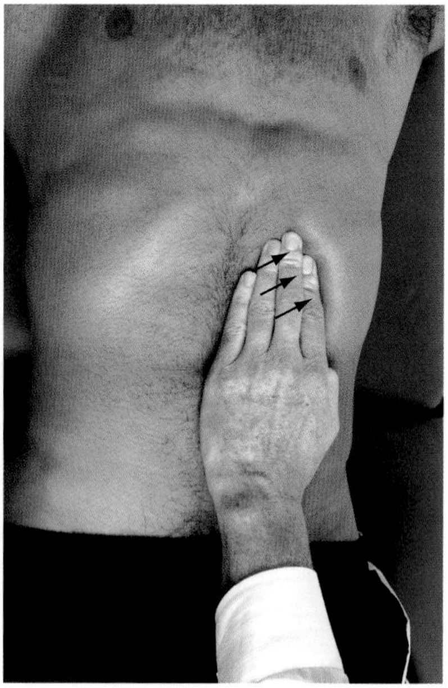

Fig. 3.4 Palpating the costal margin

Figure 3.5b. On the posterior thoracic wall, the location of the **costo-transverse joints** is clinically significant and is described at the end of the chapter.

## SKELETAL LANDMARKS IN THE LOWER ABDOMEN

With the subject lying supine, the examiner places one hand above each hip, pressing the edge of the hand downward and inward to locate the top of the **iliac crest** (Fig. 3.6). The fingers are then drawn firmly forward over the crest and a finger tip is rolled over the easily palpable **anterior superior iliac spine,** to which the inguinal ligament is attached. From here the fingers are moved firmly backward, feeling the outer edge of the crest, to reach a thickened area about 7 cm behind the spine. This is the iliac tubercle and marks the upper attachment of the iliotibial band.

Continuing posteriorly, the whole of the iliac crest can be palpated as far as the skin dimple over the **posterior superior iliac spine.**

In the medial part of the groin, two landmarks may be palpable. The first is located using deep, firm palpation, working along the medial end of the inguinal crease to the prominence of the **pubic tubercle,** where the inguinal ligament is attached. It is confirmed by rolling a finger tip

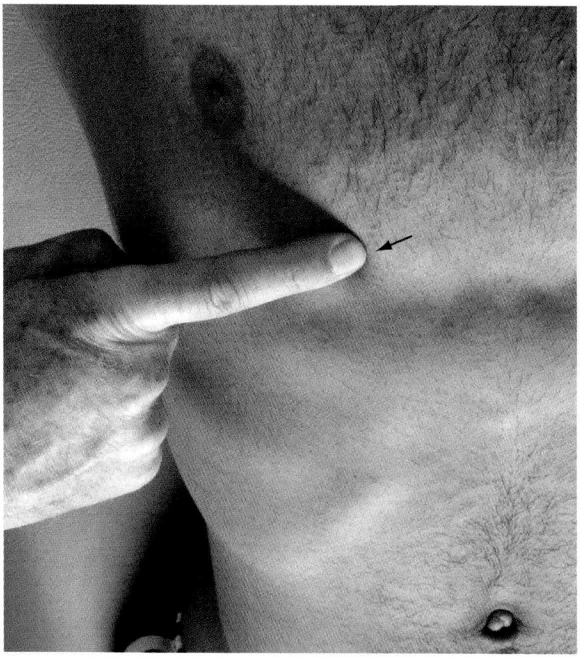

Fig. 3.5a Palpating a costo-chondral junction

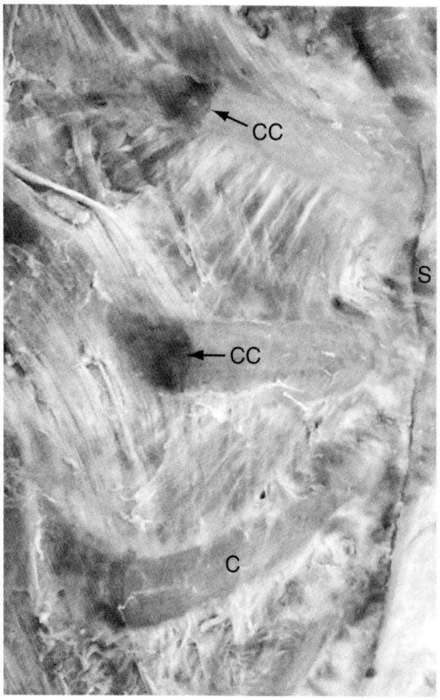


Fig. 3.5b Prosection showing costo-chondral junctions
CC = costo-chondral junctions, C = costal cartilage,
S = sternum

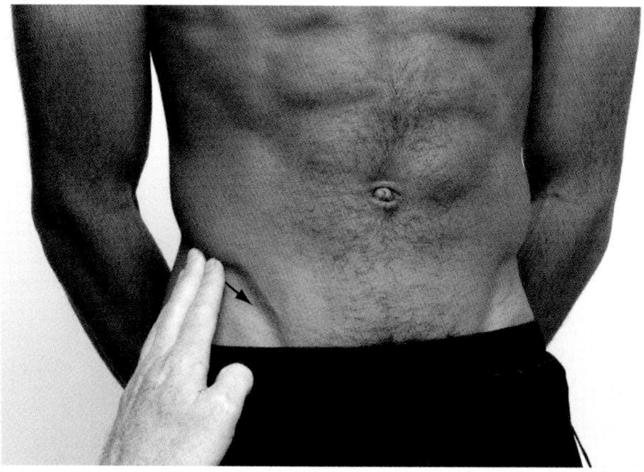

Fig. 3.6 Locating the iliac crest and tubercle

across it. In the male it can be more easily located by invaginating the lateral wall of the root of the scrotum with the index finger tip, feeling upward for the superficial inguinal ring and the tubercle just lateral to it. To locate the second landmark, the lower end of the **symphysis pubis**, deep palpation is made in the midline through the soft tissue of the pubes, with the index finger working downward to reach the point of final convergence of the subpubic arch and the finger tip being turned upward to feel the lower end of the symphysis. In the male this lies close to the root of the dorsum of the penis, and in the female close to the clitoris.

# LOCATING SOFT TISSUES

- Femoral artery

## FEMORAL ARTERY

The subject lies supine on the couch, with the thigh partially flexed and groin relaxed. With the subject's thigh passively abducted and laterally rotated, the examiner palpates with the tips of the middle fingers just below the midpoint of the inguinal crease, applying firm deep pressure to feel pulsations of the femoral artery (Fig. 3.7). Excessive pressure may obliterate the pulse.

CHAPTER

# TESTING MUSCLES

- Rectus abdominis
- Abdominal obliques
- Psoas major
- Adductors
- Transversus abdominis

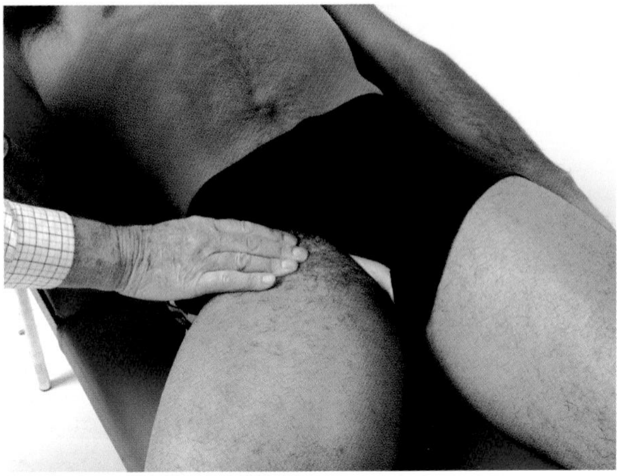

Fig. 3.7 Palpating the femoral artery

The trunk muscles fall in three groups: those attaching the upper limb to the trunk, the pectorals and serratus anterior (considered in Ch. 4); the intercostals between the ribs, which are not very accessible; and the muscles of the anterior, lateral, and posterior abdominal walls, which are more substantial. The rectus abdominis lies anteriorly on each side of the midline, whilst three muscles, the external and internal obliques and the transversus abdominis, lie more laterally, and the psoas major is on the posterior abdominal wall. Some of these muscles are shown in a prosection in Figure 3.8.

## RECTUS ABDOMINIS

To demonstrate rectus abdominis, subjects lie in crook, with the hands behind the head. They then lift their head and shoulders off the couch. In thin and muscular subjects, the recti appear as conspicuous bands, segmented above the level of the umbilicus, lying on either side of the midline and extending from the costal margin to the pubis (Fig. 3.9a). A midline groove may be palpable between them, marking the linea alba, and the lateral edge of the muscle is easily felt. Resistance may be added if the examiner presses a hand over the manubrium (Fig. 3.9b).

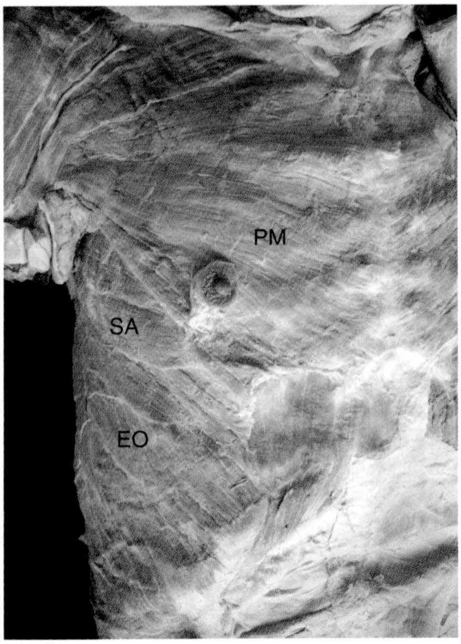


Fig. 3.8a Prosection of muscles of the anterior thoracic wall
EO = external oblique, PM = pectoralis major, SA = serratus anterior

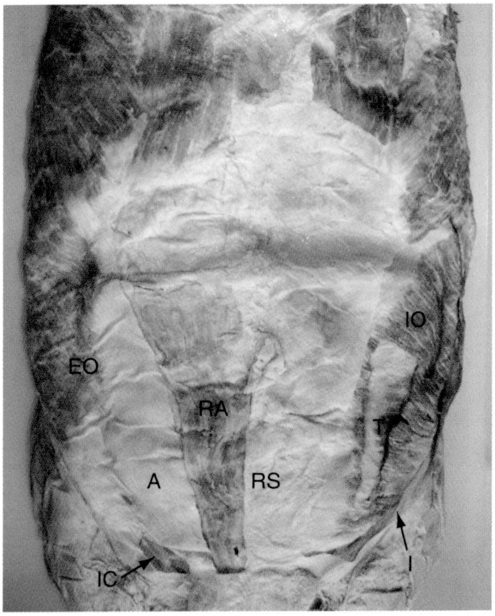


Fig. 3.8b Prosection of muscles of the anterior abdominal wall
A = external oblique aponeurosis, EO = external oblique, I = inguinal ligament, IC = inguinal canal, IO = internal oblique, RA = rectus abdominis, RS = rectus sheath, T = transversus abdominis

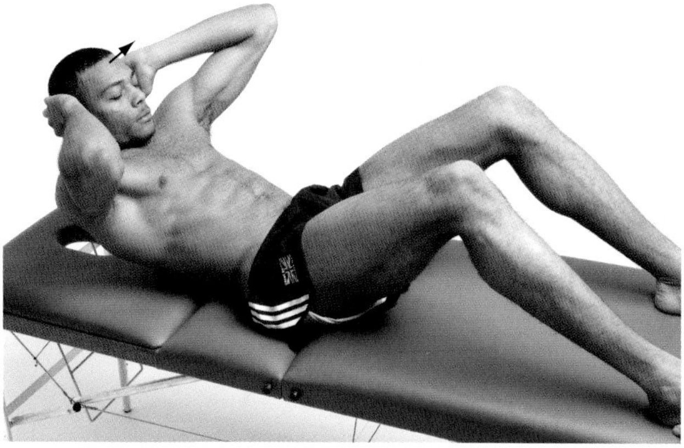

Fig. 3.9a Demonstrating and testing the rectus abdominis

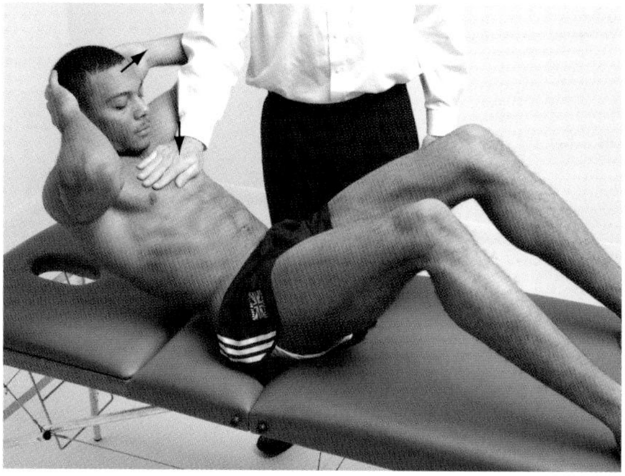

Fig. 3.9b Resisting contraction of the rectus abdominis

Weakness and mid-abdominal pain may indicate rectus abdominis strain.

## ABDOMINAL OBLIQUES

The abdominal obliques are tested with the subject standing and facing the examiner. Their actions include trunk rotation. The subject extends both arms and raises them forward and upward through 90°. The trunk is then rotated to one side, the extended arms moving with it but resisted by the examiner, who pushes against them. The test can also be performed with the subject's arms folded across the front of the chest, the examiner resisting movement by pushing against the elbow. The external oblique on one side acts with the internal oblique on the opposite side to rotate the trunk. During the movement the fibers of the external oblique may be visible passing downward and forward from the lower ribs into the abdominal wall. They can be felt contracting by holding the fingers of one hand against the chest wall in the direction of the fibers whilst rotation is being resisted. The external oblique can also be tested by asking the subject to "sit up" and twist from a crook lying position with the hands behind the head (Fig. 3.10a). Resistance to the trunk rotation can be applied using a hand over the subject's shoulder (Fig. 3.10b).

## PSOAS MAJOR

The psoas major is deep and paravertebral, and can be palpated from anteriorly, through the abdominal cavity, when the subject is positioned in crook lying with a relaxed abdomen. The tips of the examiner's index and middle fingers are placed immediately lateral to the rectus abdominis, just below the level of the umbilicus. Firm pressure directed obliquely toward the midline allows the cylindrical psoas muscle belly to be palpated (Fig. 3.11). The length of the psoas major can be tested using the modified Thomas test. Sitting on the end of the couch, subjects are asked to hold one knee to their chest and to roll on to their back. The limb is now released and the foot supported on the examiner's hip, maintaining the lumbar spine flat against the couch. The resting angle of hip extension is then measured using a goniometer or inclinometer (Fig. 3.12a). Differentiation of loss of hip extension ROM due to tightness of the rectus femoris can be assessed by attempting to flex the subject's knee passively (Fig. 3.12b). If further knee flexion ROM can be gained, then the rectus femoris is not limiting hip extension. To test the strength of the psoas in this position, the subject is asked to flex the thigh upward at the hip whilst the movement is resisted by the examiner, who pushes downward on the distal thigh (Fig. 3.13).

## ADDUCTOR GROUP

The adductor group forms three layers in the medial compartment of the thigh and is shown in a prosection in Figure 3.14. Proximally, these muscles arise from the body and rami of the pubis and distally attach to the region of the linea aspera of the femur, reaching as far as the adductor tubercle above the medial condyle of the femur. They are supplied by the obturator nerve. To test the long adductors (adductor longus, adductor magnus and gracilis), the subject lies supine with the legs extended. The examiner stands between the subject's legs and abducts the limb to be tested to approximately 45°. The subject is then asked to adduct forcefully against the outside of the

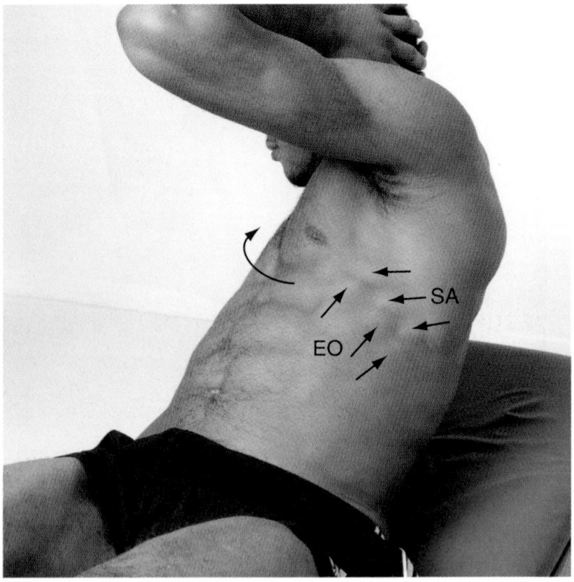


Fig. 3.10a Testing the abdominal oblique muscles
EO = external oblique, SA = serratus anterior

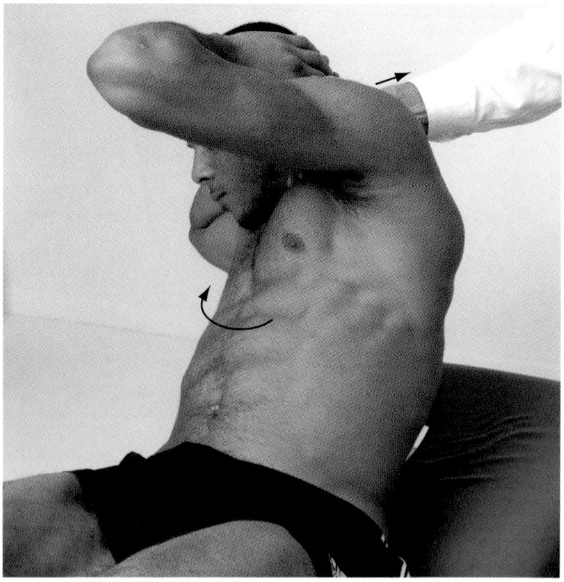

Fig. 3.10b Testing the abdominal oblique muscles with resistance

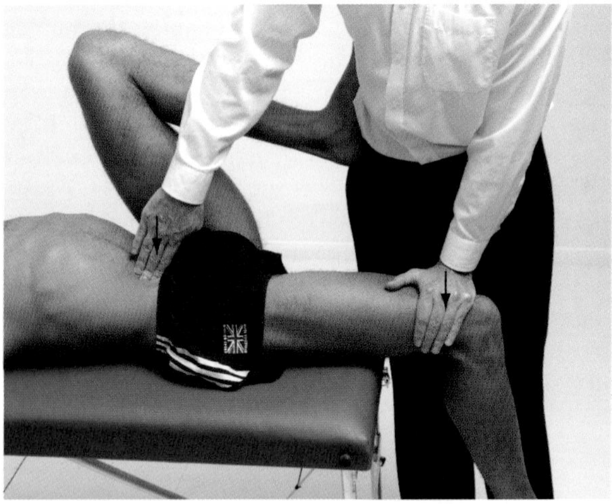

Fig. 3.11 Palpating the psoas major muscle

examiner's thigh (Fig. 3.15). The adductors can be felt contracting if the examiner palpates on the medial side of the thigh. The short adductors (adductor brevis and pectineus) can be tested with the subject lying supine, with the hips and knees sufficiently flexed to allow the feet to lie flat on the couch. Placing a clenched fist between the knees, the examiner then asks the subject to adduct them strongly (Fig. 3.16). Tears or tendonitis cause pain in the pubic region when adduction is attempted. Pain that is reproduced during a similar fist squeeze test performed with the hips and knees only slightly flexed (Fig. 3.17) may indicate **derangement of the pubic symphysis.**

## TRANSVERSUS ABDOMINIS

The transversus abdominis forms the deepest muscular layer of the lower abdominal wall. It is a horizontal forward extension having continuity with the thoraco-lumbar fascia, and is thought to play an important role in dynamic stabilization of the lumbar spine via its ability to tension the fascia and regulate intra-abdominal pressure. Insufficient tone of the transversus abdominis is manifested in the appearance of a "pot belly" and loss of the normal lumbar lordosis (Fig. 3.18a). Contraction of the transversus abdominis whilst maintaining diaphragmatic breathing results in a drawing in of the lower abdomen and restoration of the lumbar lordosis (Fig. 3.18b).

# SPECIAL TESTS

- Hernias
- Rib fracture

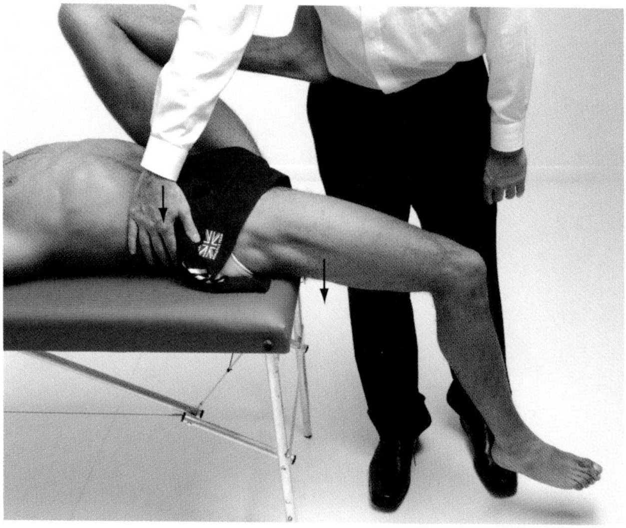

Fig. 3.12a Testing the length of the psoas major muscle (Thomas test)

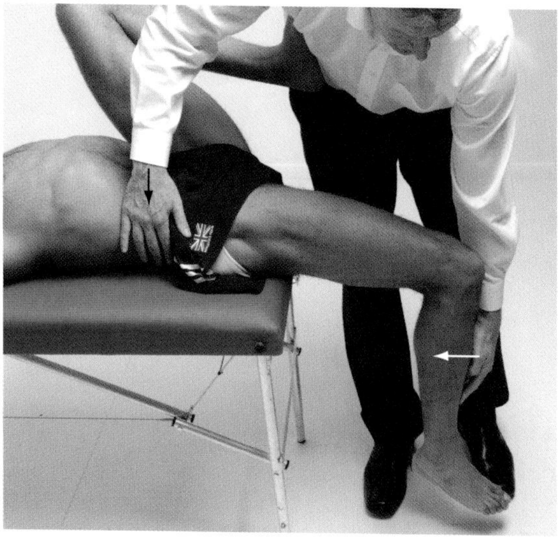

Fig. 3.12b Differentiating tightness of the psoas and rectus femoris (Thomas test)

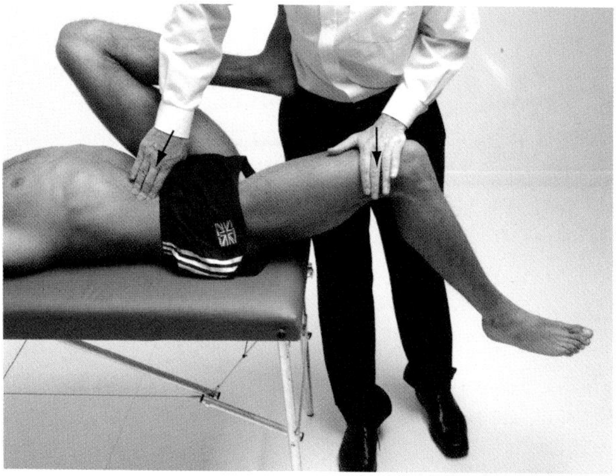

Fig. 3.13 Testing the strength of the psoas major muscle

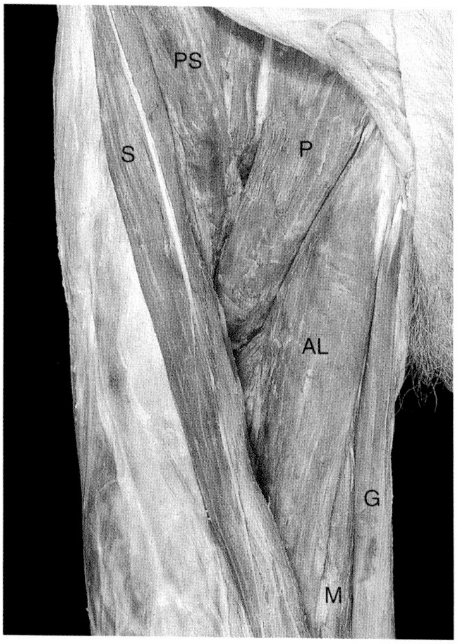


Fig. 3.14 Prosection showing the adductor group of muscles
AL = adductor longus, G = gracilis, M = adductor magnus, P = pectineus, PS = psoas major, S = sartorius (From Gosling JA, Harris PF, Whitmore I, Willan PLT. 2002 Human Anatomy, 4th edn. London: Mosby)

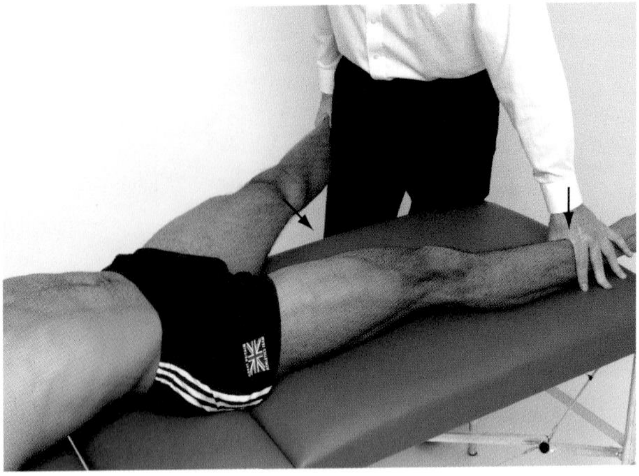

Fig. 3.15 Testing long adductors of the thigh

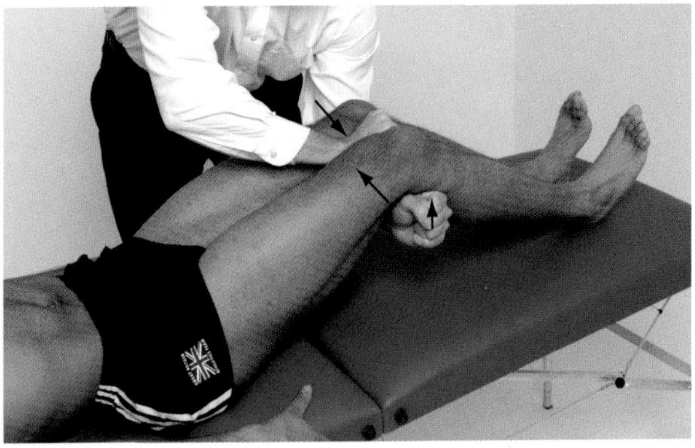

Fig. 3.17 Fist squeeze test for derangement of the pubic symphysis

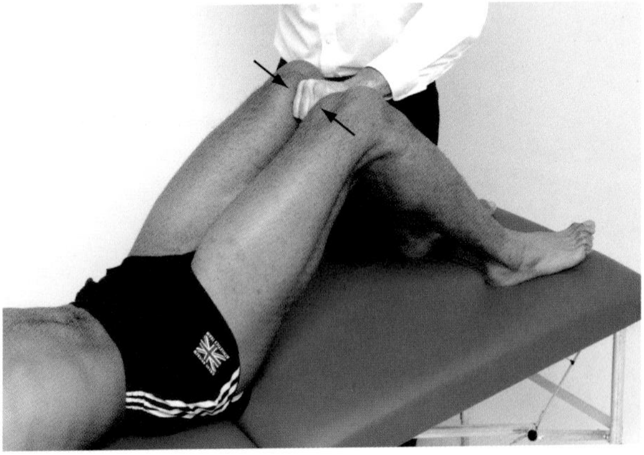

Fig. 3.16 Testing short adductors of the thigh

- Costo-transverse joints
- Obturator nerve tension test

## INGUINAL RING AND ANTERIOR ABDOMINAL WALL HERNIAS

The subject lies supine or stands facing the examiner. The groin is exposed and the subject is asked to cough, turning the head away from the examiner. A swelling may appear or increase in size. It is palpated and tested for a thrill and to ascertain whether it can be reduced; if so, its relation to the pubic tubercle is also assessed. Some sports hernias are characterized by little, if any, swelling, although the superficial inguinal ring is patent, but there is pain and tenderness above and medial to the tubercle, just lateral to the edge of the lower end of a narrow rectus abdominis.

## FRACTURED RIB(S)

The subject stands or sits facing the examiner, who places the palm of one hand over the edge of the sternum on the front of the chest, and the palm of the other diametrically opposite on the back of the chest. The chest is then compressed between the two hands, causing localized pain if there is a fracture (Fig. 3.19).

## DERANGEMENTS OF COSTO-TRANSVERSE JOINTS

These are common in activities such as rowing and racquet, throwing and combat sports. Posterior–anterior gliding is used to assess for tenderness, movement dysfunction, and mobilization of these joints. The examiner locates the angle of the rib about 7–10 cm lateral to the midline spinous processes, and uses the pads of both thumbs to apply anteriorly directed pressure (Fig. 3.20).

## SLUMP TEST (OBTURATOR NERVE BIAS)

Adverse neural tension in the obturator nerve can be assessed using a modification of the slump test described in Chapter 2. With the subject in the slump position, the examiner fully abducts the hip (Fig. 3.21). Obturator nerve tension may be present if further hip abduction can be achieved when the subject lifts the head.

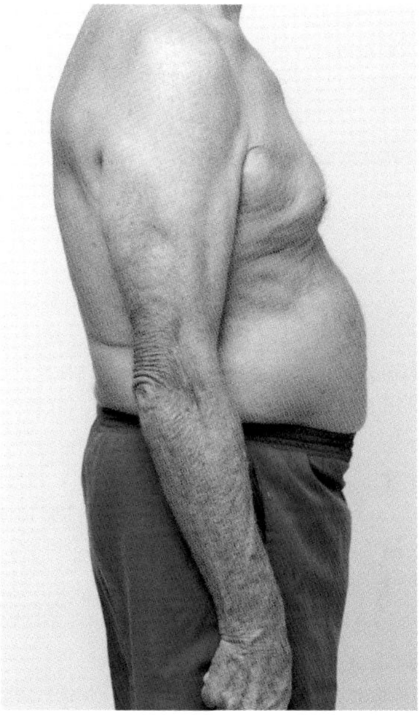

Fig. 3.18a Loss of transversus abdominis tone

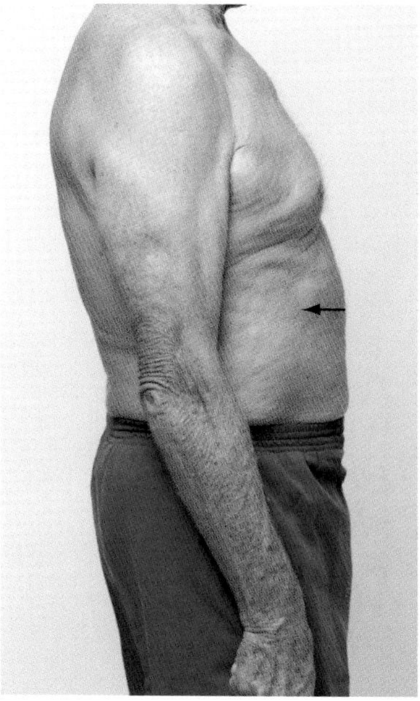

Fig. 3.18b Indrawing of the lower abdominal wall by transversus abdominis

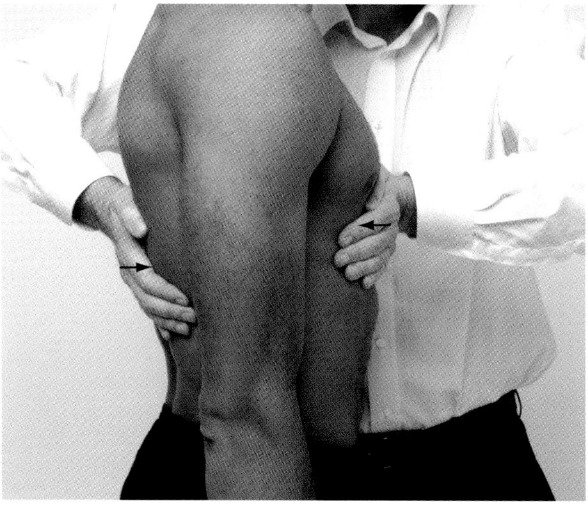

Fig. 3.19 Testing for fractured rib(s)

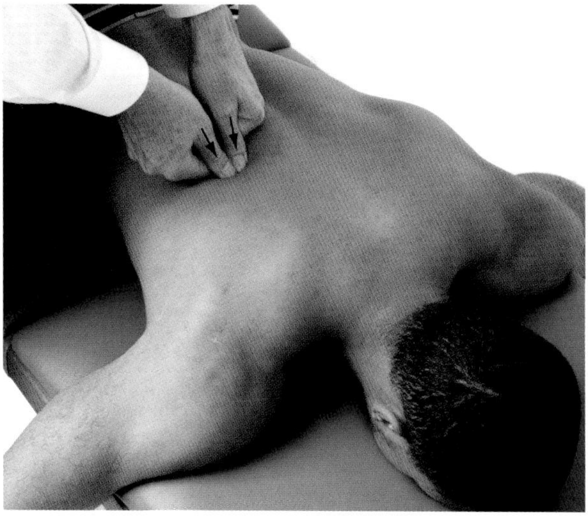

Fig. 3.20 Locating derangement in costo-transverse joints

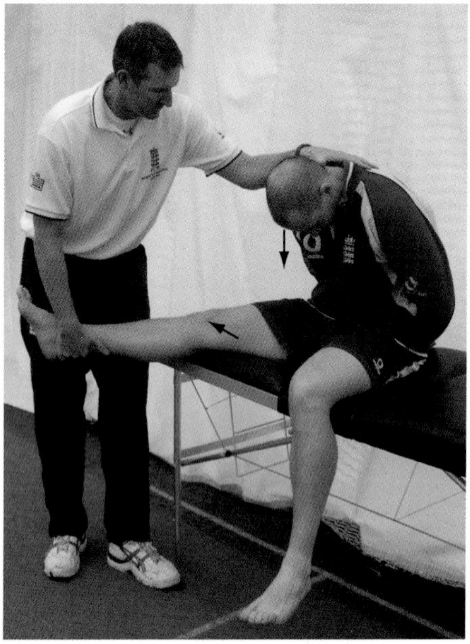

Fig. 3.21 Slump test with hip abduction (obturator nerve bias)

## FURTHER READING

Biedert RM, Warnke K, Meyer S. Symphysis syndrome in athletes: surgical treatment for chronic lower abdominal, groin and adductor pain in athletes. Clinical Journal of Sport Medicine 2003; 13:278–284.

Bradshaw C, McCrory P, Bell S, Brukner P. Obturator nerve entrapment: a cause of groin pain in athletes. American Journal of Sports Medicine 1997; 25(3):402–407.

Coris EE, Higgin II HW. First rib stress fractures in throwing athletes. American Journal of Sports Medicine 2005; 33:1400–1404.

Emery CA, Meeuwisse WH, Curl LA et al. Groin and abdominal strain injuries in the National Hockey League. Clinical Journal of Sport Medicine 1999; 9:177–183.

Flik K, Callahan LR. Delayed splenic rupture in an amateur hockey player. Clinical Journal of Sport Medicine 1998; 8:309.

Gregory PL, Biswas AC, Batt ME. Musculoskeletal problems of the chest wall in athletes. Sports Medicine 2002; 32:235–250.

Humphries D, Jamison M. Clinical and magnetic resonance imaging features of cricket bowler's side strain. British Journal of Sports Medicine 2004; 38:1–3.

Lacroix VJ, Kinnear DG, Mulder DS et al. Lower abdominal pain syndrome in National Hockey League players: a report of 11 cases. Clinical Journal of Sport Medicine 1998; 8:5–9.

Zvijac JE, Matthias RS, Hechtman KS et al. Pectoralis major tears: a correlation of magnetic resonance imaging and treatment strategies. American Journal of Sports Medicine 2006; 34:289–294.

## CASE STUDY 3 • CLINICAL PROBLEMS

**Problem 1.** *A 25-year-old male canoeist experiences a sudden, severe, right antero-lateral chest pain whilst performing strenuous paddle strokes. It continues and makes him abandon his exercise. The team physiotherapist examines him and finds a localized tender swelling along the line of the 5th rib close to the right nipple. He orders an ultrasound scan (Fig. 3.22).*

a) What is the most likely diagnosis?
b) What are the alternative diagnoses?
c) What does the scan show?
d) The attachment of which muscle is implicated in this type of injury?
e) What clinically significant costal parts can be palpated?
f) What test can be used to assess derangement of costal arches?

**Problem 2.** *A 30-year-old right-footed male footballer is experiencing right-sided lower abdominal pain when starting to sprint and when kicking the ball over a long distance. The pain radiates to his right groin and scrotum.*

a) What are three possible causes of these symptoms?
b) What other symptoms might he be experiencing?
c) What clinical tests might be used to diagnose the problem?

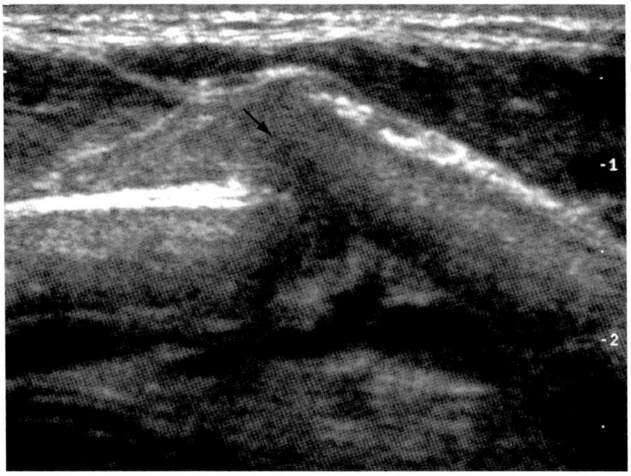


Fig. 3.22 Ultrasound image of rib injury

**Problem 3.** *A 19-year-old left-handed female tennis player feels a sudden, sharp, upper abdominal pain when attempting to serve. The pain is localized to 2 cm left of the midline and 4 cm caudal to the umbilicus, and she is unable to complete the match.*

a) What is the likely diagnosis?
b) What is one possible differential diagnosis?
c) If the symptoms are due to a muscle strain, what is the likely mechanism of injury?

**Problem 4.** *A 27-year-old right-handed male javelin thrower experiences a sharp pain in his left side following a throw in competition. He is unable to continue. Examination 24 hours later reveals tenderness over the region of the 9th rib in the mid-axillary line. Resisted trunk side-flexion and rotation to the left are also painful.*

a) What muscle is likely to have been injured?
b) In what other sports is this injury common?
c) What differential diagnoses should be considered?

**Problem 5.** *A 20-year-old male Australian Rules football player complains of right medial thigh pain that comes on approximately 10 minutes after starting to run, forcing him to stop. However, the pain subsides within 30 minutes of ceasing to run. After a series of tests, obturator nerve entrapment is diagnosed.*

a) By what mechanism and at which anatomical site is the nerve compression likely to have occurred?
b) What neurological tests might be positive?
c) Which lumbo-sacral plexus neural tension test might be positive?

4

CHAPTER

# Shoulder and arm

## INTRODUCTION

The shoulder joint forms the core of the shoulder region. Due to its mobility and wide range of movements, this joint is one of the most susceptible to injury. Additionally, the acromio-clavicular and sterno-clavicular joints at the respective ends of the clavicle have an important role in the mobility of the shoulder. Dorsally, also very important in mobility, especially in reaching and throwing, is the musculo-scapular complex mooring the scapula to the trunk. The axilla, with its muscular walls, lies between the shoulder and the upper thoracic wall, and provides passage for the main neurovascular supply from the root of the neck into the upper limb. Distal to the axilla, the arm forms the proximal part of the lever system of the

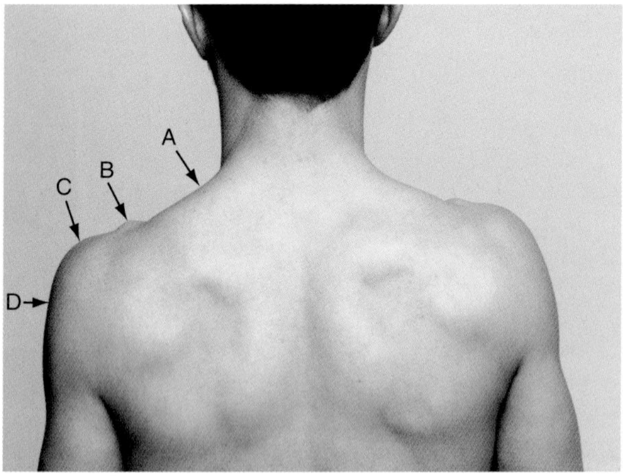


Fig. 4.1 Neck–shoulder contour from posterior
A = trapezius, B = acromio-clavicular joint, C = lateral edge of acromion, D = deltoid

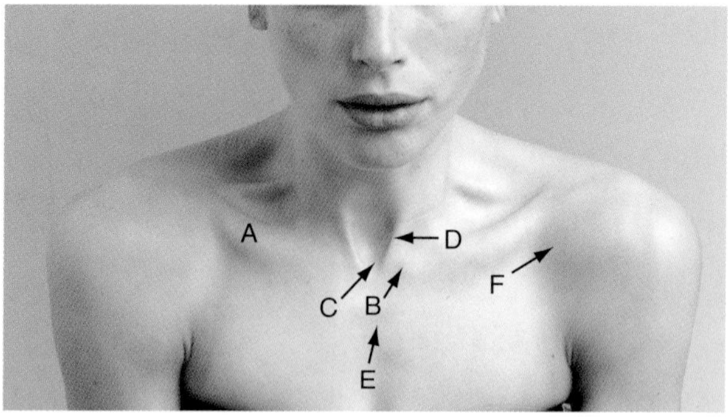


Fig. 4.2 Surface features at the root of the neck from anterior
A = clavicle (the supraclavicular and infraclavicular fossae are clearly defined), B = sterno-clavicular joint, C = upper border of manubrium, D = sterno-mastoid (the sternal and clavicular heads are each visible), E = sterno-manubrial angle, F = anterior border of deltoid

upper limb with two muscular compartments, flexor and extensor, the muscles of each being susceptible to injury.

## INSPECTION OF NORMAL CONTOURS

- Trapezius
- Deltoid
- Clavicle and scapula
- Pectoralis major
- Biceps and triceps brachii

Viewed from dorsally, the neck–shoulder contour, arising from the underlying **trapezius muscle,** forms a smooth concave curve (Fig. 4.1) downward and laterally from the side of the neck to the point of the shoulder. From the shoulder, the contour, formed by the underlying **deltoid muscle,** is smoothly convex and continues down to the lateral border of the arm. Anteriorly, the **clavicle** forms a characteristic sinuous prominence at the root of the neck, with depressions above and below it (Fig. 4.2). The medial and lateral ends of the clavicle vary in their prominence. On the back of the shoulder the triangular prominence of the **scapula,** particularly its lower half and its associated muscles, is visible, the amount of detail depending upon the extent of subcutaneous fat and thickness of the muscles covering it.

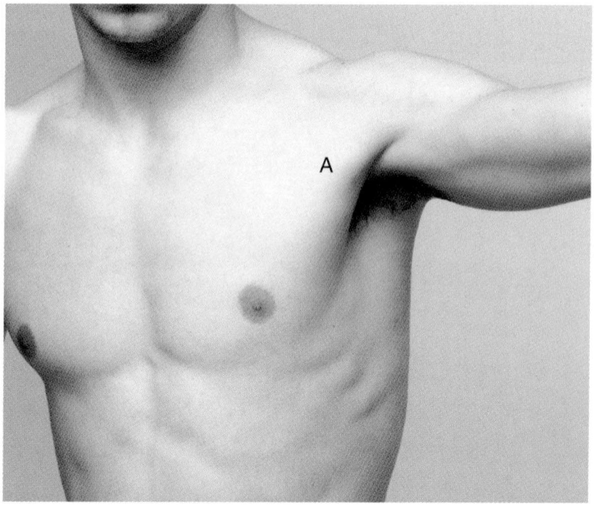


Fig. 4.3 Anterior wall of the axilla
A = pectoralis major. Note: serrations of serratus anterior also visible

The **pectoralis major** and underlying pectoralis minor contribute to the fullness over the anterior chest wall, being particularly visible in the male, and more laterally to the anterior axillary fold (Fig. 4.3). On the front of the arm the **biceps brachii** forms a prominence, on each side of which is a furrow, the medial being the more important.

On the posterior aspect of the arm there is an elongated prominence due to the underlying **triceps brachii.**

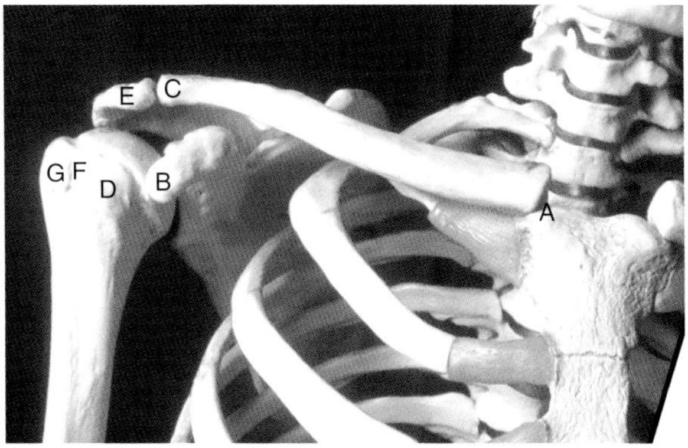


Fig. 4.4 Bony landmarks on the shoulder skeleton from the front
A = sterno-clavicular joint, B = coracoid process, C = lateral end of clavicle articulating with acromion, D = lesser tuberosity, E = anterior border of acromion, F = bicipital groove of humerus, G = greater tuberosity

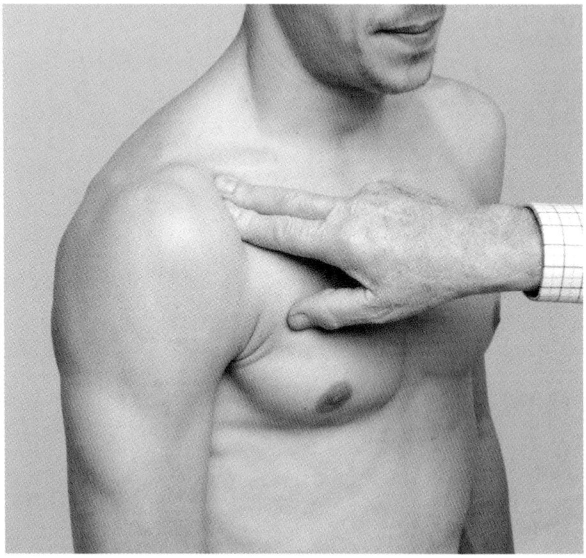

Fig. 4.5 Palpating the coracoid process

# LOCATING BONY LANDMARKS

- Clavicle
- Scapula
- Subacromial groove
- Humerus: greater and lesser tuberosity
- Bicipital groove

Palpable bony landmarks on the anterior aspect of the shoulder are indicated on the skeleton in Figure 4.4.

## THE CLAVICLE

The clavicle is best palpated starting from the medial rounded end, where it forms the lateral boundary of the suprasternal notch. The finger is passed laterally along the anterior subcutaneous border of the medial half of the shaft, noting the anterior convexity. Continuing laterally, the clavicle changes direction, becoming convex posteriorly. The lateral end of the clavicle terminates at the shoulder as a flattened edge, which is felt as a ridge rising above the level of its articulation with the acromion.

## THE SCAPULA

Several parts of the scapula are palpable. If two finger tips are rolled over it, the **coracoid process** can be felt as an oblique prominence about 2 cm below the lateral part of the clavicle, just beneath the anterior border of the deltoid muscle (Fig. 4.5). It can be confirmed by feeling it rotate whilst the arm is abducted. The bony points that are palpable on the posterior aspect of the shoulder are summarized on the skeleton in Figure 4.6. The **acromion** is best located by firm palpation of its lateral edge, where it forms a distinct ridge at the summit of the shoulder (Fig. 4.7). As the lateral edge of the acromion is traced posteriorly, it abruptly turns medially, the change in direction being marked by a sharp angular point, easily palpable. This is an important landmark, which can be used as a guide when injecting into the subacromial space (Fig. 4.8). As palpation is continued medially from the posterior border of the acromion, this leads on to the **spine.** Using firm palpation, the spine can be traced medially to its termination at the medial border of the scapula. The **medial border** can be felt starting at the **superior angle** and continuing down to the easily palpable **inferior angle** (Fig. 4.9). This can be confirmed by palpating over the angle as it moves laterally whilst the limb is abducted to lie above the head. The lateral border is difficult to define, being covered by the teres major and latissimus dorsi muscles. The **scapula** can be balloted by pressing two finger tips firmly backward on the coracoid process, at the same time using the other hand to grip the inferior angle to push the scapula upward. This is painful in the presence of a fracture.

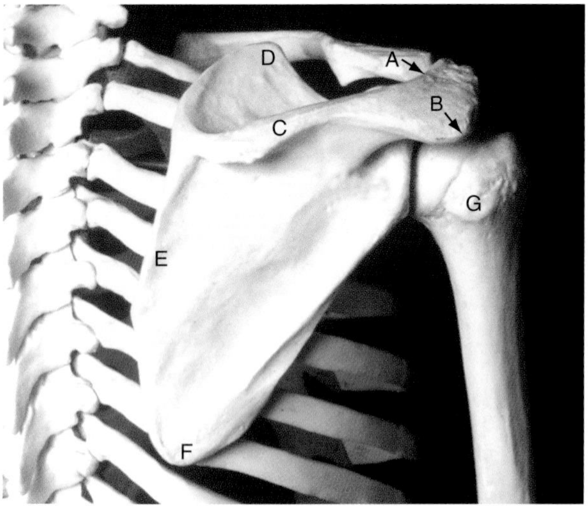


Fig. 4.6 Bony landmarks on the shoulder skeleton from the back
A = acromio-clavicular joint, B = posterior angle of acromion, C = spine of scapula, D = superior angle of scapula, E = medial (vertebral) border of scapula, F = inferior angle of scapula, G = inferior facet on greater tuberosity (teres minor attachment)

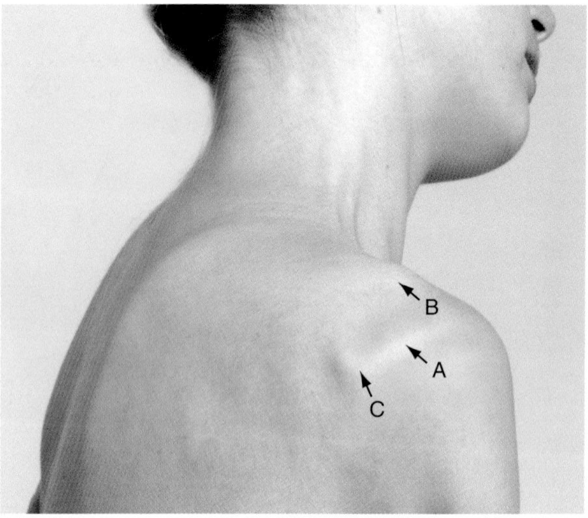


Fig. 4.7 Surface features of the shoulder from laterally
A = lateral edge of acromion, B = lateral end of clavicle and acromio-clavicular joint, C = posterior angle of acromion

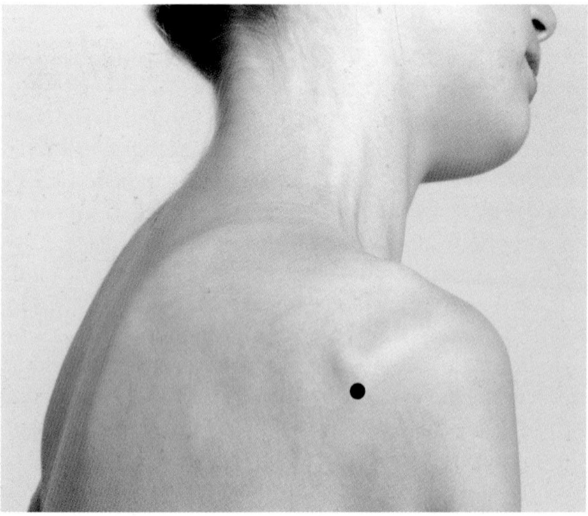

Fig. 4.8 Site for injecting into the subacromial space (black dot)

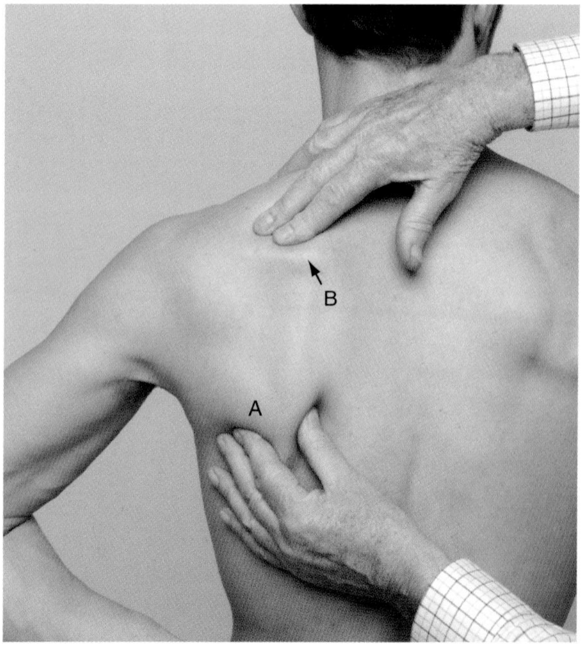


Fig. 4.9 Palpating the inferior angle of the scapula and supraspinous fossa
A = teres major, B = spine of scapula

## SUBACROMIAL GROOVE

Immediately below the lateral edge of the acromion, a distinct **groove** can be felt, with the deltoid muscle relaxed, by applying firm palpation over the soft tissues (Fig. 4.10). This overlies the **subacromial space** (Fig. 4.11).

## HUMERUS: GREATER AND LESSER TUBEROSITY

Continuing below the groove on the lateral surface of the shoulder and using a firm massaging motion with the finger tips, the resistance of the **greater tuberosity** of the humerus can be felt through the deltoid muscle (Figs 4.12 and 4.13). Lateral to the coracoid process, under cover of the deltoid, the rounded prominence of the **lesser tuberosity** of the humerus can be palpated (Fig. 4.14). It is confirmed by flexing the elbow to 90° and then passively rotating the arm at the shoulder externally and internally.

## BICIPITAL GROOVE

The bicipital groove with the **tendon of the long head of the biceps** is palpable immediately lateral to the lesser tuberosity (Figs 4.14 and 4.15). This is confirmed by

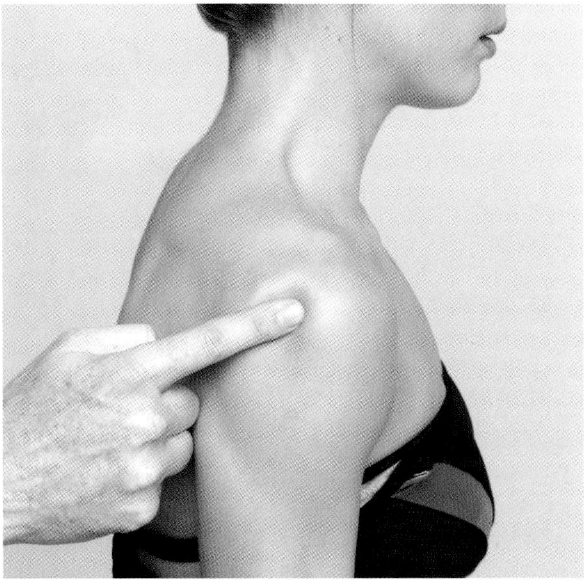

Fig. 4.10 Palpating the subacromial groove

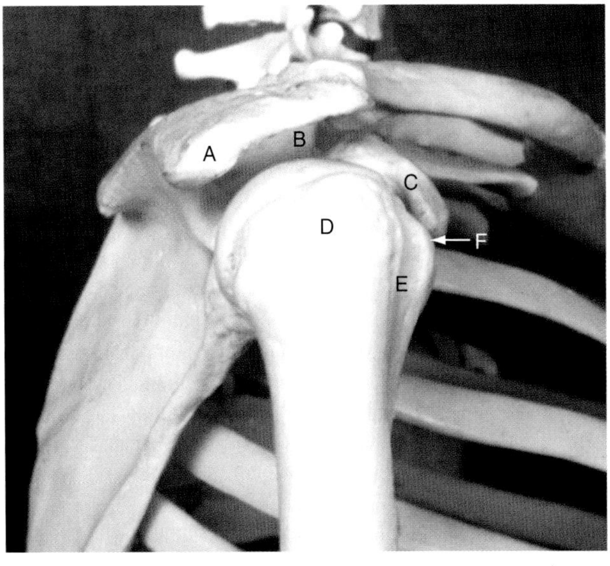


Fig. 4.11a Bony points on the lateral side of the skeleton of the shoulder
A = posterior angle of acromion, B = subacromial space, C = coracoid process, D = greater tuberosity, E = bicipital groove of humerus, F = lesser tuberosity

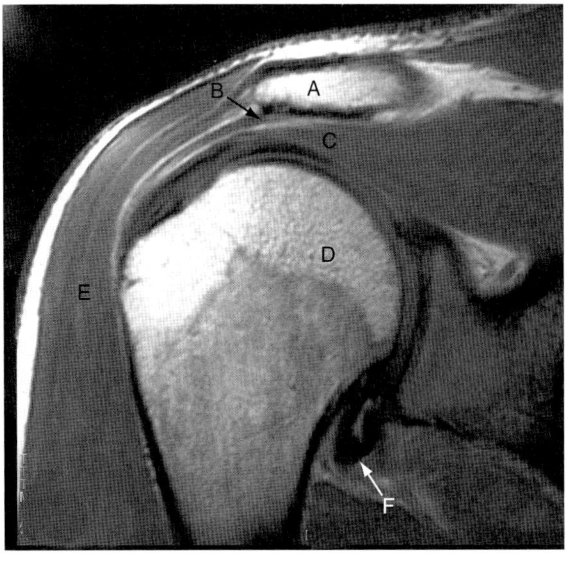


Fig. 4.11b MRI scan of the shoulder showing the subacromial space
A = acromion, B = subacromial bursa, C = supraspinatus, D = humeral head, E = deltoid, F = inferior fold in capsule in adduction

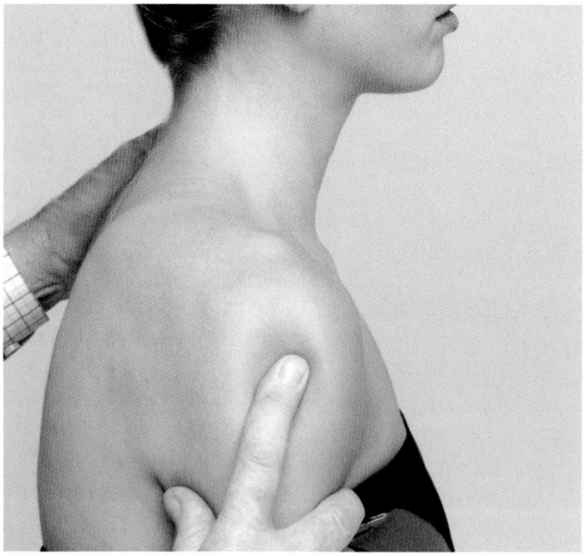

Fig. 4.12 Palpating the greater tuberosity of the humerus

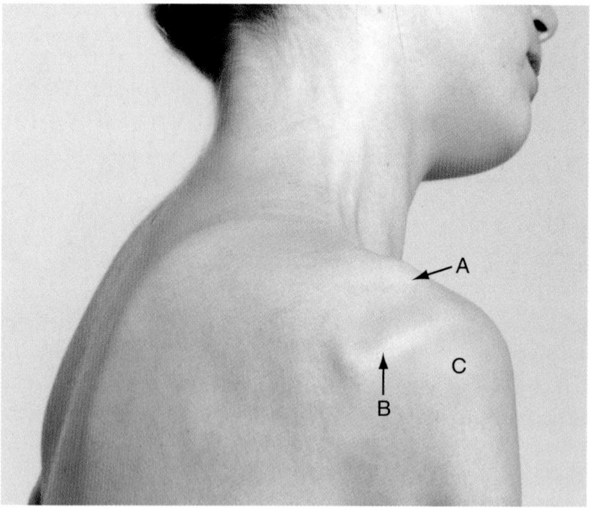


Fig. 4.13 Surface features of the shoulder from laterally
A = acromio-clavicular joint, B = lateral edge of acromion,
C = greater tuberosity of humerus

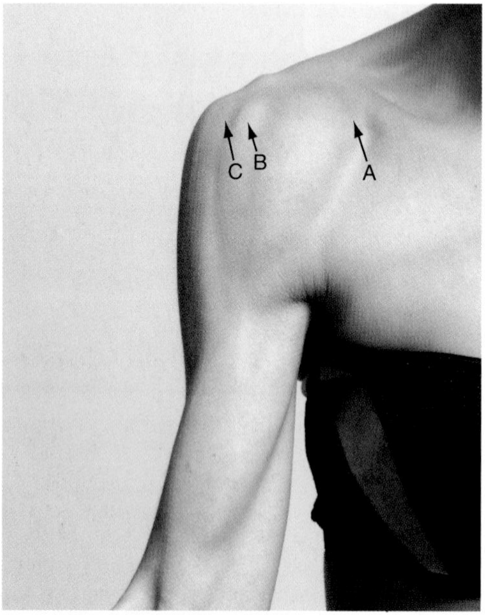


Fig. 4.14 Surface features on the front of the shoulder
A = coracoid process, B = lesser tuberosity, C = bicipital groove of humerus

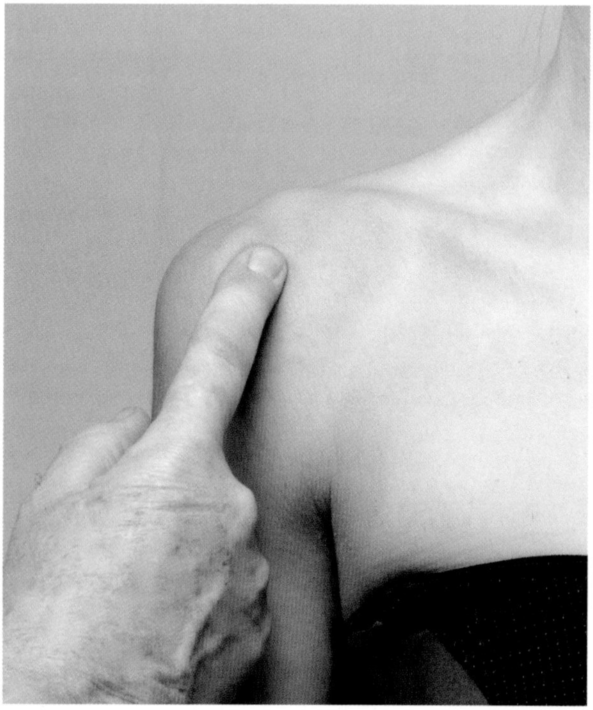

Fig. 4.15 Palpating the bicipital groove

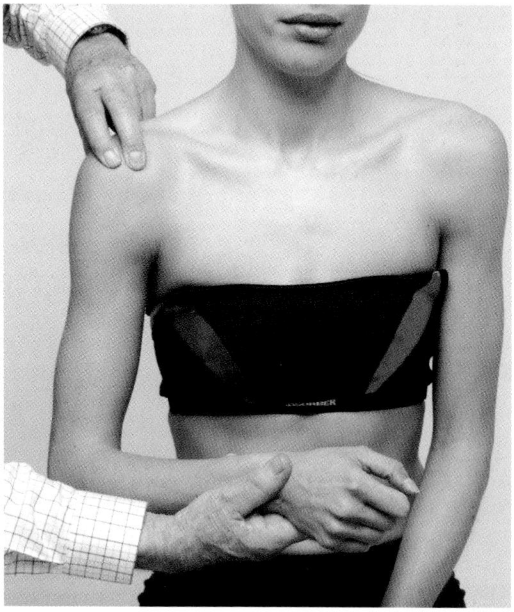

Fig. 4.16 Palpating the shoulder to confirm anterior bony landmarks by internal and external rotation at the shoulder joint

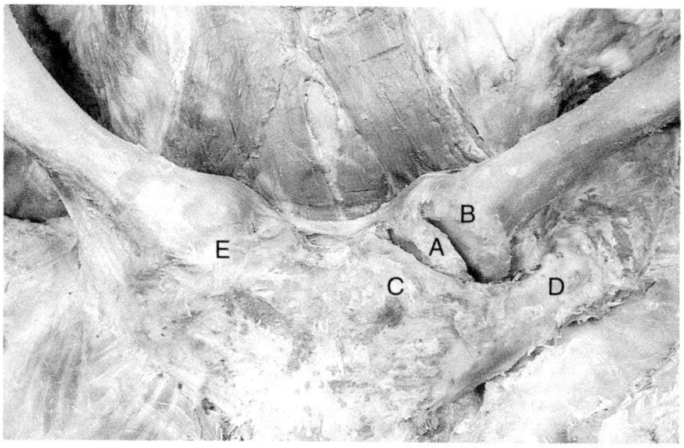


Fig. 4.17 Prosection of the sterno-clavicular joint A = the conspicuous intra-articular disc, particularly important in facilitating clavicular spin, B = clavicle, C = manubrium, D = 1st costal cartilage, E = capsule (From Gosling JA, Harris PF, Whitmore I, Willan PLT. 2002 Human Anatomy, 4th edn. London: Mosby)

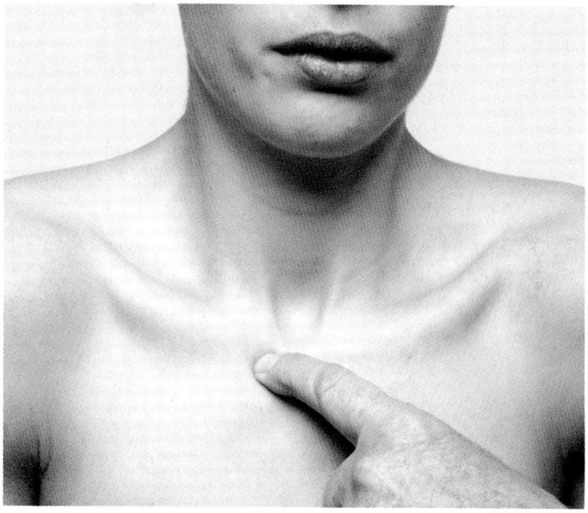

Fig. 4.18 Palpating the sterno-clavicular joint

palpating over the groove whilst passively rotating the arm internally and externally at the shoulder with the elbow flexed to 90° (Fig. 4.16). Alternatively, the groove can be located lying medial to the anterior border of the greater tuberosity, and the tendon confirmed by feeling it tense when the subject attempts to flex the fully extended limb against resistance to 60°.

# JOINTS LINES AND MOVEMENTS

- Sterno-clavicular
- Acromio-clavicular
- Gleno-humeral

## STERNO-CLAVICULAR JOINT

The basic structure of the sterno-clavicular joint is shown in Figure 4.17. Its intra-articular disc facilitates clavicular spin. With the index finger tip over the medial end of the clavicle, the groove marking the sterno-clavicular joint line can be located (Fig. 4.18). Whilst the groove is being palpated, the subject is asked to abduct the fully extended limb through 180°, starting with the limb fully dependent at the subject's side. As the limb is raised, hinge movement up to 30° accompanies elevation of the lateral end of the clavicle (Fig. 4.19a and b), and with further elevation the medial end of the clavicle can be felt to rotate at the joint line, indicating clavicular spin. This rotation can be confirmed by palpating the anterior surface at the medial end of the bone. By relaxing tension in the coraco-clavicular ligament, spin allows further clavicular elevation, which increases from 30 to 60° (Fig. 4.19c and d) and is vital for further rotation of the scapula (up to 60°) in achieving maximum abduction at the shoulder.

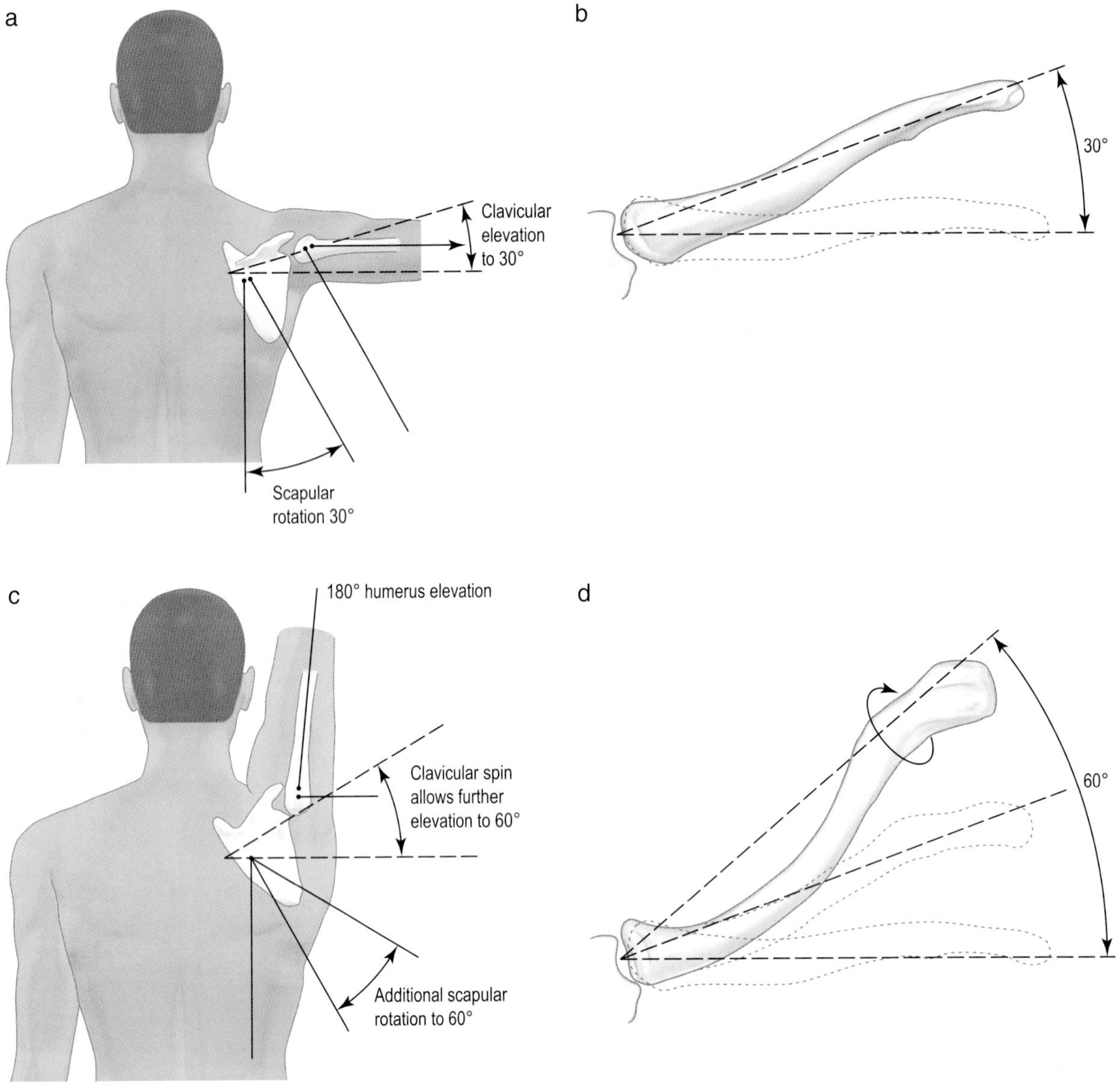


**Fig. 4.19** Diagram showing movements of the clavicle during abduction of the arm at the shoulder
**a and b** 30° rotation of scapula is accompanied by 30° elevation of the clavicle. **c and d** Clavicular spin allows a further 30° of clavicular elevation together with an additional 30° of scapula rotation
Redrawn from *Joint motion: method of measuring and recording.* Edinburgh: E&S Livingstone, 1965 (with the permission of the American Academy of Orthopedic Surgeons, reprinted with their permission by the British Orthopaedic Association)

## ACROMIO-CLAVICULAR JOINT

To identify the **acromio-clavicular joint**, the finger tip is glided over the lateral end of the clavicle on to the upper surface of the acromion to locate the groove marking the joint line (Figs 4.6, 4.7 and 4.20). The joint is confirmed when the examiner palpates over it whilst passively abducting the limb beyond 90°, producing a hinge movement as the acromion angles on the end of the clavicle. Additionally, gliding movements can be felt by palpating over the joint line whilst the partially flexed and abducted limb is gripped and swung passively forward and backward on the arc of a circle, whose fulcrum is the clavicle.

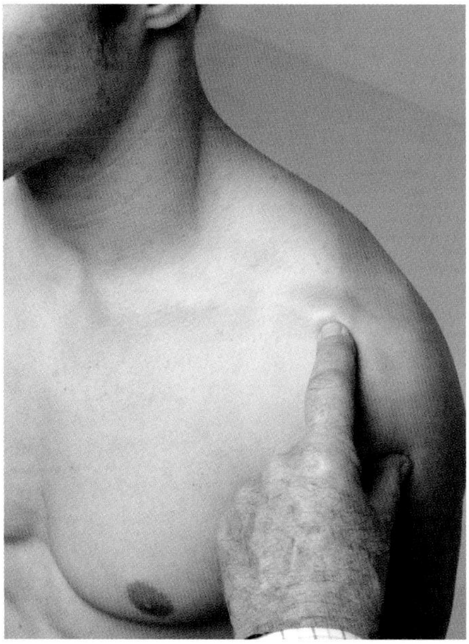

Fig. 4.20 Palpating the acromio-clavicular joint

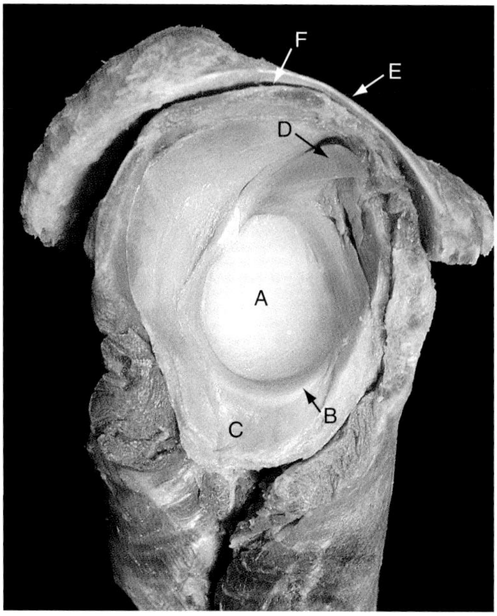


Fig. 4.21 Prosection of the shoulder joint with the humerus removed and viewing it "en face"
A = glenoid fossa, B = glenoid rim, C = capsule, D = long head of biceps, E = coraco-acromial ligament and arch, F = subacromial space (From Gosling JA, Harris PF, Whitmore I, Willan PLT. 2002 Human Anatomy, 4th edn. London: Mosby)

### SHOULDER (GLENO-HUMERAL) JOINT

The basic structure of the shoulder joint, when the glenoid is viewed "en face," is shown in Figure 4.21. Since the humeral head lies under cover of the coraco-acromial arch, the joint line is not palpable except for the lower part lying deeply in the axilla. With the subject supine or sitting, the examiner holds the extended limb away from the side of the trunk, with the axillary muscles relaxed. If the examiner inserts the finger tips firmly upward into the depths of the axilla whilst the limb is being passively abducted and adducted, movement of the humeral head can be felt.

With the subject standing, the following **primary movements** can be tested and demonstrated, actively or passively, starting with the limb fully extended in the resting position at the side of the body. If the examiner grasps the wrist, the limb can be **abducted** through **90°** whilst the scapula is stabilized to prevent rotation, or upward to **180°** allowing scapula movement (Fig. 4.22). In testing **adduction,** the extended limb can be swung up to **75°** across the front of the trunk toward the opposite side. Forward and upward **flexion** can reach up to **180°**, whilst backward extension can reach up to **60°**. With the subject's arm held to the side, the elbow flexed to 90°, and the hand supported in the mid-prone position, the examiner grasps the wrist and can either **medially or laterally rotate** the arm through 90° (Fig. 4.23). Medial rotation is also tested by asking subjects to reach behind their back, placing the dorsum of the hand against the body wall and trying to reach the scapula.

## TESTING MUSCLES

- Trapezius, deltoid
- Rotator cuff group
- Latissimus dorsi, teres major
- Pectoralis major, serratus anterior
- Biceps brachii, triceps brachii

### TRAPEZIUS

The wide extent of the muscle is shown in Figure 4.24. Its actions include elevation and backward bracing of the shoulder, and it is also involved in scapular rotation when the arm is raised above the head. The upper and middle fibers can be seen and felt to contract using the following procedures. Standing behind the subject, the examiner

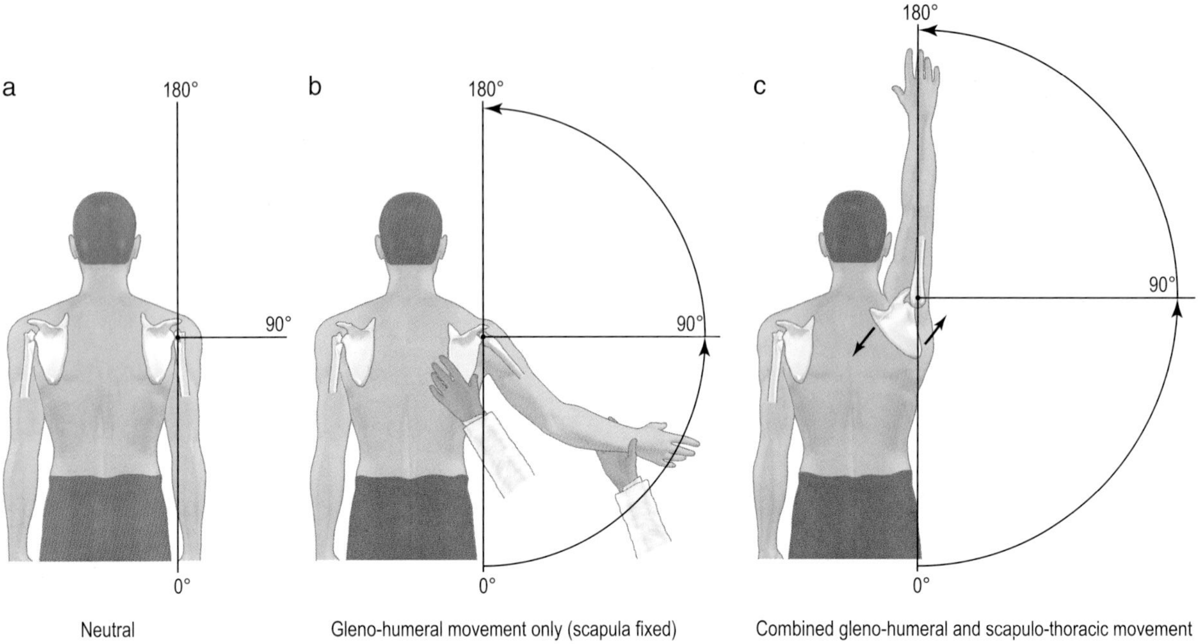


**Fig. 4.22** Diagram showing the range of abduction movements at the shoulder joint
**a** Neutral. **b** Gleno-humeral movement only (scapula fixed). **c** Gleno-humeral + scapulo-thoracic movement combined
Redrawn from *Joint motion: method of measuring and recording.* Edinburgh: E&S Livingstone, 1965 (with the permission of the American Academy of Orthopedic Surgeons, reprinted with their permission by the British Orthopaedic Association)

places a hand above each shoulder and with firm downward pressure resists the subject's attempts to shrug the shoulders upward; upper fibers are also demonstrated by placing a hand over the back of the head and resisting the subject's attempts to extend the head backward. The middle fibers are demonstrated by the examiner placing a hand behind each shoulder and resisting the subject's attempts to brace the shoulders backward (Fig. 4.25).

## DELTOID

This muscle forms the smooth convex contour along the lateral border of the arm distal to the point of the shoulder, resembling an epaulette covering the shoulder joint. It is the principal abductor of the arm at the shoulder joint. To test its action the examiner faces the subject, whose extended upper limb lies at the side of the trunk. The subject attempts to abduct the arm against strong resistance by the examiner. The middle multi-pennate fibers may be seen contracting (Fig. 4.26). The anterior fibers of the deltoid attached to the lateral part of the clavicle can be demonstrated by the examiner resisting forward flexion of the arm at the shoulder, whilst the posterior fibers attached to the spine of the scapula (see Fig. 4.30 below) become conspicuous when the examiner resists extension of the arm at the shoulder joint.

## ROTATOR CUFF GROUP

Supraspinatus, infraspinatus, teres minor and subscapularis comprise the rotator cuff group and are shown in Figures 4.27–4.29. They are intimately attached to the capsule of the shoulder joint and have a major role in its stability, in addition to their roles as prime movers.

### SUPRASPINATUS

The examiner stands behind the subject, who attempts to abduct the arm from the side against resistance. By palpating above the spine of the scapula and keeping the trapezius relaxed during the early stage of abduction, the examiner can feel the supraspinatus tense through it.

### INFRASPINATUS AND TERES MINOR

The subject stands with the arm to the side, the elbow flexed to 90° and hand mid-prone. The examiner stands behind the subject and resists attempts to rotate laterally at the shoulder by pressing against the dorsum of the hand. Palpation below the spine of the scapula confirms tension in the infraspinatus and teres minor.

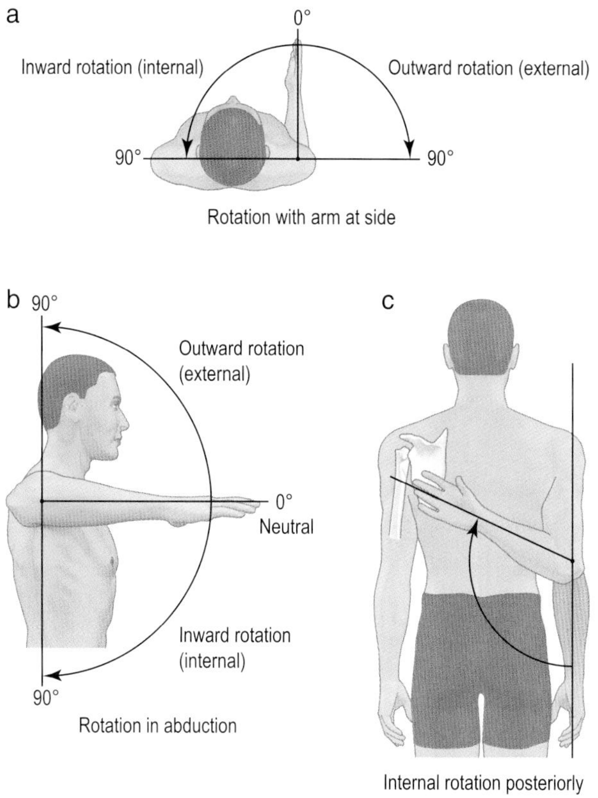

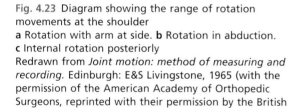

Fig. 4.23 Diagram showing the range of rotation movements at the shoulder
**a** Rotation with arm at side. **b** Rotation in abduction. **c** Internal rotation posteriorly
Redrawn from *Joint motion: method of measuring and recording.* Edinburgh: E&S Livingstone, 1965 (with the permission of the American Academy of Orthopedic Surgeons, reprinted with their permission by the British Orthopaedic Association)

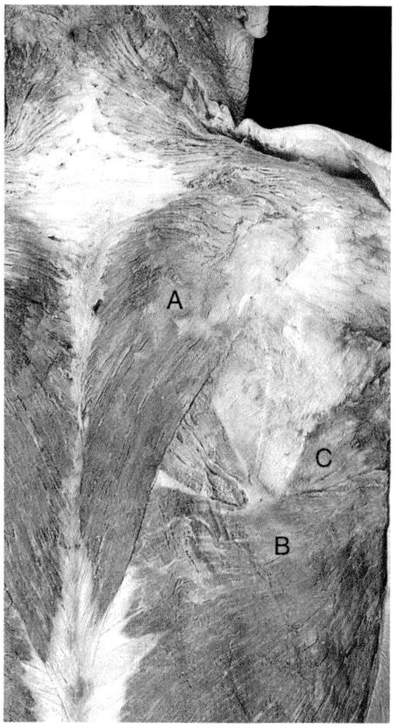


Fig. 4.24 Prosection showing dorsal trunk muscles, trapezius and latissimus dorsi
A = trapezius, B = latissimus dorsi, C = teres major (From Gosling JA, Harris PF, Whitmore I, Willan PLT. 2002 Human Anatomy, 4th edn. London: Mosby)

## SUBSCAPULARIS

Subscapularis produces medial rotation at the shoulder and can be tested in a similar manner to infraspinatus and teres minor, except that the examiner resists medial rotation by pressing against the palm of the subject's hand. Because it lies deeply beneath the scapula, the muscle cannot be seen or felt when it contracts.

## LATISSIMUS DORSI AND TERES MAJOR

To demonstrate these muscles, the examiner stands behind the subject. Keeping the limb straight, the subject flexes it forward to about 45° and abducts it to about 45°. With the examiner pushing strongly forward against the forearm, the subject attempts to pull the limb backward and inward. The teres major is seen to contract in the lower

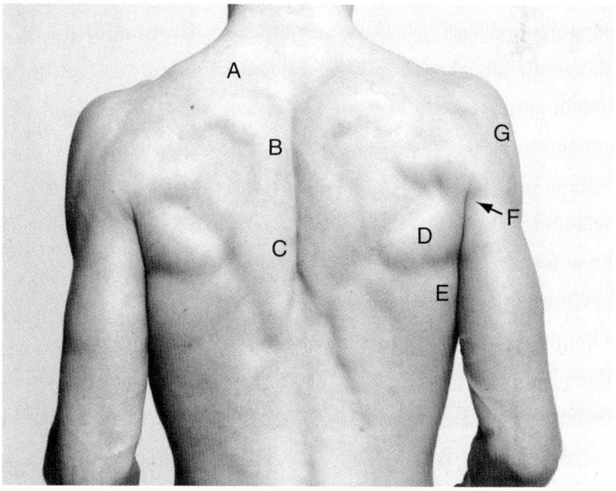


Fig. 4.25 Muscles on the dorsum of the shoulder
A = upper fibers of trapezius, B = middle fibers of trapezius C = lower fibers of trapezius, D = teres major, E = latissimus dorsi, F = long head of triceps, G = deltoid

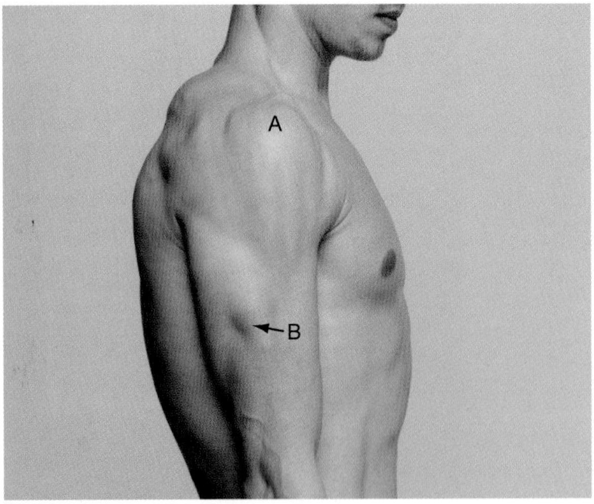


Fig. 4.26 Surface features of the lateral side of the shoulder and arm
A = deltoid (the intramuscular septa are visible), B = lateral head of triceps

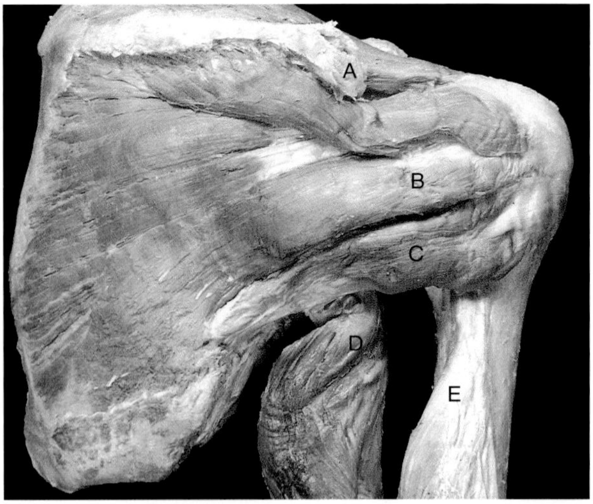


Fig. 4.27 Prosection of the shoulder from posterior showing the rotator cuff muscles
A = supraspinatus, B = infraspinatus, C = teres minor, D = long head of triceps, E = lateral head of triceps (From Gosling JA, Harris PF, Whitmore I, Willan PLT. 2002 Human Anatomy, 4th edn. London: Mosby)

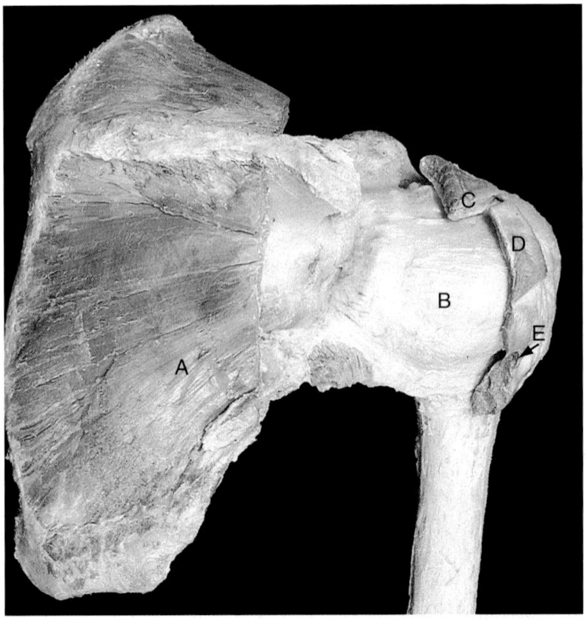


Fig. 4.28 Prosection of the shoulder from anterior showing subscapularis and attachments of the rotator cuff muscles
A = infraspinatus (muscle belly), B = capsule, C–E = rotator cuff (C = supraspinatus, D = infraspinatus, E = teres minor) (From Gosling JA, Harris PF, Whitmore I, Willan PLT. 2002 Human Anatomy, 4th edn. London: Mosby)

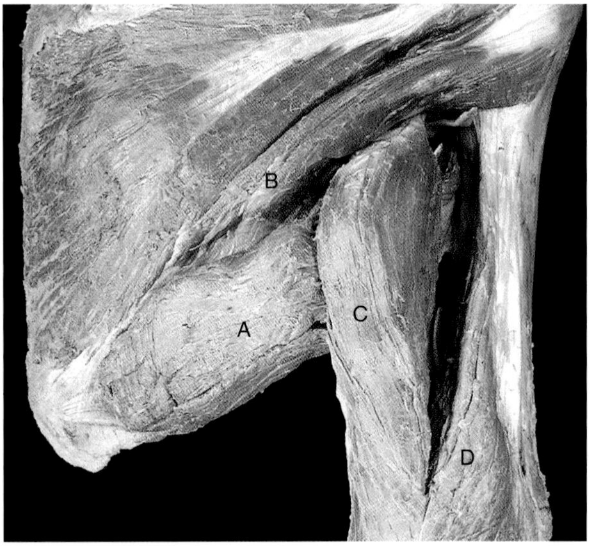


Fig. 4.29 Prosection of the shoulder from posterior showing teres major with the long and lateral heads of triceps
A = teres major, B = teres minor, C = long head of triceps, D = lateral head of triceps (From Gosling JA, Harris PF, Whitmore I, Willan PLT. 2002 Human Anatomy, 4th edn. London: Mosby)

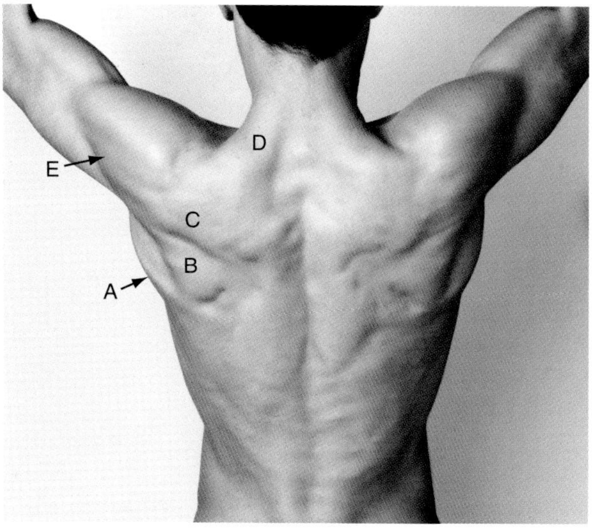


Fig. 4.30 Muscles on the posterior aspect of the shoulder and trunk
A = latissimus dorsi, B = teres major, C = infraspinatus, D = trapezius: upper fibers, E = deltoid: posterior fibers

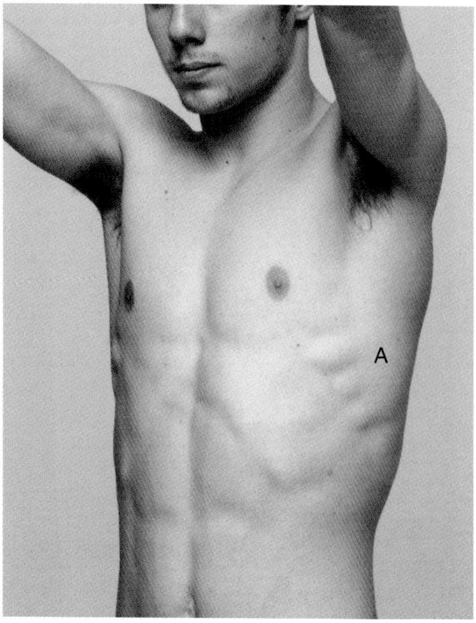


Fig. 4.31 Muscles on the lateral thoracic wall
A = serratus anterior (the individual serrations are clearly visible)

border of the posterior axillary wall, and the latissimus dorsi can be felt contracting if the palm of the hand is placed on the dorso-lateral side of the trunk just below the level of the axilla. Its extensive lower border may be visible passing downward and medially on to the trunk. Surface features of dorsal muscles in the shoulder region are shown in Figure 4.30.

## PECTORALIS MAJOR

This muscle is demonstrated with the examiner facing the subject, who is asked to place a hand on his or her hip and push strongly downward and inward. The pectoralis major can be seen to contract (pectoralis minor is deep) in the anterior wall of the axilla, and felt to be contracting if the tensed anterior axillary wall is gripped firmly between fingers and thumb. The surface features are shown in Figure 4.3.

## SERRATUS ANTERIOR

The subject stands facing a wall with both arms outstretched and the palms of the hands against the wall. The subject is asked to press forward strongly. The muscle is seen to contract where it covers the ribs forming the medial wall of the axilla, and can be felt to be tense if the fingers are placed over the ribs. The typical serrations can be clearly seen in a muscular subject (Fig. 4.31).

## BICEPS BRACHII

The two heads of the biceps have different proximal attachments, as shown in Figure 4.32. The long head is the more important and can be located in the bicipital groove of the humerus (Figs 4.4 and 4.14). To demonstrate the muscle, the subject stands facing the examiner. With the arm to the side, the elbow flexed to 90° and the hand pronated, the subject attempts to supinate whilst the examiner grasps the hand firmly and resists this movement. The biceps can be seen to contract (Fig. 4.33), and its tensed tendon is palpated deeply in the distal part of the cubital fossa as it descends to its attachment on the radial tuberosity. The sharp edge of the bicipital aponeurosis can be felt as it crosses medially to attach over the common flexor origin on the front of the medial epicondyle of the humerus.

Biceps can also be seen and felt to contract when the subject faces the examiner, with the arm to the side and flexed to 90°, and attempts further flexion at the elbow whilst this is resisted by the examiner. Locating the long head in the bicipital groove has already been described.

## TRICEPS BRACHII

The triceps is shown in the prosection in Figure 4.34a. The subject slightly abducts the arm at the shoulder and flexes

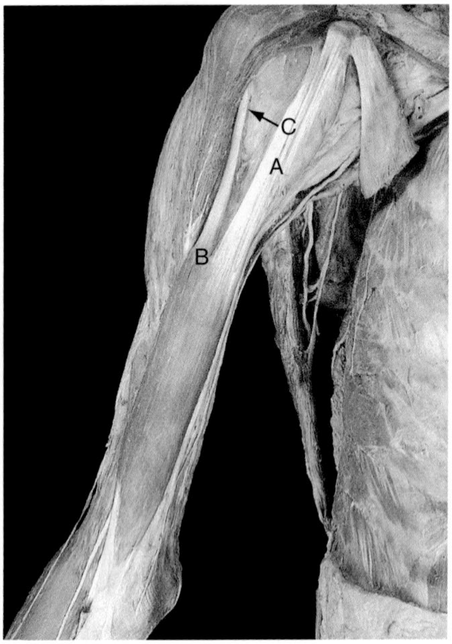


Fig. 4.32 Prosection showing the biceps muscle and its two heads
A = short head of biceps, B = long head of biceps, C = tendon in bicipital groove entering capsule (From Gosling JA, Harris PF, Whitmore I, Willan PLT. 2002 Human Anatomy, 4th edn. London: Mosby)

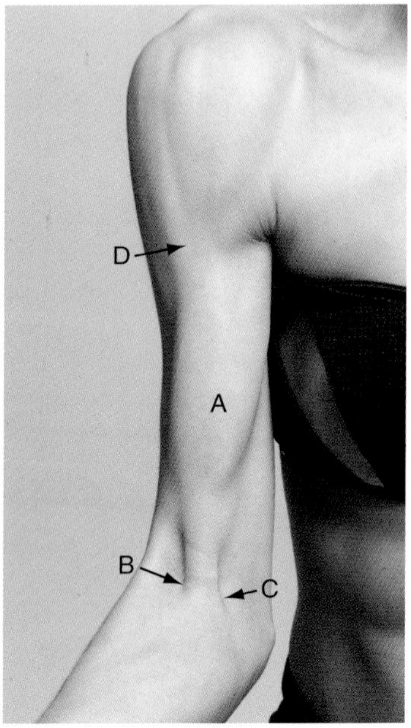


Fig. 4.33 Biceps brachii flexing the elbow joint
A = belly of biceps, B = biceps tendon, C = bicipital aponeurosis, D = position of tendon of long head (confirm by palpation when flexing the shoulder)

the elbow to at least 90°. Further extension is attempted but resisted by the examiner pushing strongly against the back of the forearm. If a finger is placed in the groove just above the olecranon when the triceps contracts, the tendon can be felt to tense. In the upper part of the arm the long and lateral heads may be visible (Fig. 4.34b) and are palpable when the muscle is made to contract.

# LOCATING ARTERIAL PULSATION

- Brachial artery

The subject faces the examiner with the arm slightly abducted and elbow extended to approximately 160°. The furrow on the medial side of the biceps is located and palpated about the midpoint of the arm by applying direct pressure in a postero-lateral direction or by encircling the arm in a grip with the finger tips in the furrow. The pulsating brachial artery can be compressed against the shaft of the humerus.

# SPECIAL TESTS

- Shoulder joint
- Subacromial impingement
- Rotator cuff
- Acromio-clavicular joint
- Biceps brachii

These techniques are primarily designed to test for impingement, capsule laxity, tears and strains. As with all instability tests, the unaffected side should be tested first and compared to findings on the affected side.

## SHOULDER JOINT

To test pure gleno-humeral movement, the scapula should be fixed by the examiner grasping the lower part of the scapula firmly between fingers and thumb (Fig. 4.35).

### APPREHENSION TEST FOR ANTERIOR DISLOCATION OF THE SHOULDER

Standing, the subject places the palm of the hand on the back of the head. The examiner stands behind the subject, placing one hand on the front of the subject's elbow. The other hand is positioned so it can apply an anteriorly directed force on the back of the upper end of the subject's humerus (Fig. 4.36). A positive test is elicited if the subject reports apprehension or steps

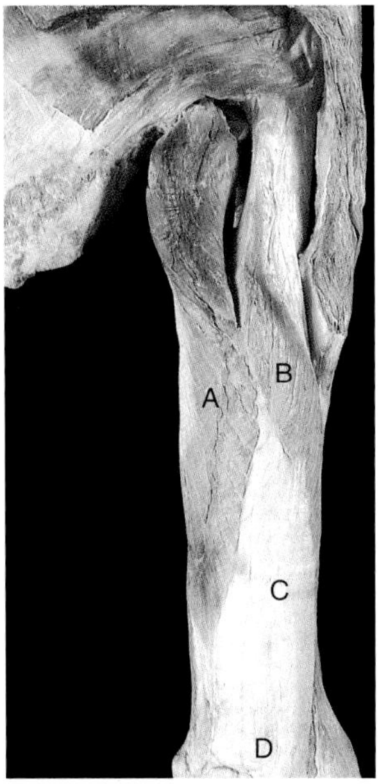


Fig. 4.34a Prosection showing triceps and its three heads
A = long head, B = lateral head, C = medial head, D = triceps tendon (From Gosling JA, Harris PF, Whitmore I, Willan PLT. 2002 Human Anatomy, 4th edn. London: Mosby)

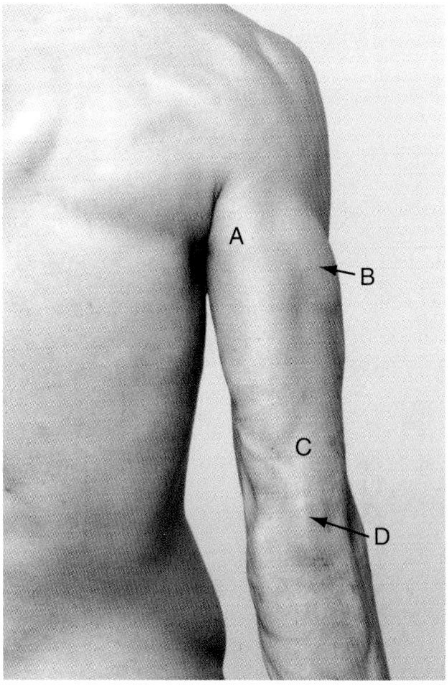


Fig. 4.34b Muscles on the posterior aspect of the arm
A = long head of triceps, B = lateral head of triceps, C = medial head of triceps, D = tendon of triceps

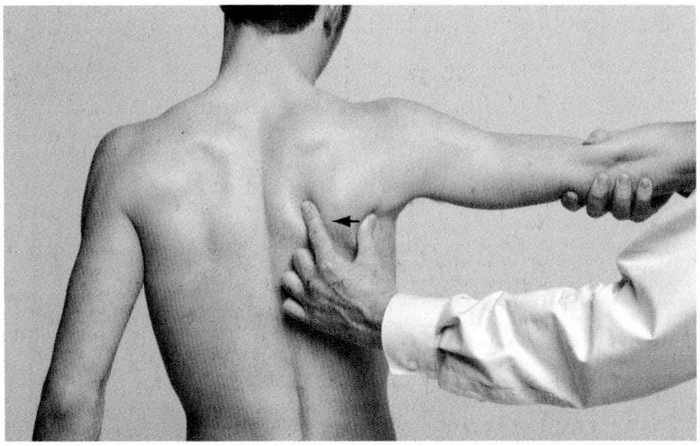

Fig. 4.35 Fixing the scapula when testing pure abduction at the shoulder joint

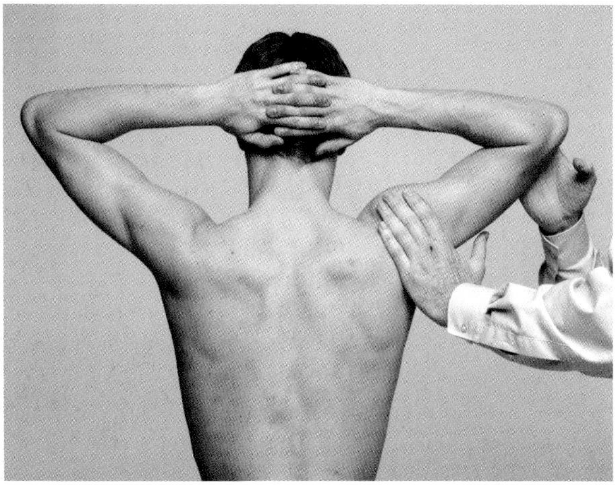

Fig. 4.36 Anterior apprehension test for instability of the shoulder joint
Backward pressure is applied on the elbow and forward pressure on the shoulder

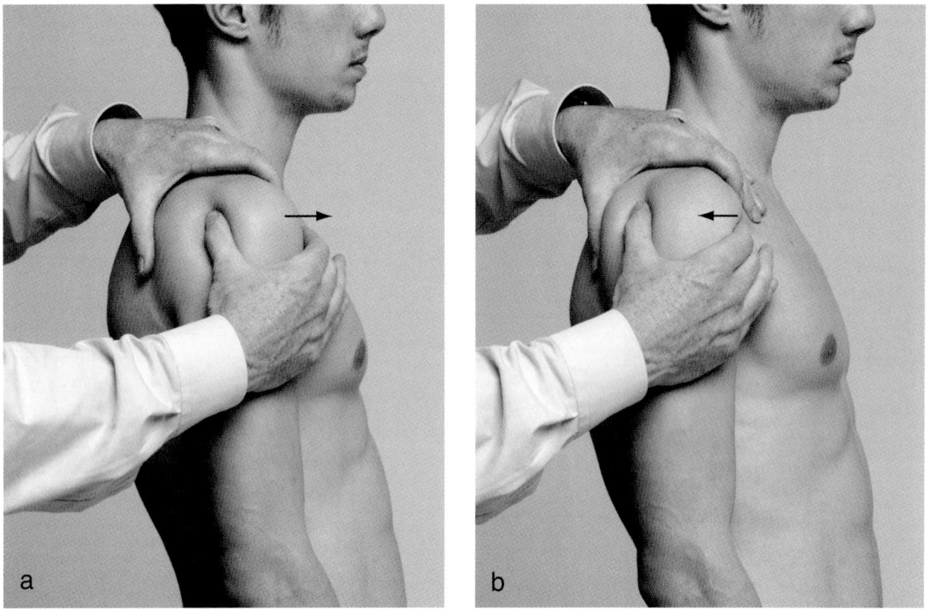


Fig. 4.37 Drawer test for instability of the shoulder joint
**a** Anterior drawer. **b** Posterior drawer

forward to avoid subluxation or dislocation of the joint.

## TESTS FOR SHOULDER LAXITY

The subject may be seated or standing during the following two tests.

### *Drawer test*

With one hand, the examiner grasps the lateral end of the subject's clavicle and acromion. The humeral head is gripped firmly with the examiner's other hand and the examiner attempts to move the humerus in the anteroposterior plane (Fig. 4.37).

### *Sulcus test*

With one hand stabilizing the subject's shoulder from above, the examiner uses the other hand to grip the subject's extended upper limb just above the elbow and applies downward traction (Fig. 4.38). A visible groove (sulcus) appears just below the lateral edge of the acromion if the capsule is lax.

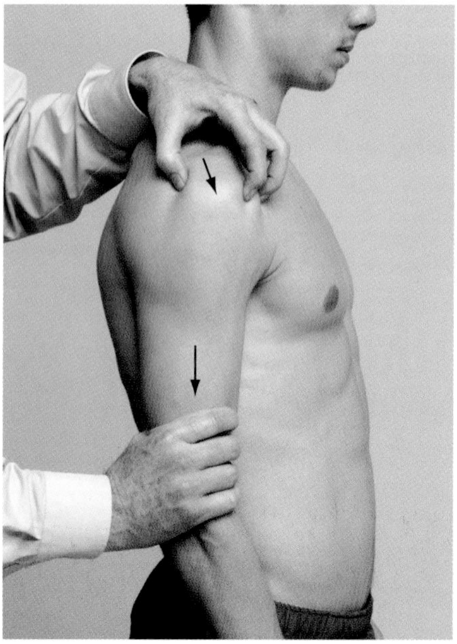

Fig. 4.38 Sulcus test for laxity of the shoulder joint capsule

## TESTS FOR SUBACROMIAL IMPINGEMENT

### NEER'S TEST

The examiner stands beside the subject and stabilizes the scapula with one hand. With the subject's upper limb fully extended at his or her side and the forearm pronated, the examiner grasps the wrist and passively elevates the limb forward and upward. Pain at the end of range will be reported by patients with impingement. Subtle symptoms may be elicited by gentle overpressure (Fig. 4.39).

### HAWKINS–KENNEDY TEST

The subject forward-flexes the injured shoulder to 90° and the elbow to a right angle in the horizontal plane, with the hand hanging downward at the wrist. The examiner faces the subject, guiding his or her hand below the subject's forearm at the same time as supporting it, to grasp the ipsilateral shoulder from above. The examiner uses the other free hand to grip the dorsum of the subject's wrist and apply downward pressure on it, internally rotating the shoulder (Fig. 4.40). Patients with impingement will have pain with this maneuver.

### RELOCATION TEST

This is a test for anterior instability or secondary, internal, gleno-humeral joint impingement. Secondary impingement, due to abutment of the humeral head against the glenoid labrum and/or underside of the supraspinatus tendon, is common in players of overhead sports such as tennis and throwing sports. The subject is supine with the shoulder abducted to 90° and elbow flexed to 90°. The examiner grips the subject's distal forearm and passively rotates the shoulder externally, noting the range at which pain or apprehension occurs (Fig. 4.41a). The test is repeated with the examiner applying an anterior to posterior pressure on the humeral head (Fig. 4.41b), to center it in the glenoid fossa during the maneuver. Subjects with instability or secondary impingement will have their symptoms relieved or will tolerate a markedly increased range of external rotation whilst the pressure on the humeral head is maintained.

## TESTS FOR ROTATOR CUFF MUSCLES

### "EMPTY CAN" OR JOBE'S TEST FOR SUPRASPINATUS TEAR

The examiner stands at one side of the subject, who actively abducts the extended upper limb to 90° and horizontally adducts to 30°. The shoulder is then internally rotated by the subject pointing the thumb downward (mimicking the motion of emptying a can). Insufficient strength to maintain the arm in this position may indicate rupture of the supraspinatus. The examiner can then test the strength of the supraspinatus by trying to push the limb downward by applying firm pressure over the dorsum of the forearm (Fig. 4.42). Weakness and pain may indicate a partial tear of the supraspinatus.

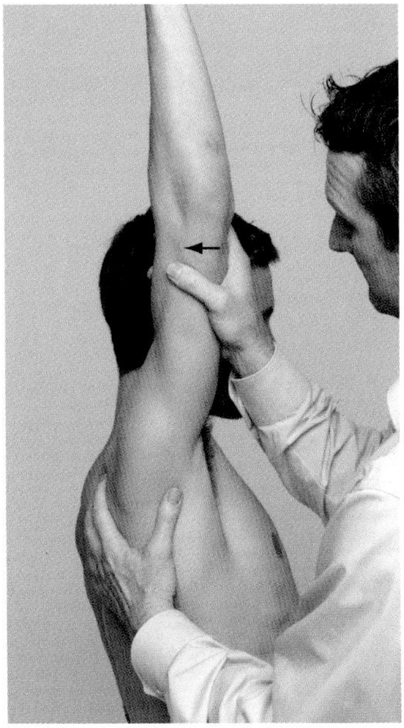

Fig. 4.39 Neer's test for subacromial impingement

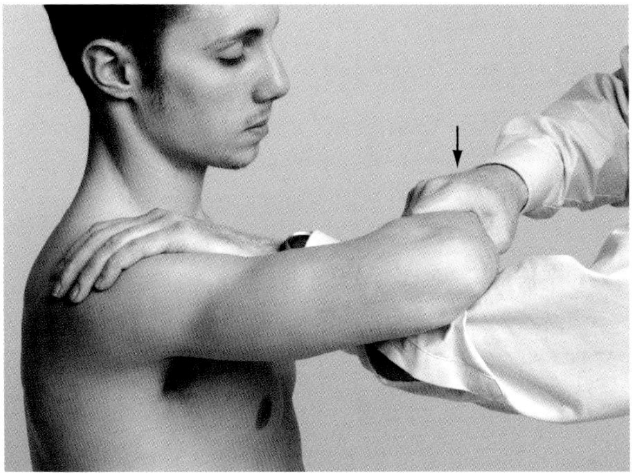

Fig. 4.40 Hawkins–Kennedy test for subacromial impingement

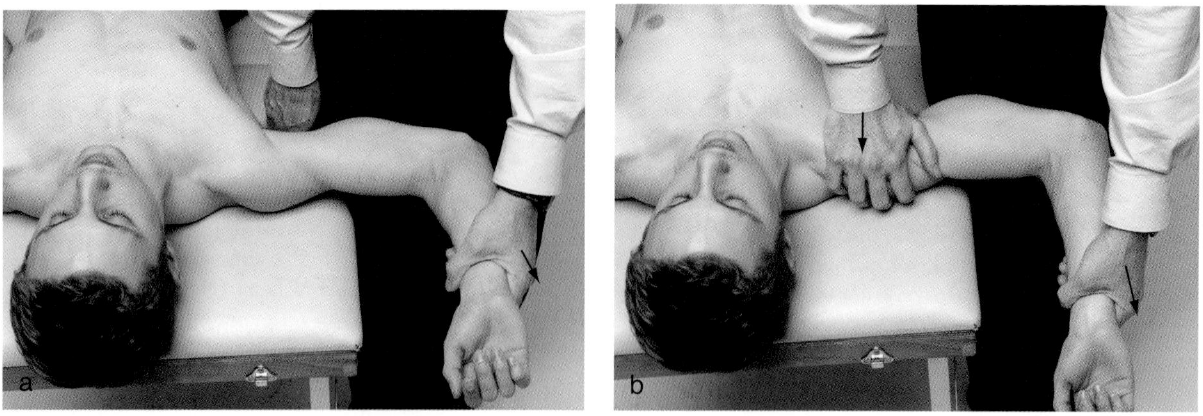

Fig. 4.41 Relocation test for secondary impingement
**a** Shoulder external rotation. **b** Shoulder external rotation plus relocation of the humeral head

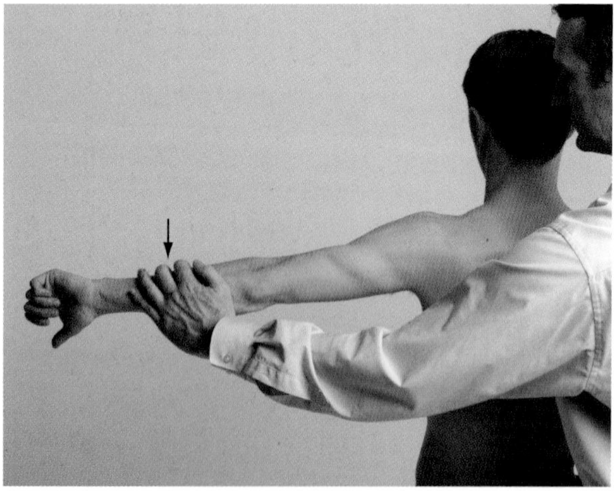

Fig. 4.42 Test for rotator cuff strain ("empty can" test)

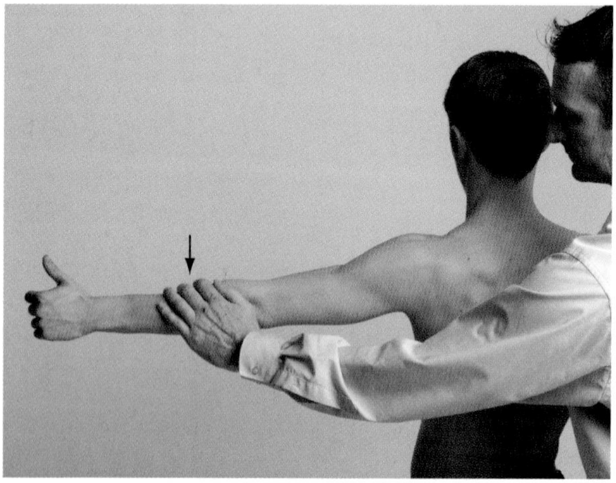

Fig. 4.43 Test to distinguish between supraspinatus and deltoid injury ("full can" test)

## "FULL CAN" TEST

The "full can" test can be used to distinguish deltoid strain from supraspinatus tendinopathy. The subject stands and actively abducts the extended limb to 90°, with the thumb pointing upward. This is followed by further abduction and extension at the shoulder, which is resisted by the examiner. The anterior deltoid fibers are seen to contract if intact (Fig. 4.43).

## TESTS FOR DISRUPTION OF THE SUBSCAPULARIS

### *"Lift-off" (Gerber's) test*

Subjects stand with their back to the examiner, with the dorsum of the hand placed against the lower part of the back. The subject then attempts to bring the hand away from the back whilst the examiner resists the movement (Fig. 4.44).

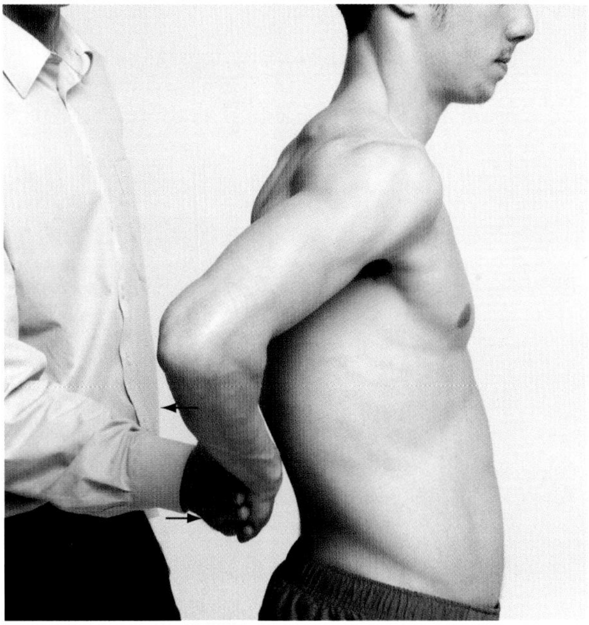

Fig. 4.44 Gerber's "lift-off" test for subscapularis strain

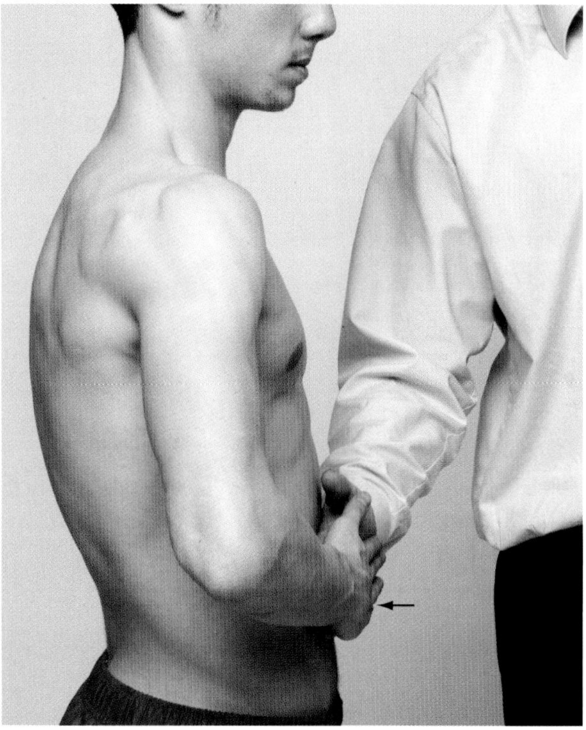

Fig. 4.45 "Belly press" sign for damage to subscapularis

### *"Belly press" test*

This is an alternative test for subjects who cannot attain the position for the lift-off test. The subject stands and presses the palm of the hand firmly against the examiner's hand placed on the upper abdominal wall. The examiner looks for any posterior movement of the elbow during this maneuver (Fig. 4.45).

## ACROMIO-CLAVICULAR JOINT STRESS TESTS

Two maneuvers may be used to stress the acromio-clavicular joint.

### "MONKEY GRIP" TEST

The subject stands or sits facing the examiner, then grips the hands together under the chin by locking the flexed fingers together. The subject then attempts to pull the hands apart whilst maintaining the fingers in a tight lock (Fig. 4.46). Acromio-clavicular joint pain indicates a positive test.

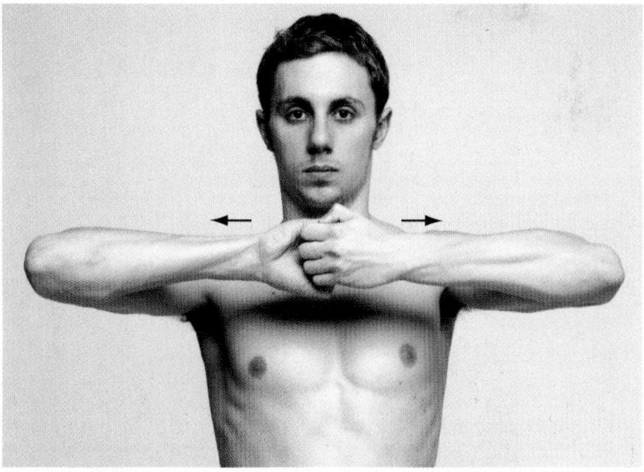

Fig. 4.46 "Monkey grip" test for damage to the acromio-clavicular joint

### SCARF TEST

The subject faces the examiner and forward-flexes the arm to 90°. The examiner assists the subject to adduct the arm horizontally whilst bending the elbow acutely so that the hand and wrist lie over the opposite shoulder. The examiner then applies firm backward pressure over the elbow (Fig. 4.47). This may elicit pain in the joint.

## BICEPS BRACHII

These two tests can be used to assess for strain or rupture of the biceps.

### YERGASON'S TEST

The subject stands facing the examiner, with the limb fully extended at the elbow and forearm pronated. The subject attempts to flex the elbow to 90° and at the same time tries to bring the forearm into supination, both movements being resisted by the examiner (Fig. 4.48).

### SPEED'S TEST

This test is particularly suitable for testing the long head. The subject faces the examiner, with the elbow extended and forearm supinated. The subject tries to flex the limb to 90° against resistance (Fig. 4.49).

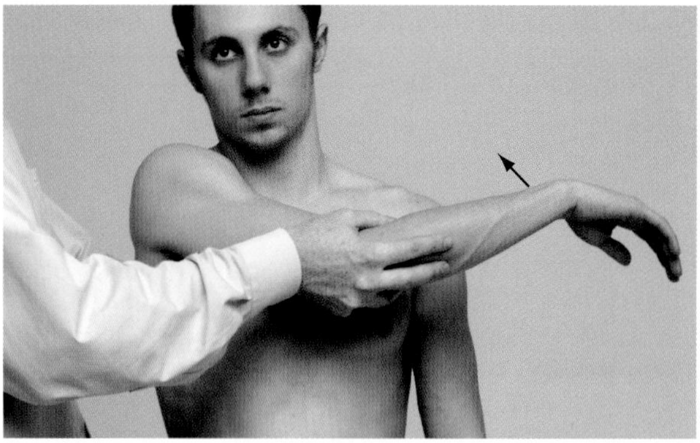

**Fig. 4.47** Scarf test for damage to the acromio-clavicular joint

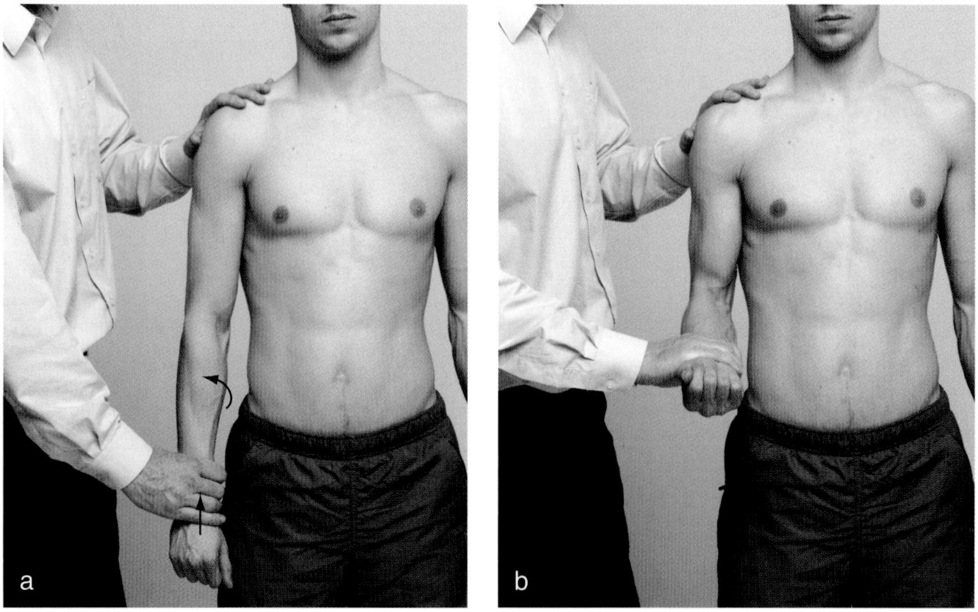


**Fig. 4.48** Yergason's test for biceps brachii strain
**a** Elbow extension and forearm pronation. **b** Resisted elbow flexion and forearm supination

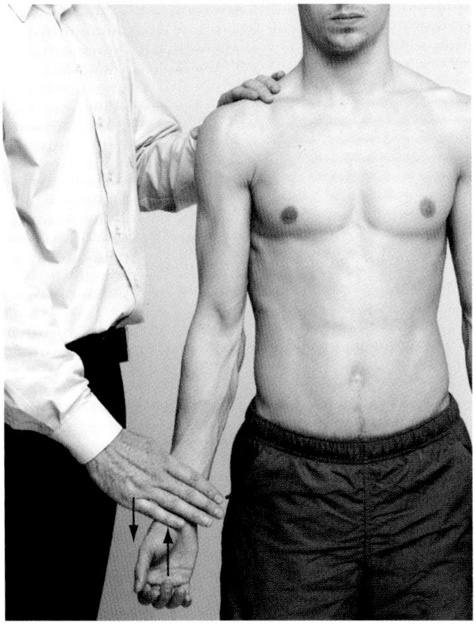

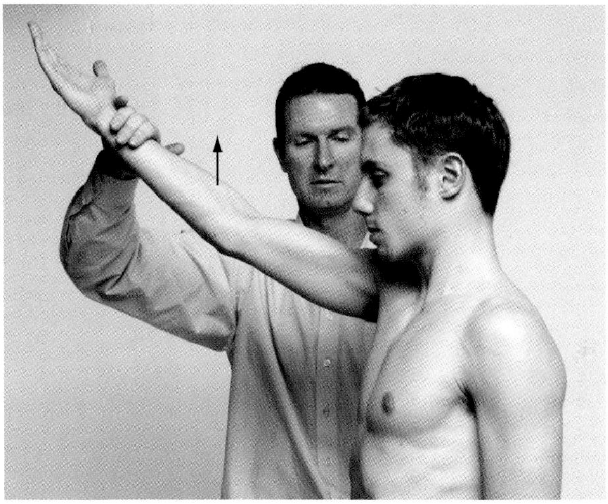

Fig. 4.49 Speed's test for injury to the long head of biceps brachii

## FURTHER READING

Burkhart SS, Morgan CD, Kibler WB. The disabled throwing shoulder: spectrum of pathology. Part 1: Pathoanatomy and biomechanics. Arthroscopy 2003; 19(4):404–420.

Mair SD, Isbell WM, Gill TJ et al. Triceps tendon ruptures in professional football players. American Journal of Sports Medicine 2004; 32:431–434.

Safran MR. Nerve injury about the shoulder in athletes. Part 1: Suprascapular nerve and axillary nerve. American Journal of Sports Medicine 2004; 32:803–819.

Tarkin IS, Morganti CM, Zillmer DA et al. Rotator cuff tears in adolescent athletes. American Journal of Sports Medicine 2005; 33:596–601.

Tennent DT, Beach WR, Meyers JF. A review of the special tests associated with shoulder examination. Part 1: The rotator cuff tests. American Journal of Sports Medicine 2003; 31(1):154–159.

Tennent DT, Beach WR, Meyers JF. A review of the special tests associated with shoulder examination. Part 2: Laxity, instability and superior labral anterior and posterior (SLAP) lesions. American Journal of Sports Medicine 2003; 31:301–307.

Weiland DE, MacGillivray JD. Isolated supraspinatus muscle paralysis after shoulder dislocation. American Journal of Sports Medicine 2003; 31:462–464.

Zvijac JE, Matthias RS, Hechtman KS et al. Pectoralis major tears: correlation of magnetic resonance imaging and treatment strategies. American Journal of Sports Medicine 2006; 34:289–294.

CHAPTER

## CASE STUDY 4 • CLINICAL PROBLEMS

**Problem 1.** *A 28-year-old female sprint canoeist complains of shoulder pain when she lifts the paddle out of the water. She cannot recall a specific injury but is now beginning to experience symptoms when reaching for the seatbelt in her car and combing her hair.*

a) What is the likely diagnosis?
b) What structures should be palpated?
c) Which manual tests should be performed?

**Problem 2.** *An 18-year-old male rugby player dislocated his shoulder 3 months earlier when he was tackling an opposition player during a match. The shoulder was relocated at the local hospital and was immobilized in a sling for 3 weeks. He is now apprehensive about reaching overhead with the affected arm as he feels the shoulder will "come out of the joint." There is also mild weakness of shoulder abduction.*

a) What structures are likely to have been damaged?
b) Which manual tests should be performed?

**Problem 3.** *A 25-year-old downhill mountain bike racer falls off his bicycle at high speed and describes landing on the point of his right shoulder. He is concerned because his shoulder is now painful to move and there is a palpable deformity across the top of the shoulder.*

a) Which joint should be palpated?
b) What is the most likely diagnosis?
c) What are three differential diagnoses?

**Problem 4.** *A 33-year-old American football quarterback has a painful throwing shoulder and is diagnosed as having a SLAP lesion.*

a) What does the term "SLAP lesion" signify?
b) The tendon attachment of which muscle is implicated in this injury?
c) Which manual tests can be used to assess this muscle?

**Problem 5.** *A 65-year-old veteran athlete felt a sudden tearing sensation in his shoulder during a javelin competition 3 months ago. He now has difficulty reaching behind his back to thread his trouser belt. An ultrasound scan reveals a ruptured rotator cuff tendon.*

a) The tendon of which rotator cuff muscle is likely to have been ruptured?
b) What two muscle tests can be used to confirm the diagnosis?

**Problem 6.** *A 30-year-old male international butterfly swimmer complains of left shoulder pain when midway through the "pull" phase of his swimming stroke. An ultrasound scan of his shoulder (Fig. 4.50) reveals a tear in the tendon of a rotator cuff muscle. The swimmer's doctor feels the tear is secondary to repetitive impingement of the tendon.*

a) The tendon of which muscle has been torn?
b) Which test can be used to determine the strength of the muscle?
c) Which impingement test most closely replicates the position of the shoulder during the mid-"pull" phase of the swimming stroke?

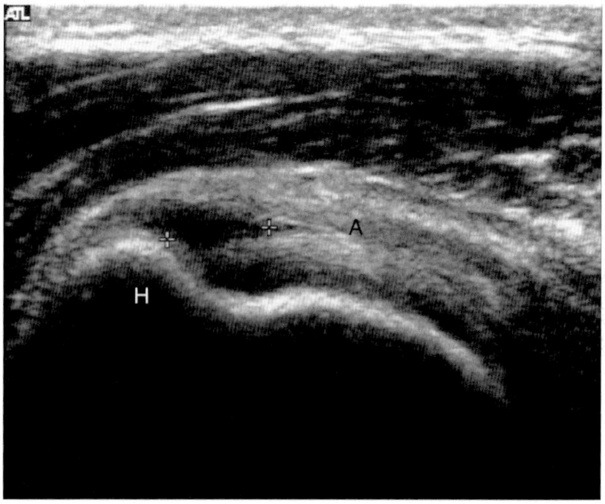


Fig. 4.50 Ultrasound scan of the shoulder showing a tear in a rotator cuff muscle
The tear lies between the two white crosses. A = rotator cuff muscle, H = upper border of humeral head

CHAPTER 5

# Elbow and forearm

## INTRODUCTION

The elbow forms the link between two lever systems, the arm proximally and the forearm distally. The elbow joint and the proximal radio-ulnar joint in their continuity comprise the core of the region. Anteriorly, a space, the cubital fossa, is traversed by the brachial artery with the median nerve close to it, both descending to reach the ventral (flexor) compartment of the forearm. The radial nerve also crosses the fossa more laterally, passing distally toward the neck of the radius. The ulnar nerve is not in the fossa but passes postero-medially, very close to the epicondyle and the elbow joint itself. The regions of the epicondyles provide origins for common flexor and extensor muscle groups. Posteriorly, there is less soft tissue.

The point of the elbow is formed by the olecranon process of the ulna, with the triceps tendon attaching to it. The forearm has two long bones, the radius and ulna, connected by the interosseous membrane at its core and dividing it into two main compartments: the more bulky anterior (flexor) compartment innervated by the median and ulnar nerves, and the smaller posterior (extensor) compartment innervated by the radial nerve.

## INSPECTION OF NORMAL CONTOURS

- Carrying angle
- Common flexor origin
- Common extensor origin
- Biceps brachii
- Olecranon process
- Epicondyles
- Ulna: subcutaneous border

Viewed from ventrally (Fig. 5.1), the forearm, extended and supinated, is seen to incline laterally at the elbow **(carrying angle)** and there is an overall widening of the limb in the region of the elbow. Medially is a fullness due to the underlying medial epicondyle, enhanced by the muscles arising from the **common (superficial) flexor origin** on the front of the epicondyle. Laterally, the contour is slightly convex with a less conspicuous fullness caused by the lateral epicondyle with the overlying **common extensor origin** and presence of the brachioradialis muscle. Proximally, descending from the lower part of the arm, is a distinct ventral bulge due to the underlying belly of the **biceps brachii,** which tapers as it converges into the fossa. It is enhanced by slight flexion of the elbow. Over the center of the fossa, the roof is slightly depressed. Posteriorly, the contours vary according to the position of the elbow. When this is fully extended, a central prominence marks the underlying **olecranon process** of the ulna. Proximal to this, transverse skin creases overlie the olecranon fossa, and a broad midline fullness tapering toward the olecranon marks the lower end of **triceps** and its tendon. The **epicondyles** form prominences on the medial and lateral borders at the widest point of the elbow, where they lie subcutaneously. With the subject's elbow fully flexed and the dorsum of the forearm facing the examiner, a distinct groove is visible passing from the elbow obliquely down to the wrist (Fig. 5.2). It marks the **subcutaneous border of the ulna.**

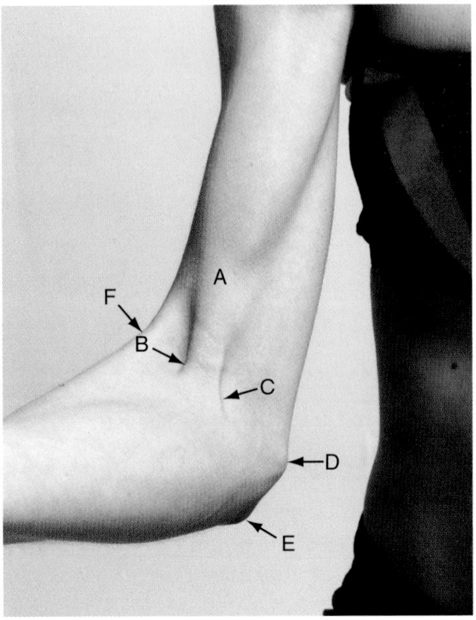


Fig. 5.1 Frontal view of the elbow and forearm
A = biceps brachii, B = biceps tendon, C = biceps aponeurosis (passing medially over common flexor tendon), D = medial epicondyle, E = olecranon tip, F = brachioradialis

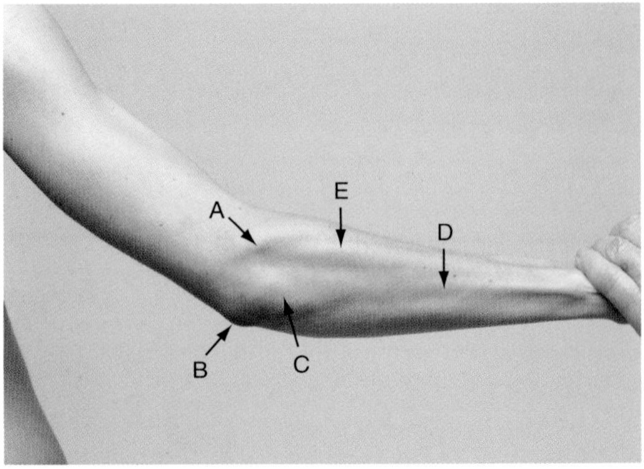


Fig. 5.2 Posterior view of elbow and forearm
A = lateral epicondyle with common extensor tendon, B = medial epicondyle, C = subcutaneous surface of olecranon, D = posterior subcutaneous border of ulna, E = extensor carpi ulnaris

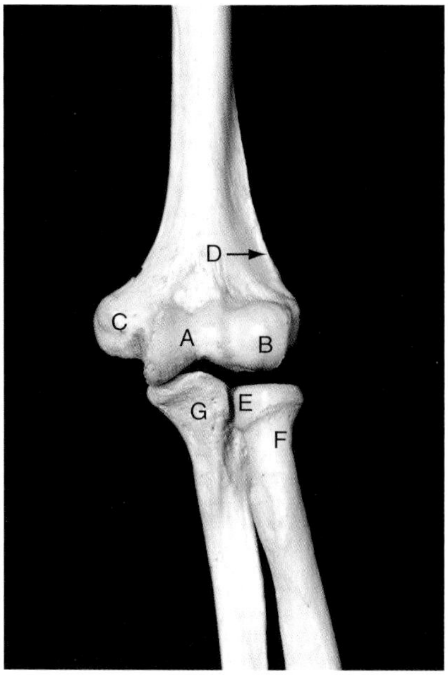


Fig. 5.3a Frontal view of the skeleton of the elbow and forearm
A = trochlea, B = capitulum, C = medial epicondyle, D = lateral supracondylar ridge, E = radial head, F = radial neck, G = coronoid process

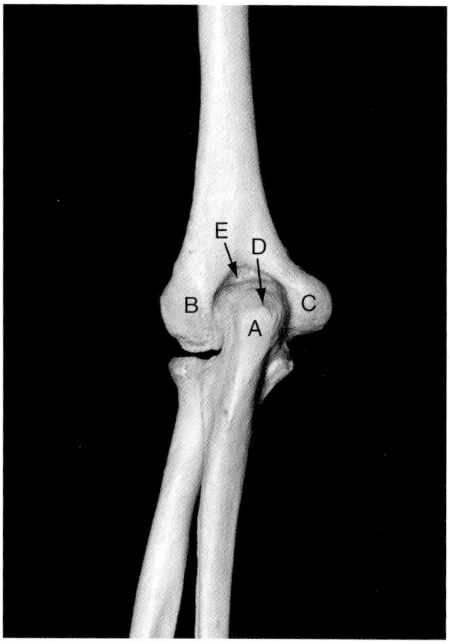


Fig. 5.3b Posterior view of the skeleton of the elbow and forearm
A = subcutaneous surface of olecranon, B = lateral epicondyle of humerus, C = medial epicondyle, D = site of triceps tendon attachment, E = olecranon fossa

# LOCATING BONY LANDMARKS

- Medial and lateral epicondyles
- Olecranon process and shaft of ulna
- Head of radius

Bony landmarks are shown on the skeleton of the elbow in Figure 5.3, and on radiographs of the elbow in Figures 5.6 and 5.7 below.

## MEDIAL AND LATERAL EPICONDYLES, AND HEAD OF RADIUS

The subject faces the examiner with the elbow fully extended and forearm supinated. On the medial side of the elbow the **medial epicondyle** is very conspicuous (Fig. 5.4a), and can be easily palpated or gripped between the examiner's index finger and thumb. Palpating the posterior and lateral side of the forearm with the subject's elbow slightly flexed, the examiner slides the index and middle finger tips firmly upward toward the elbow to locate a distinct **groove** marking the junction between the **head of radius** and **lateral epicondyle** (Fig. 5.4b). The head is confirmed when it rotates as the examiner passively supinates and pronates the forearm. As the index finger slides upward beyond the groove, the posterior surface of the lateral epicondyle is felt to be well defined, although generally this epicondyle is much less evident than on the

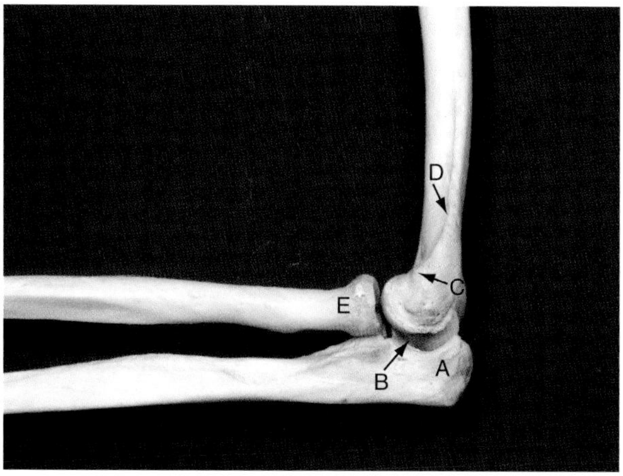


Fig. 5.3c Lateral view of the skeleton of the elbow
A = olecranon, B = trochlear notch, C = lateral epicondyle, D = lateral supracondylar ridge, E = radial neck

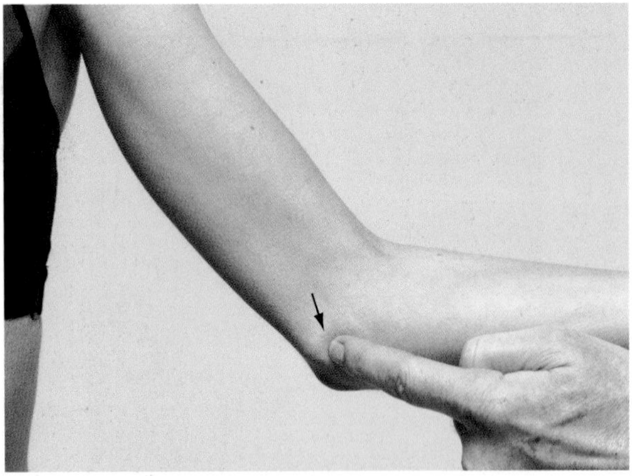

Fig. 5.4a Palpating the medial epicondyle (arrow)

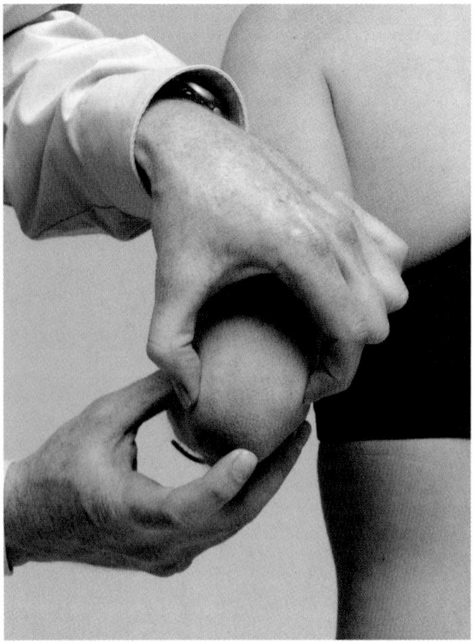

Fig. 5.5 Locating the three landmarks forming the bony triangle
The tips of the finger and thumb grasp the epicondyles and the index finger of the lower hand is on the tip of the olecranon

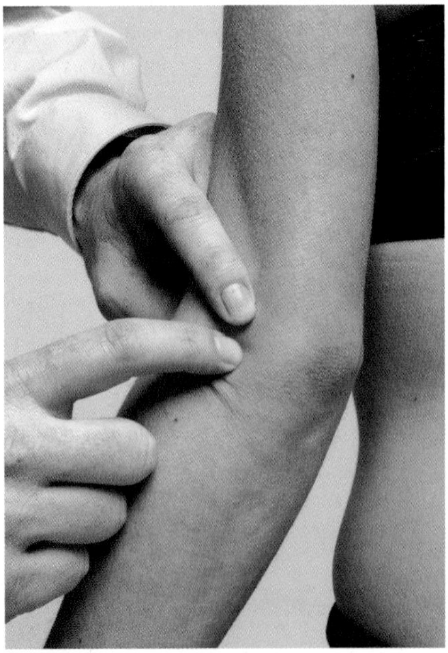

Fig. 5.4b Palpating the lateral epicondyle and radial head
The upper finger lies on the epicondyle and the lower finger in the groove between the radial head and epicondyle

medial side. On both sides, with the subject maintaining slight elbow flexion and the examiner using firm pressure, the finger tip can be passed upward from the epicondyles on to the **supracondylar ridges,** which are confirmed by rolling the finger tips across them. The lateral ridge is particularly conspicuous.

## OLECRANON PROCESS AND SHAFT OF RADIUS

Standing, the subject turns their back to the examiner and holds their forearm slightly abducted and very slightly flexed, allowing the examiner to palpate the **olecranon process.** The sides of the process can be gripped between finger and thumb, whilst the upper border and posterior subcutaneous surface can be palpated with the index finger tip. The superficial olecranon bursa overlies the posterior subcutaneous surface, and is commonly injured in sport when the elbow strikes the ground. Confirmation is sought that three bony landmarks, comprising the olecranon process and the two epicondyles, form a symmetrical triangle (Fig. 5.5), whose configuration may be disturbed by trauma to the elbow. The examiner continuing palpation distally from the posterior surface of the olecranon, the **subcutaneous border of the ulna** can be traced down to its head, which is located at the wrist. This border marks the boundary between flexor and extensor compartments. The **shaft of the radius** is less evident but can be located if the examiner firmly grips the mid-forearm by wrapping fingers and thumb around its circumference, the fingers being on the radial border, and asks the subject to alternate between supination and pronation.

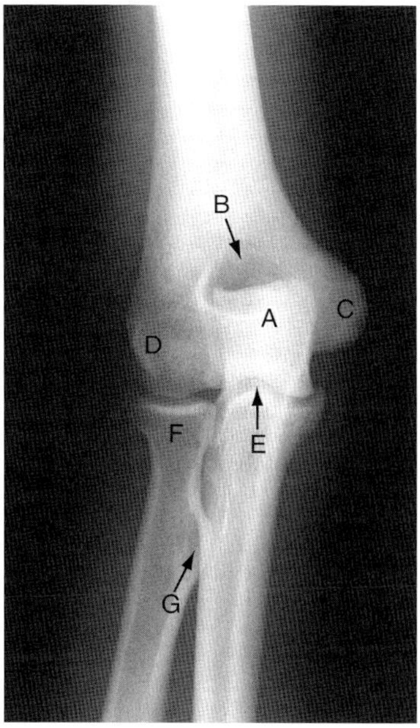


Fig. 5.6 Radiograph of the frontal view of the elbow
A = olecranon, B = olecranon fossa, C = medial epicondyle, D = lateral epicondyle, E = joint line, F = radial head, G = radial tuberosity

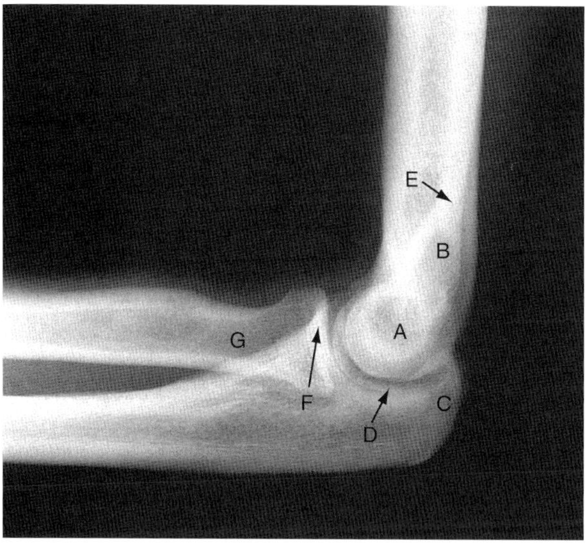


Fig. 5.7 Radiograph of the lateral view of the elbow
A = trochlea, B = medial epicondyle, C = olecranon, D = trochlear notch and joint line, E = supracondylar ridge, F = coronoid process, G = radial neck

## LOCATING THE ELBOW JOINT LINE

Some radiological features of the articulating surfaces are shown in Figures 5.6 and 5.7.

Due to the articulating features of this joint, it is difficult to locate a joint line. The sulcus marking the junction between the radial head and capitulum with the adjacent lateral epicondyle is the most obvious and has already been palpated. With the subject presenting the forearm supinated and fully extended, the examiner palpates carefully and firmly behind the elbow to locate depressions, one medial and one lateral, on each side of the olecranon adjacent to each epicondyle. Whilst the subject flexes and extends the elbow, the moving edges of the articulating trochlea can be felt.

## LOCATING SOFT TISSUES

- Biceps tendon and aponeurosis
- Triceps tendon
- Brachioradialis
- Common flexor origin
- Common extensor origin
- Pronator teres
- Outcropping muscles
- Brachial artery
- Nerves: ulnar, median and radial
- Collateral ligaments: radial and ulnar

Features of the cubital fossa and posterior aspect of the elbow and forearm are shown in the prosections in Figures 5.8 and 5.9.

### BICEPS TENDON AND APONEUROSIS

The biceps tendon and aponeurosis are considered in Chapter 4. Recall that the tendon is palpated passing distally and deeply down the middle of the fossa, whilst resisting further flexion of the partially flexed elbow. In this position, the sharp proximal border of the aponeurosis, passing medially across the common flexor origin onto the medial epicondyle, can also be defined by rolling the index and middle finger tips against it.

### TRICEPS TENDON

The triceps tendon can also be revisited here. If the index and middle fingers are placed across the groove just above the upper border of the olecranon, the groove disappears

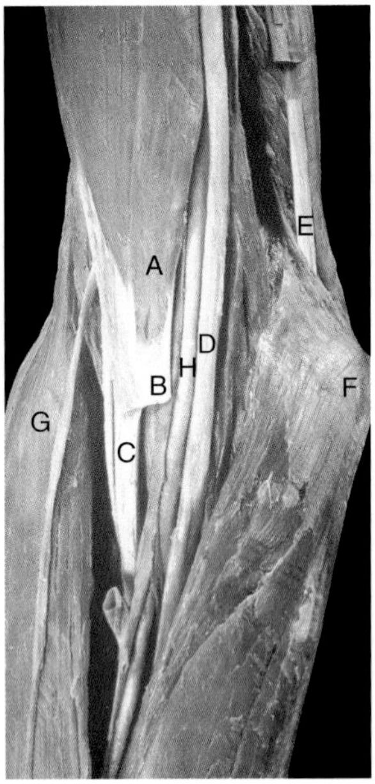


Fig. 5.8 Prosection of the anterior aspect of the elbow
A = biceps brachii, B = biceps aponeurosis, C = biceps tendon, D = median nerve, E = ulnar nerve, F = common flexor origin on medial epicondyle, G = brachioradialis, H = brachial artery (From Gosling JA, Harris PF, Whitmore I, Willan PLT. 2002 Human Anatomy, 4th edn. London: Mosby)

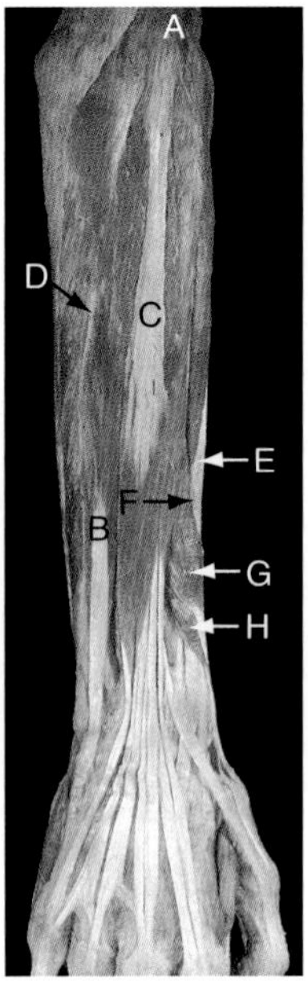


Fig. 5.9 Prosection of the posterior aspect of the elbow
A = common extensor origin on lateral epicondyle, B = extensor carpi ulnaris, C = extensor digitorum, D = subcutaneous border of ulna, E = extensor carpi radialis longus, F = location of intersection with outcropping muscles, G = abductor pollicis longus, H = extensor pollicis brevis (From Gosling JA, Harris PF, Whitmore I, Willan PLT. 2002 Human Anatomy, 4th edn. London: Mosby)

as the underlying tendon is felt to tense when the muscle contracts to extend the elbow.

## BRACHIORADIALIS AND THE RADIAL NERVE

To locate the **brachioradialis,** the subject faces the examiner with the forearm in the mid-prone position and elbow flexed to 90°. The muscle mass forms an elevation on the radial side just below the elbow, which the examiner's finger and thumb can grip and move from side to side. When further flexion of the elbow is resisted, the contracting brachio-radialis is clearly visible (Fig. 5.10a). The **radial nerve** enters the cubital fossa deep to the upper medial edge of this muscle (Fig. 5.10b).

## COMMON FLEXOR ORIGIN

To locate the common flexor origin, the subject presents the supinated forearm with elbow extended, allowing the examiner to palpate the fullness anterior and distal to the medial epicondyle (Fig. 5.11). With the tips of the index and middle fingers, the underlying muscles can be felt to contract as the subject alternately flexes and extends the fingers.

## COMMON EXTENSOR ORIGIN

With the subject maintaining the same position and repeating extension of the wrist and fingers, the examiner palpates *anterior* and immediately distal to the lateral epicondyle (Fig. 5.12) to locate the common extensor origin. The extensor origin can be felt to tense with extension of the fingers.

## PRONATOR TERES

The pronator teres is palpable if the examiner grips the subject's wrist in the mid-prone position and resists further pronation, whilst using the fingers of the other hand to feel deeply along the medial boundary of the cubital fossa. The muscle can be felt contracting and may be visible (Fig. 5.13) distally and laterally toward its attachment on the lateral surface of the radius.

## OUTCROPPING MUSCLES

To locate the deep outcropping muscles (extensor pollicis longus and brevis, abductor pollicis longus) passing distally toward the thumb, the subject pronates the forearm

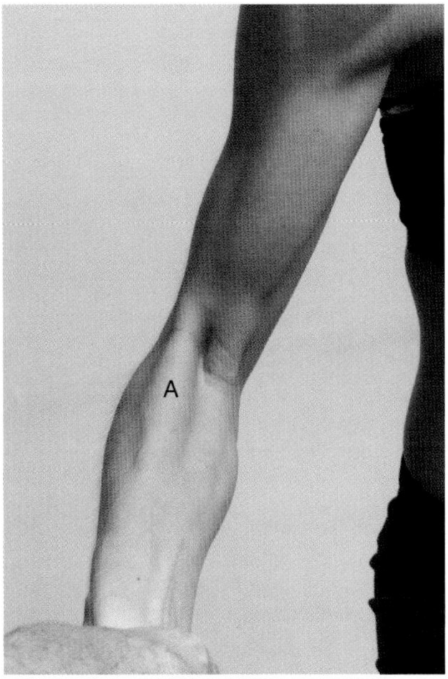


Fig. 5.10a Demonstrating the brachioradialis muscle (A)

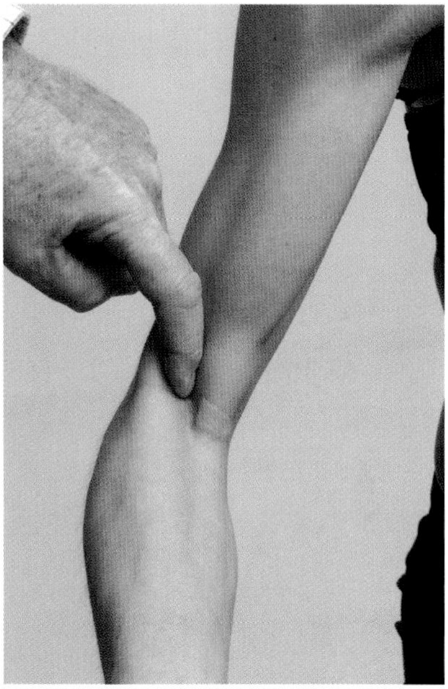

Fig. 5.10b Locating the radial nerve in the cubital fossa
Palpation is deep to the brachioradialis

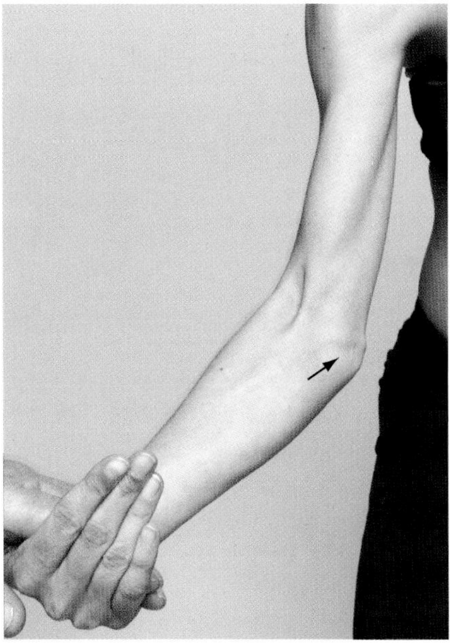

Fig. 5.11 Locating the common flexor origin (arrow)

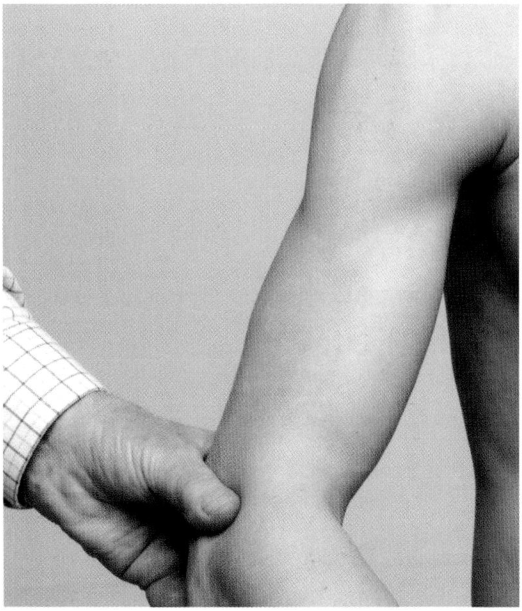

Fig. 5.12 Locating the common extensor origin
Palpation is anterior to the lateral epicondyle

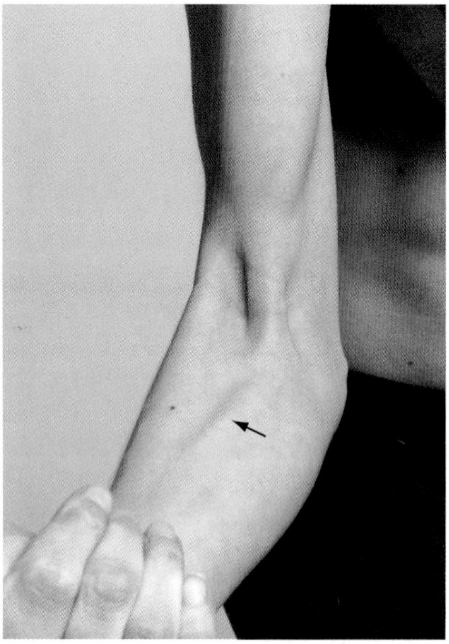

Fig. 5.13 Locating the pronator teres
Pronation is resisted, making the muscle prominent (arrow)

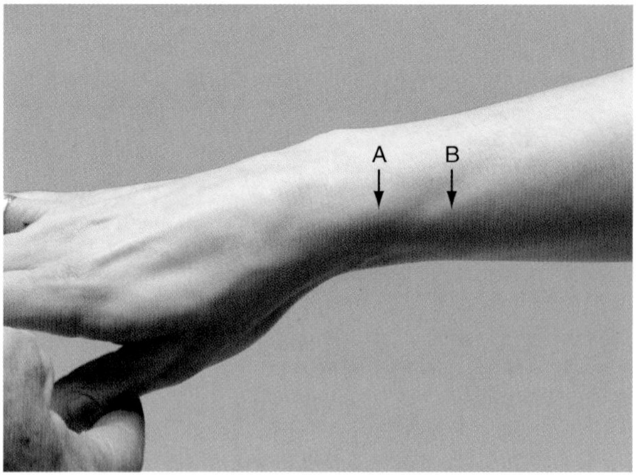


Fig. 5.14 Locating the deep outcropping muscles of the forearm
The groove between A and B marks the location of the intersection. A = outcropping muscles to the thumb, B = extensor carpi radialis longus

with the elbow extended, enabling the examiner to palpate over the radial margin in the distal third of the forearm using the tips of the index and middle fingers. When the subject strongly extends and abducts the thumb, the examiner feels the muscles tense obliquely around the radial margin accompanied by a visible fullness (Figs 5.14 and 6.20).

## BRACHIAL ARTERY

To access the brachial artery and its pulsations, the subject's elbow is extended and the limb partially abducted, allowing the examiner to apply firm deep pressure using the middle and index fingers in the furrow of the cubital fossa just above and medial to the bicipital aponeurosis (see Fig. 5.1).

## NERVES: MEDIAN AND ULNAR

The **median nerve** lies adjacent to the artery. The **ulnar nerve** is easily palpated behind the medial epicondyle (Fig. 5.15). The subject faces the examiner, with the limb slightly abducted, the forearm supinated, and the elbow flexed to about 90°. Using the tip of the index finger, the examiner feels for the cord-like nerve, which can be rolled in the groove between the posterior surface of the medial epicondyle and the olecranon. This procedure may cause discomfort.

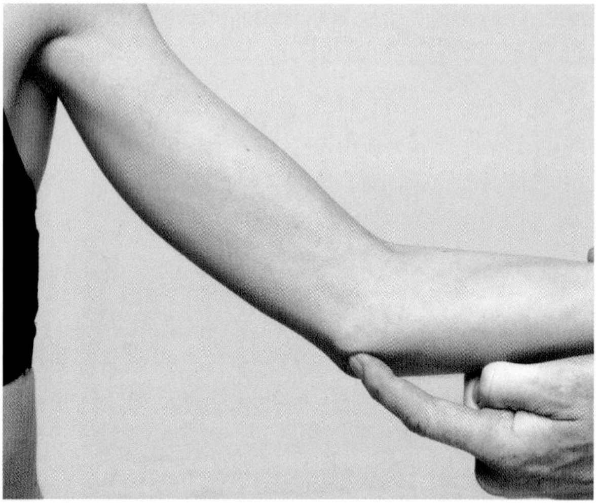

Fig. 5.15 Palpating the ulnar nerve
The finger tip is inserted behind the medial epicondyle

## COLLATERAL LIGAMENTS: RADIAL AND ULNAR

The examiner can locate the collateral ligaments by palpating tension in them whilst grasping the forearm and passively changing the position of the elbow, alternating between flexion and extension of the joint. To feel the **ulnar ligament,** the examiner places the tip of the index finger deeply into the groove between the posterior part

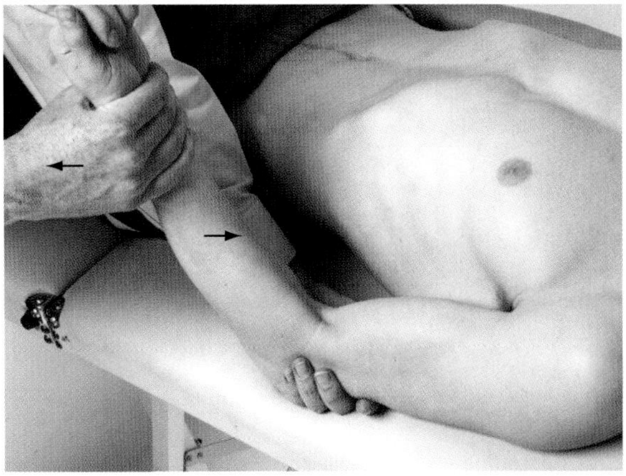

Fig. 5.16a Strength test for biceps brachii

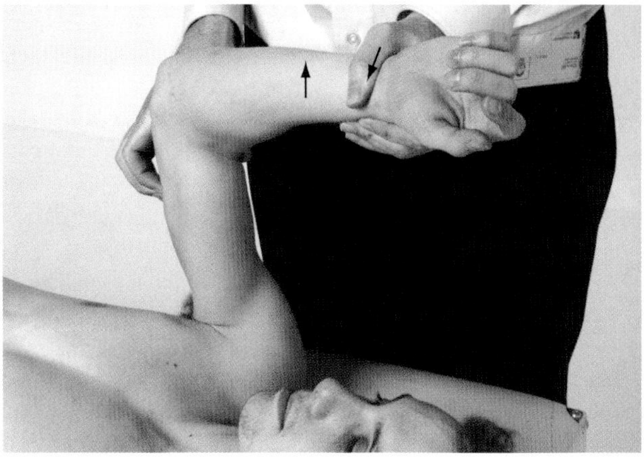

Fig. 5.16b Strength test for triceps brachii

of the medial epicondyle and the medial surface of the olecranon. To feel the **radial collateral ligament,** the index finger is inserted into the groove between the head of the radius and the lateral epicondyle on the lateral border of the forearm.

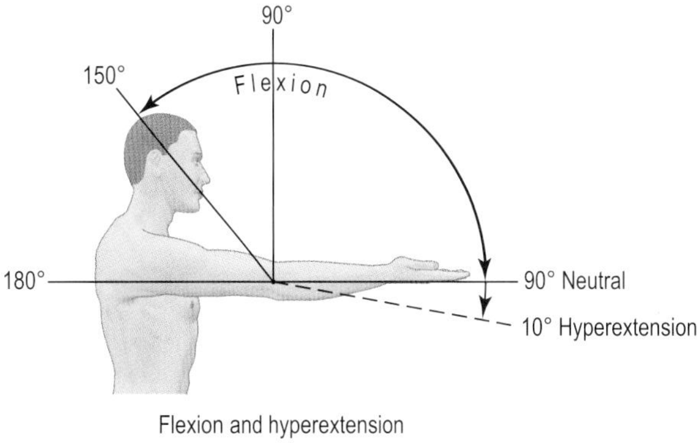


Fig. 5.17 Range of movements at the elbow
Redrawn from *Joint motion: method of measuring and recording.* Edinburgh: E&S Livingstone, 1965 (with the permission of the American Academy of Orthopedic Surgeons, reprinted with their permission by the British Orthopaedic Association)

# TESTING MUSCLES AND MOVEMENTS

- Biceps brachii and brachialis
- Triceps
- Supinators
- Pronators
- Range of movements

The principal movements are flexion and extension. The subject stands facing the examiner, with the forearm supinated, and raises the extended limb forward to about 90°. Active movements produced by the **biceps** and **brachialis** are tested by asking the subject to flex (bend) the forearm as far as possible. The **triceps** extends the elbow and is tested by asking the subject to straighten the elbow maximally from the fully flexed position. Supination at the proximal radio-ulnar joint is produced by **biceps** and **supinator,** and pronation by **pronator teres** and **quadratus.** The movements are tested with the subject seated and resting the elbow and extended forearm on a table in the mid-prone position. The subject is asked to turn the limb so that the palm faces the table and then in the opposite direction so that the dorsum of the hand lies flat on the table. All of these movements are also tested against resistance by the examiner.

## STRENGTH TEST FOR BICEPS AND TRICEPS

The subject is seated, facing forward with the arms to the side and elbows flexed to 90° or lies supine. Standing behind the chair, the examiner reaches downward and tests the biceps by gripping the forearms above the wrists and pushing downward whilst resisting the subject's attempts to bend the elbows (Fig. 5.16a). Conversely, to assess the triceps, the examiner grasps the forearms similarly but pulls upward whilst asking the subject to straighten the elbows (Fig. 5.16b).

## RANGE OF MOVEMENTS

Whilst testing the muscles, the examiner assesses the range of joint movements achieved. Ranges are shown in Figures 5.17 and 5.18. Starting with the limb fully extended and

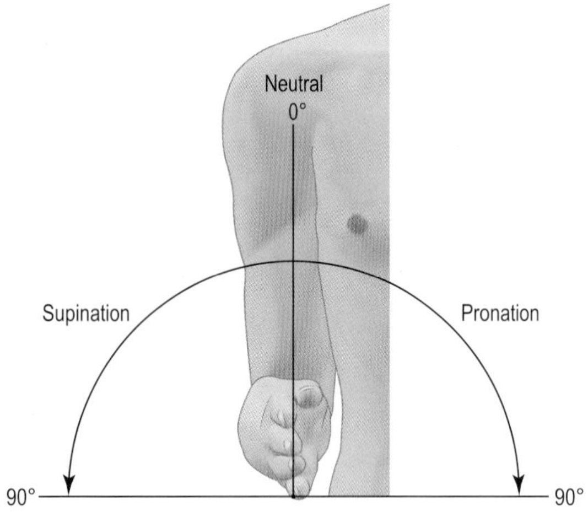


Fig. 5.18 Range of supination and pronation movements of the forearm
Movements involve the proximal and distal radio-ulnar joints and the radio-ulnar syndesmosis
Redrawn from *Joint motion: method of measuring and recording.* Edinburgh: E&S Livingstone, 1965 (with the permission of the American Academy of Orthopedic Surgeons, reprinted with their permission by the British Orthopaedic Association)

supinated, the total range of flexion is about **150°**. Some subjects can achieve a small amount of hyperextension in the order of approximately **10°**. Starting with the forearm in the mid-prone position, full supination and pronation traverse **90°** in each direction.

# TESTING REFLEXES

- Biceps
- Supinator
- Triceps

## BICEPS JERK

Cord segments and nerve roots involved are C5 and C6. The subject is seated facing the examiner, with the elbow relaxed and partially flexed. The examiner supports the bend of the elbow with one hand, using the thumb to locate the partially stretched tendon anteriorly in the cubital fossa. The percussion hammer is applied briskly over the thumb stretching the tendon.

## BRACHIORADIALIS ("SUPINATOR") JERK

Cord segments and nerve roots involved are C5 and C6. The subject adopts the same position as for the biceps reflex, except that the forearm is in the mid-prone position and supported on a table with the elbow partially flexed. The examiner percusses the tendon located about two-thirds down the length of the anterior border of the forearm.

## TRICEPS JERK

Cord segments and nerve roots involved are C7 and C8. The examiner stands behind the subject, who is seated with the arm abducted about 60° and the relaxed elbow flexed to a right angle, supported in this position by the examiner's hand on the under surface of the elbow. The triceps tendon is palpated just above the olecranon and percussed briskly.

# SPECIAL TESTS

- Collateral ligaments
- Ulnar collateral ligament 90/90 stress test
- Valgus stress test
- Common extensor tendinopathy
- Common flexor tendinopathy

## STRESSING COLLATERAL LIGAMENTS

The subject lies supine, with the elbow to be tested extended and the forearm supinated (Fig. 5.19). Facing the subject, the examiner grasps the wrist with one hand. To test the **medial** (ulnar) ligament, the examiner applies firm pressure medially over the lateral side of the elbow, at the same time using the other hand to lever the wrist laterally. Conversely, to test the **lateral** (radial) ligament, the examiner applies firm pressure over the medial side of the elbow in a lateral direction, whilst levering the forearm in a medial direction.

## ULNAR COLLATERAL LIGAMENT (UCL) 90/90 STRESS TEST

The oblique and anterior bands of the UCL of the elbow, frequently strained or ruptured by throwing maneuvers, can be tested as follows. The subject lies supine, with the shoulder abducted and externally rotated to 90° (Fig. 5.20). The examiner stands facing the subject and grips the subject's wrist with one hand, whilst supporting the mid-humerus with the other so as to prevent further external rotation of the shoulder. The examiner then exerts a valgus force on the elbow by pushing the subject's forearm toward the floor. Medial elbow pain and/or laxity may indicate strain or rupture of the anterior or oblique band of the UCL.

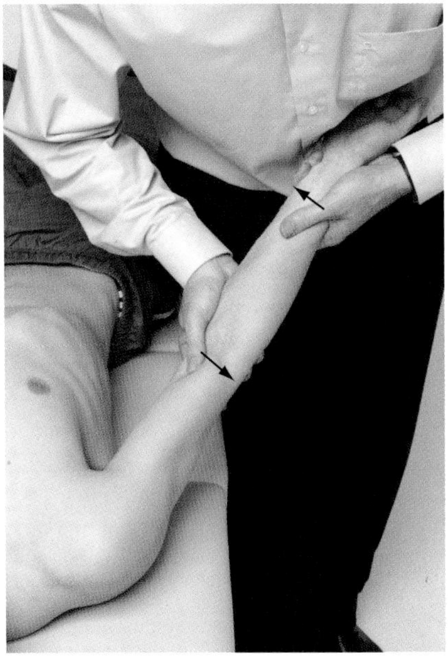

Fig. 5.19a Stressing the lateral (radial) collateral ligament of the elbow

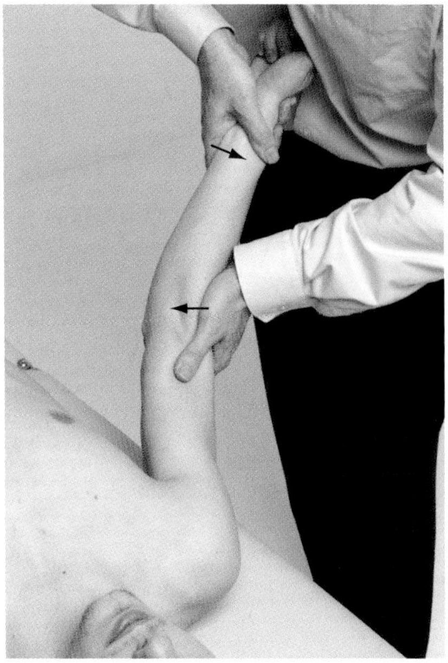

Fig. 5.19b Stressing the medial (ulnar) collateral ligament of the elbow

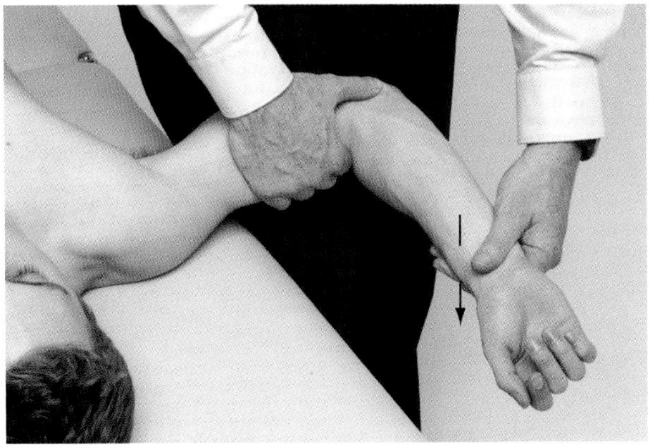

Fig. 5.20 Ulnar collateral ligament 90/90 stress test

## THE MOVING VALGUS STRESS TEST

To perform the moving valgus stress test, the examiner applies and maintains a constant moderate valgus torque to the fully flexed elbow and then quickly extends the elbow. The test is positive if the medial elbow pain is reproduced at between 120° and 70° of elbow flexion.

## COMMON EXTENSOR ORIGIN TENDINOPATHY

The subject is seated, with the arm partially abducted and flexed to approximately 90°, the palm facing downward, and the wrist flexed. Maintaining firm pressure over the dorsum of the hand, the examiner asks the subject to dorsiflex the hand at the wrist. Pain may be experienced at the lateral epicondyle. The test can be focused to assess tendinopathy in the extensor carpi radialis brevis (ECRB) by keeping the wrist in a neutral position whilst the subject attempts to extend first the index then the middle finger against resistance (Fig. 5.21). Lateral elbow pain with resisted middle digit extension is indicative of ECRB tendinopathy.

## COMMON FLEXOR ORIGIN TENDINOPATHY

The subject is seated, with the arm slightly abducted, elbow extended and forearm supinated (Fig. 5.22). Subjects are asked to make a fist around the examiner's index and middle fingers, squeezing them tightly. They are then asked to perform resisted wrist flexion. Pain may be experienced at the medial epicondyle.

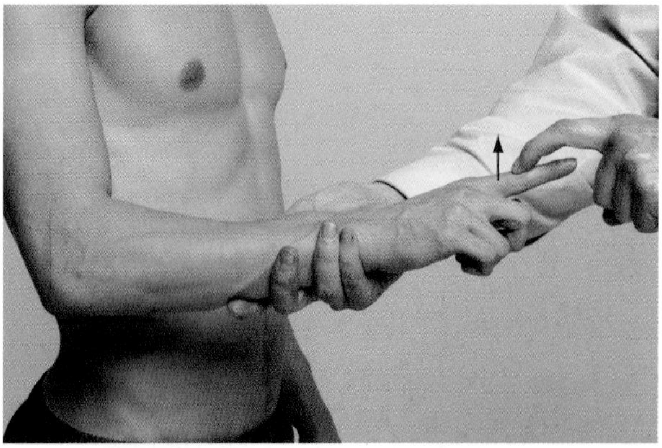

Fig. 5.21a Testing for common extensor origin tendinopathy
Extending the index finger against resistance tests extensor carpi radialis longus

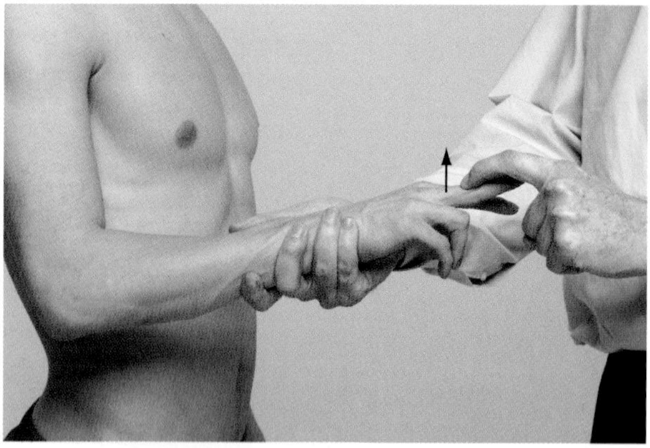

Fig. 5.21b Testing for common extensor origin tendinopathy
Extending the middle finger against resistance tests extensor carpi radialis brevis

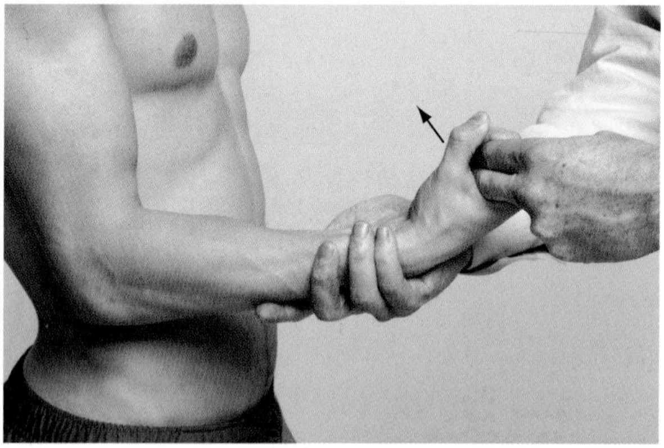

Fig. 5.22 Testing for common flexor origin tendinopathy
Wrist flexion against resistance tests the common flexor origin

## FURTHER READING

Benjamin HJ, Briner WW. Little League elbow. Clinical Journal of Sport Medicine 2005; 15:37–40.

Cain EL, Dugas JR, Wolf RS, Andrews JR. Elbow injuries in throwing athletes: a current concepts review. American Journal of Sports Medicine 2003; 31:621–635.

Capasso G, Testa V, Cappabianca S et al. Recurrent dislocation of the ulnar nerve in athletes: a report of two cases. Clinical Journal of Sport Medicine 1998; 8:56–58.

Conrad JM, Stanitski CL. Osteochondritis dissecans: Wilson's sign revisited. American Journal of Sports Medicine 2003; 31:777–778.

Hamilton BH, Colsen E, Brukner P. Stress fracture of the ulna in a baseball pitcher. Clinical Journal of Sport Medicine 1999; 9:231–232.

Holtzhausen LM, Noakes TD. Elbow, forearm, wrist and hand injuries among sport rock climbers. Clinical Journal of Sport Medicine 1996; 6:196–203.

Mata SG, Ovejero AH, Grande MM. Bilateral chronic exertional compartment syndrome of the forearm in two brothers. Clinical Journal of Sport Medicine 1999; 9:91–94.

## CASE STUDY 5 • CLINICAL PROBLEMS

**Problem 1.** *A 20 year-old international javelin thrower experiences a sudden, severe pain at the medial elbow during a throw in competition. She is unable to continue.*

a) What is the likely diagnosis?
b) What is the mechanism of injury?
c) What are two possible differential diagnoses?
d) How is this injury normally managed?

**Problem 2.** *A 35-year-old recreational tennis player complains of lateral elbow pain that has gradually worsened over the last 4 months. It is aggravated by backhand shots.*

a) The tendon of which muscle is commonly implicated in the above scenario?
b) How is this tendon tested?
c) What term is used to describe the "non-inflammatory" pathological condition that affects the tendon?
d) Suggest at least two alterations this player could make to equipment and technique that might alleviate the symptoms.

**Problem 3.** *A 60-year-old male golfer describes sharp medial elbow pain when miss-hitting a shot "fat," i.e. when the ground is struck hard when a shot is played.*

a) What is this condition commonly known as?
b) What structures might be injured?
c) What is the mechanism of injury?

**Problem 4.** *A judo player notices a soft swelling the size of a golf ball affecting the posterior elbow following a bout.*

a) What is the likely diagnosis?
b) What condition needs to be excluded?

**Problem 5.** *A 12-year-old baseball pitcher has just started practicing throwing "curve balls." He has developed medial elbow pain.*

a) What is the common name given to this condition?
b) Name at least three pathological processes that might contribute to this young pitcher's symptoms.

**Problem 6.** *A 12-year-old female gymnast falls off the uneven bars and breaks her fall with her left arm. Her elbow is slightly flexed when the hand impacts with the ground and she immediately experiences severe elbow pain. On examination, there is deformity of the elbow with posterior and proximal displacement of the olecranon process.*

a) What is the likely diagnosis?
b) What possible associated injuries need to be excluded?
c) What are three possible complications of this injury?

**Problem 7.** *A 25-year-old male outfielder in cricket has a 6-week history of low-grade medial elbow pain with throwing. During one throw yesterday he felt a sharp pain in his medial elbow, after which subsequent throws caused considerable pain. An MRI scan conducted today reveals a partial tear of the humeral attachment of the ulnar collateral ligament with edema surrounding the tear (Fig. 5.23).*

a) Which clinical tests could be used to confirm the MRI findings?
b) What are two differential diagnoses and what clinical tests could be used to exclude them?

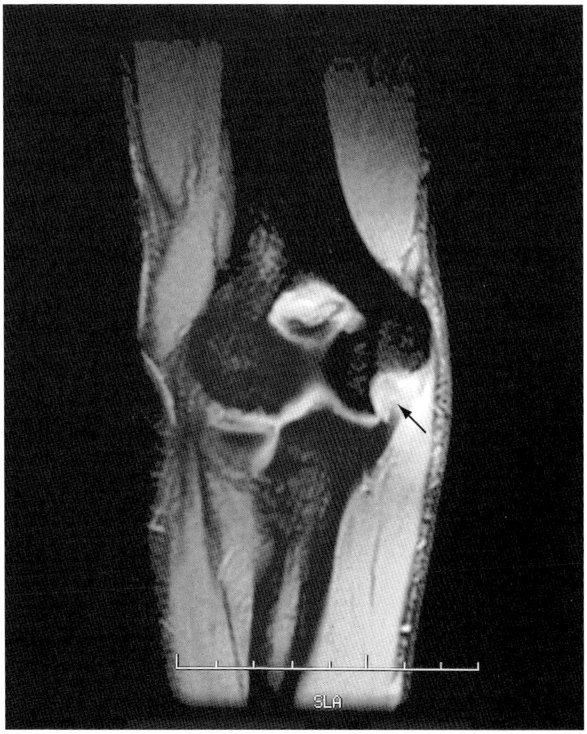


Fig. 5.23 MRI scan of elbow joint showing tear and edema of medial collateral ligament (arrow)

6

CHAPTER

# Wrist and hand

## INTRODUCTION

The wrist lies at the junction of the forearm, the penultimate segment in the lever system of the upper limb, with the hand, the terminal segment, specialized for the important and exclusive functions of touching and gripping. The wrist is a complex of joints, including the distal radio-ulnar, the wrist joint itself, and the carpal joints, all of them synovial, facilitating and enhancing the gripping actions of the hand. Long flexor and extensor tendons, restrained by retinacula, cross the ventral and dorsal aspects of the wrist. Some are attached to carpals and metacarpals, controlling movements and position of the wrist, essential for an effective power grip, whilst others continue more distally into the digits to control their movements. The small intrinsic muscles arising in the palm of the hand have a major role in forming functional arches in the hand and refining the specialized movements of the thumb and fingers expressed in the various forms of grip, of which there are three basic types: power, precision, and hook. Combinations of these types are used in a wide variety of sports. Because of its terminal position in the limb, the hand is particularly vulnerable to injury.

## INSPECTION OF NORMAL CONTOURS

- Skin creases: wrist, palm, fingers
- Palmar aponeurosis
- Head of ulna
- Extensor tendons
- Metacarpal heads

The distal part of the forearm tapers at the wrist, the most slender part of the limb. Beyond the wrist the hand broadens into the palm in the form of a truncated triangle with medial and lateral diverging borders. Distally, the palm gives way to the divergent thumb on the radial side and to the four fingers, index, middle (the neutral and longest digit), ring, and little finger, on the ulnar side.

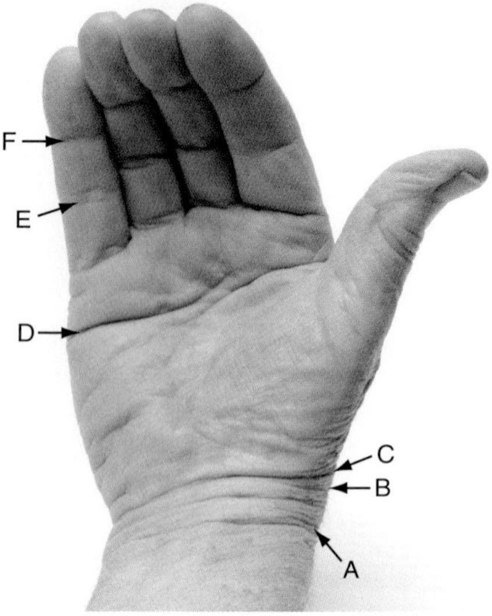


**Fig. 6.1** Transverse skin creases in the wrist, palm, and fingers
A = limit of flexor tendon sheaths, B = line of wrist joint, C = proximal limit of flexor retinaculum, D = line of metacarpo-phalangeal joint, E = line of proximal interphalangeal joint, F = line of distal interphalangeal joint

### VENTRAL (PALMAR) ASPECT

When the wrist and hand are viewed from ventrally and slight flexion of the **wrist** is used, **three transverse skin creases** (Fig. 6.1) appear. The most distal crease marks the proximal border of the flexor retinaculum, the middle crease overlies the wrist joint, and the proximal crease marks the proximal limit of the ulnar and radial synovial sheaths enclosing the long flexor tendons to the thumb and fingers as they approach the carpal tunnel.

Inspection of the palm shows the prominent thenar eminence with the underlying intrinsic thenar muscles on the radial side, and the less prominent hypothenar eminence on the ulnar side. Keeping the fingers straight and partially flexing the **hand** produces **transverse skin creases** (Fig. 6.1), of which the distal marks the line of the metacarpo-phalangeal joints. By extending the fingers maximally and viewing the palm in "skyline" contour, longitudinal depressions appear in the skin extending toward the roots of the fingers. Conversely, in the intervals between these depressions, the skin bulges, coinciding with the webs of the fingers. Palpation confirms that the depressions have underlying firm tissue which constitutes the **digital slips of the palmar aponeurosis** (Fig. 6.2), whilst the bulges are soft due to fat extruding from the underlying mid-palmar space.

Flexion of the **fingers** emphasizes **three transverse skin creases** on their palmar aspects. The distal and intermediate creases mark the line of the **distal and proximal interphalangeal joints,** but the proximal do not overlie joints. The thumb has only one transverse crease and it marks the interphalangeal joint.

### DORSAL ASPECT

Dorsally and close to the ulnar border of the proximal part of the wrist is a rounded swelling made more prominent by palmar flexion of the wrist. This is the **head of the ulna.** Just beyond the wrist, longitudinal subcutaneous ridges diverge, made more visible by strongly extending the wrist and fingers. These can be traced on to the dorsum of each finger and the thumb, and are caused by the underlying **long extensor tendons.** Flexion of the fingers to make a tight fist emphasizes the prominence of the knuckles due to the underlying **heads of the metacarpals** (Fig. 6.3).

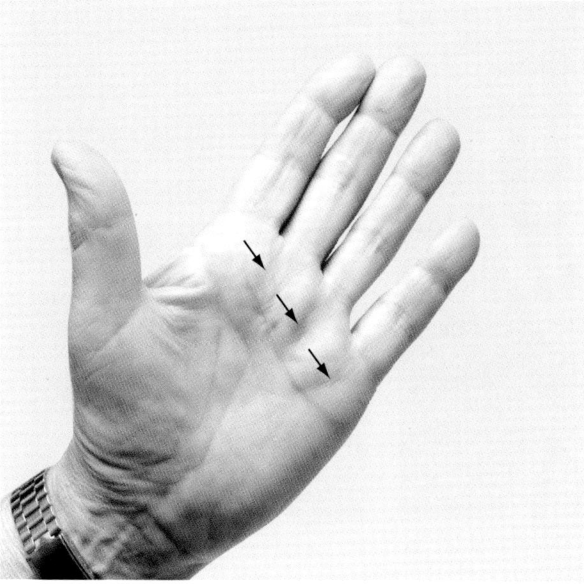

Fig. 6.2 Location of the digital slips of the palmar aponeurosis in the palm
The arrows indicate grooves overlying the slips. Intervening bulges between the grooves are due to fat in the mid-palmar space

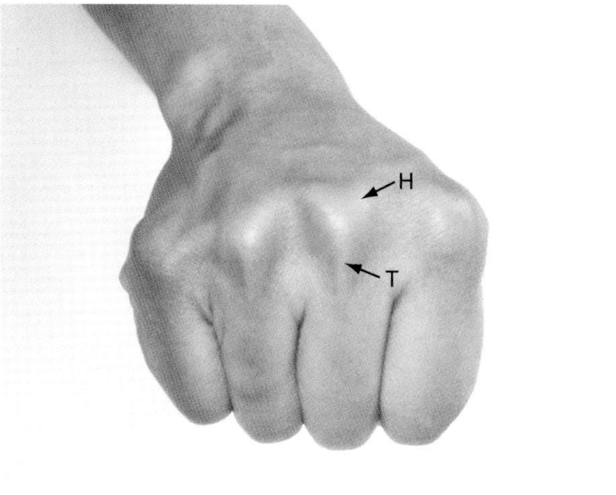


Fig. 6.3 Heads of metacarpals demonstrated by making a fist
H = head of metacarpal, T = extensor tendon overriding metacarpal head

# LOCATING BONY LANDMARKS

- Ulna:
  Head
  Styloid process
- Radius:
  Styloid process
  Dorsal tubercle
- Carpals:
  Scaphoid
  Triquetrum
  Lunate
  Pisiform
  Trapezium
- Metacarpals
- Phalanges

Some bony features of the wrist and hand are emphasized in the photographs of the skeleton of the wrist and hand in Figure 6.4a and b. These are also shown on the radiograph (Fig. 6.4c).

## RADIUS AND ULNA

The examination is facilitated with the subject seated and elbow flexed. The forearm is pronated, with the elbow and forearm supported on a flat surface and wrist relaxed. Using an index finger tip, the examiner locates the **radial styloid process** (Fig. 6.5) in the anatomical "snuff box," applying upward pressure toward the radius. The **ulnar styloid** is more difficult to feel. The index finger of the opposite hand locates the tip just distal to the ulnar head in a groove lying on the deep aspect of the extensor carpi ulnaris tendon, which itself grooves the medial side of the head (Fig. 6.5). Its location is facilitated by palpating in the groove whilst the wrist is passively moved, alternating between radial and ulnar deviation using deep firm pressure. Once the two processes have been located, their relative levels are compared, the radial styloid lying more distally. On the dorsum of the wrist, the conspicuous **head of the ulna** is easily palpable (Fig. 6.6).

## CARPALS

Keeping a finger tip on the head and flexing the wrist, the examiner then moves the finger distally off the ulna into the groove which appears below it. Firm pressure on the far side of the groove locates the proximal carpus: in particular, the **triquetrum** (Fig. 6.7). From the triquetrum, palpation continuing laterally and flexion of the wrist

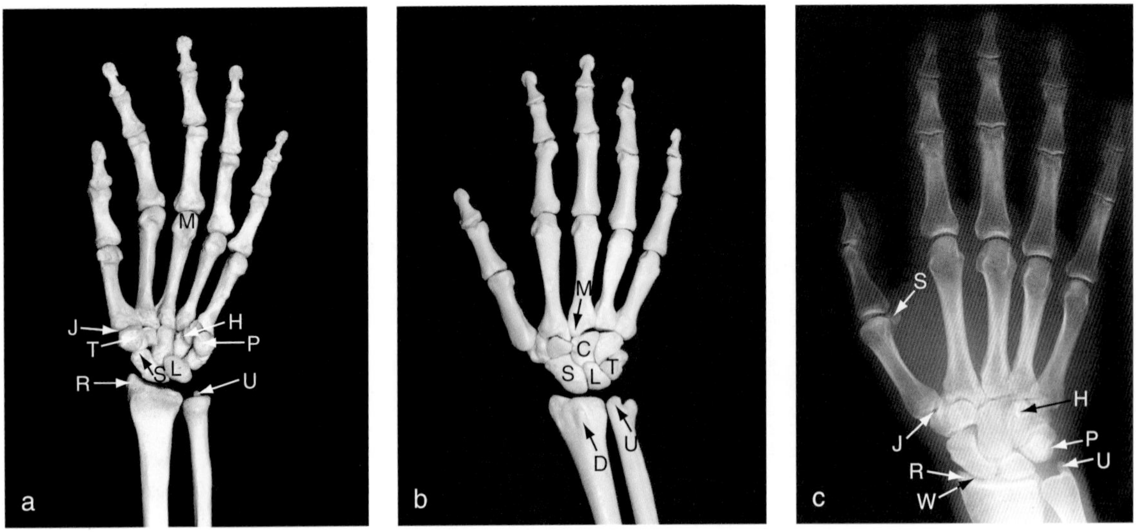


Fig. 6.4a Bones of the wrist and hand: palmar aspect
H = hook of hamate, J = first carpo-metacarpal (trapezium) joint, L = lunate, M = metacarpal head, P = pisiform, R = radial styloid process, S = scaphoid, T = ridge of trapezium, U = ulna: styloid process
Fig. 6.4b Bones of the wrist and hand: dorsal view
C = capitate, D = dorsal radial tubercle, L = lunate, M = styloid process, base of third metacarpal, S = scaphoid, T = triquetrum, U = ulnar head
Fig. 6.4c Frontal radiograph of the wrist and hand
H = hook of hamate, J = first carpo-metacarpal joint, P = pisiform, R = styloid process of radius, S = sesamoid bone, U = styloid process of ulna, W = cavity of wrist joint

increasing, the groove separating the triquetrum from the **lunate** becomes evident, enabling location of the lunate, although this is not as easily palpable as the triquetrum. On the lateral side of the wrist, palpation with a finger tip using a massaging motion over the dorsum of the radius reveals the **dorsal tubercle** (Fig. 6.8), with the tendon of extensor pollicis longus winding around it. Passing the finger distally in line with the dorsal tubercle and with the subject's wrist in neutral extension, the examiner can palpate a groove marking the distal end of the radius, which gives way to the **dorsum of the scaphoid** (Fig. 6.9). This is best confirmed using firm pressure over it whilst the subject makes circumduction movements with the hand. The **scaphoid** can also be palpated by inserting the finger tip deeply into the distal part of the anatomical "snuff box," using firm pressure with the finger pointing toward the root of the thumb.

On the ventral aspect of the wrist and palm there are several bony landmarks. The **tubercle of the scaphoid** lies close to the distal skin crease of the wrist and the root of the thumb. It is palpated by finding the tendon of flexor carpi radialis, with the wrist slightly extended, and tracing it into the palm. Near the base of the thumb it passes over a bony prominence, the tubercle of the scaphoid, which is easily felt (Fig. 6.10). More difficult to define is the **ridge of the trapezium** (Fig. 6.11), just distal to the tubercle and in line with the tendon of flexor carpi radialis. It is located at the middle of the root of the thenar eminence. The examiner grasps the subject's hand between the fingers and thumb, applying firm deep pressure with his or her own thumb to explore the root of the thenar eminence. On the ulnar side of the wrist close to the distal skin crease, the **pisiform** can be palpated (Fig. 6.12). This is best achieved by slight flexion of the wrist to identify the tendon of flexor carpi ulnaris and then following it into the hand. The pisiform is located as a rounded hard swelling in the tendon. If it is gripped by the examiner between finger and thumb and the wrist then pronated and supported hanging in passive flexion, maintaining the grip on the pisiform, it can be displaced from side to side lying in the tendon. The **hook of the hamate,** lying adjacent to Guyon's canal, is amongst the most difficult carpal bones to locate. It lies about 1 cm distal and lateral to the pisiform and is best located by very deep pressure with the pad of the thumb. It can only be felt in a very thin hand.

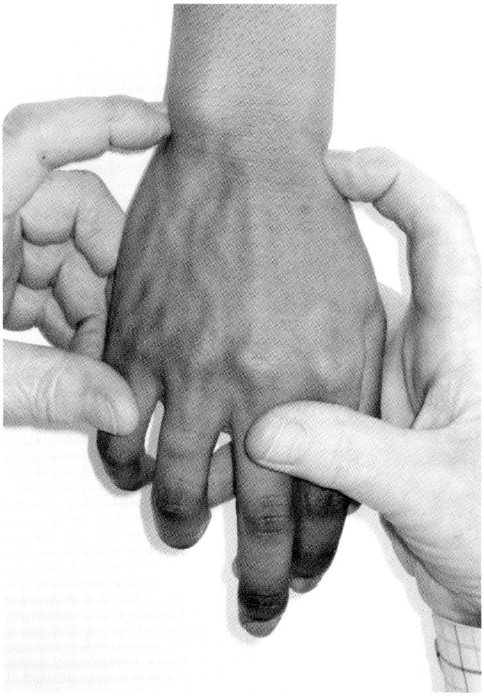

Fig. 6.5 Locating the radial and ulnar styloid processes
The tips of the index fingers are used to locate them. Note the radial styloid is the more distal

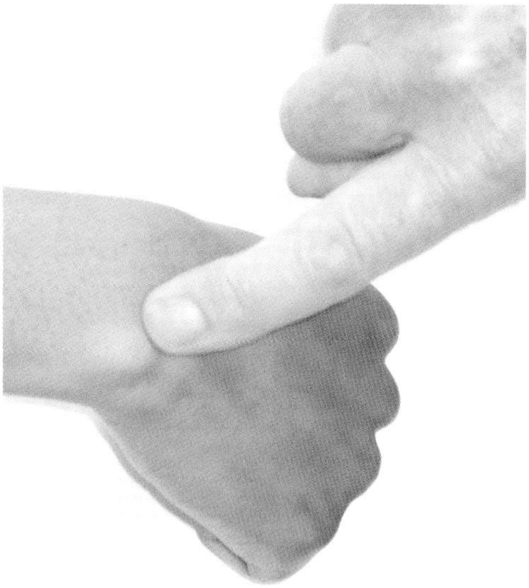

Fig. 6.6 Locating the head of the ulna on the dorsum of the wrist
Wrist flexion increases its prominence

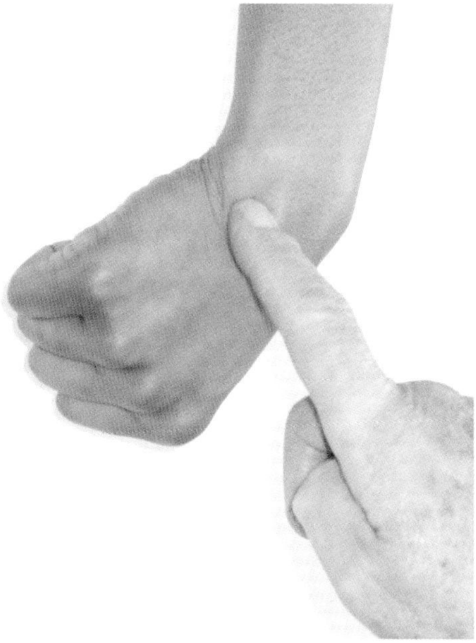

Fig. 6.7 Locating the triquetrum from dorsally
Wrist flexion assists palpation

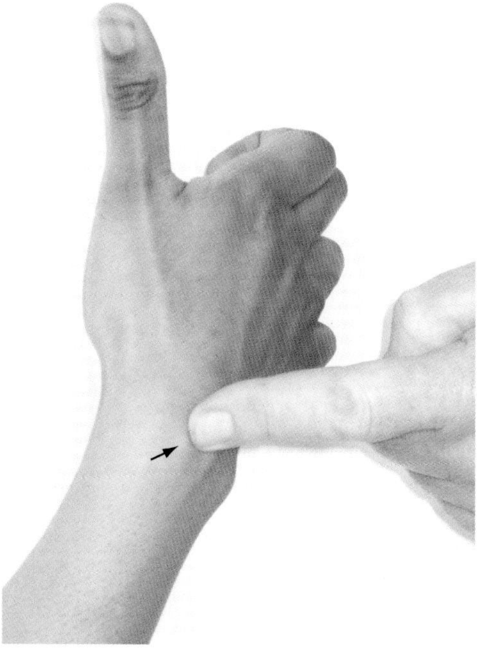

Fig. 6.8 Locating the dorsal radial tubercle
Thumb extension reveals the tendon of extensor pollicis longus, which leads toward the tubercle (arrow) around which it winds

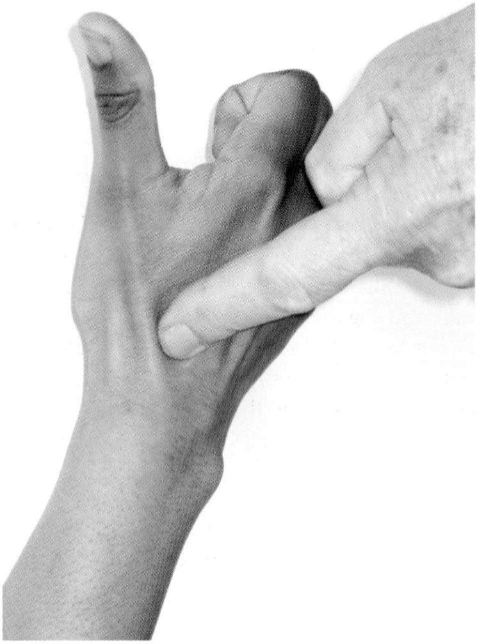

Fig. 6.9 Palpating the dorsum of the scaphoid

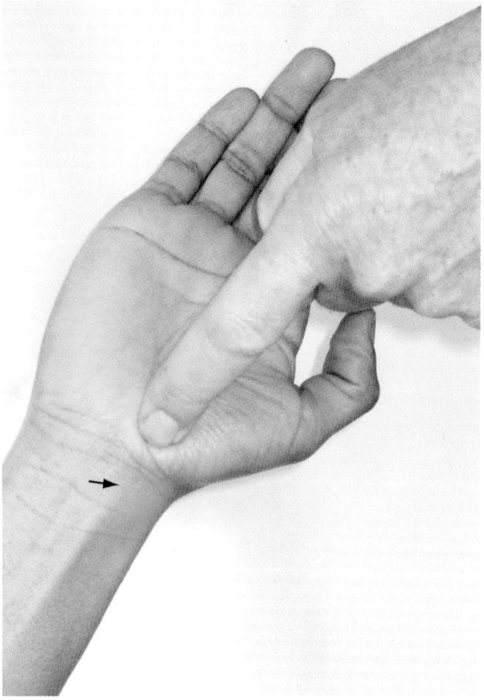

Fig. 6.10 Palpating the scaphoid tubercle
The tendon of flexor carpi radialis (arrow) is in direct line with the tubercle which it crosses

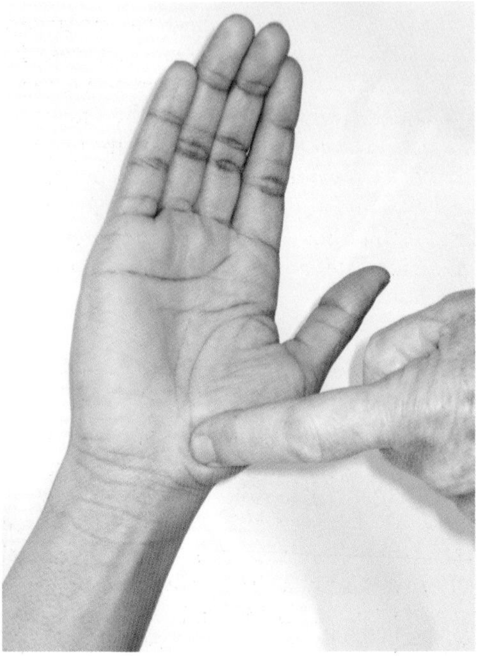

Fig. 6.11 Locating the tubercle (ridge) of the trapezium
Palpation is at the middle of the root of the thenar eminence, distal to and in line with the scaphoid

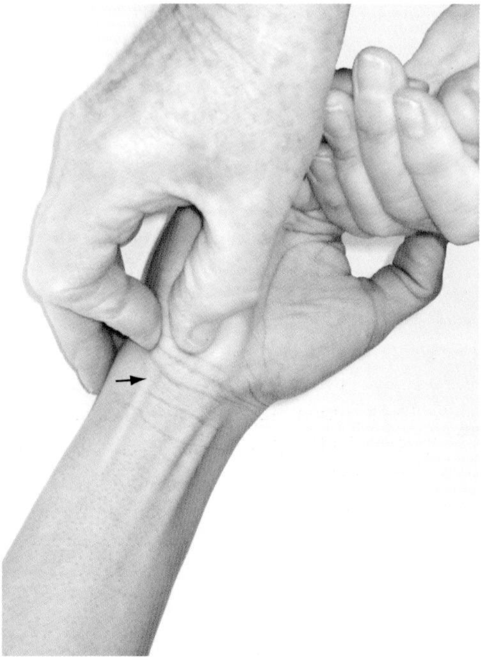

Fig. 6.12 Palpating the pisiform
The tendon of flexor carpi ulnaris (arrow) leads directly to the pisiform

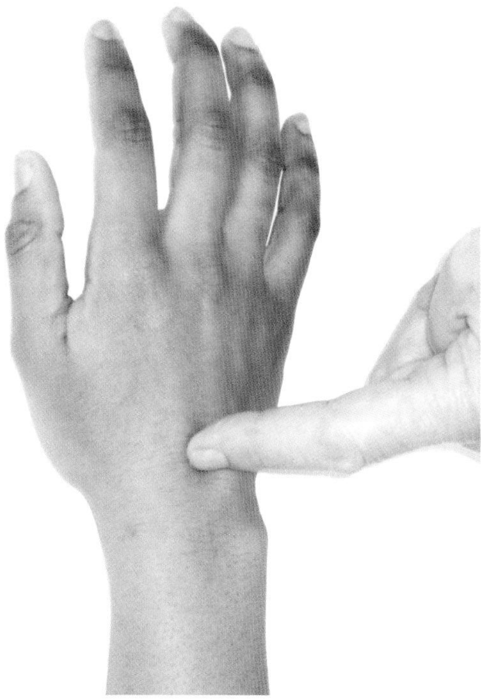

Fig. 6.13 Palpating the capitate and the base of the third metacarpal

## METACARPALS

The remaining skeleton in the hand and fingers is best examined from the dorsal aspect. The flattened dorsal surfaces of the **shafts** of the **metacarpals** can be palpated along their entire length with the thin extensor tendons overlying them. The **heads of metacarpals** 2–4 are easily palpated between finger and thumb, especially if the fingers are fully flexed to make a fist. If the hand is slightly flexed and palpation continued proximally along the shafts, the **bases** of the **second** and **third metacarpals** are located with the finger tip in the deep groove overlying them. Palpation in the groove immediately proximal to the base of the third metacarpal locates the **capitate** bone (Fig. 6.13). It is enhanced by slight dorsiflexion of the wrist.

## PHALANGES

The dorsum, sides of the shafts, and the heads of all the phalanges except the distal can be palpated using the tips of the index finger and thumb.

# LOCATING JOINT LINES

- Wrist
- First carpo-metacarpal
- Metacarpo-phalangeal
- Interphalangeal

## WRIST JOINT

The joint can be accessed from each side and dorsally, but is obscured ventrally by several layers of tendons. With the wrist relaxed, the examiner grips it firmly between fingers and thumb, using the pad of the thumb to palpate deeply in the "snuff box" to locate the tip of the styloid process, and then moving it dorsally to locate the groove between the edge of the radius and the scaphoid whilst at the same time flexing and extending the wrist. Continuing across the wrist, the groove marking the dorsum of the distal radio-ulnar joint can be felt and emphasized by making slight circumduction movements. The joint line medially is easily located by palpating the distal edge of the head of the ulna and then palmar-flexing the wrist to feel the groove between the ulna and the triquetrum, which can be emphasized by circumduction whilst palpating the groove.

## FIRST CARPO-METACARPAL JOINT

The saddle joint between the metacarpal and trapezium is one of the most important in the hand since much of the movement of opposition of the thumb occurs there.

The examiner feels for the base of the extended metacarpal in the "snuff box." Then, bringing the palpating pad of his or her thumb out of the box on to the ulnar side of the metacarpal base, the examiner feels for the groove marking the joint line (Fig. 6.14), which is confirmed by making circumduction movements with the thumb.

## METACARPO-PHALANGEAL (MCP) AND INTERPHALANGEAL (IP) JOINTS

These are accessible from dorsally. The examiner grips each side of the metatarsal head between finger and thumb in a precision grip and also locates the long extensor tendon as it crosses the **MCP joint.** Steadily flexing each joint, the finger reaches a critical point where the metacarpal head becomes conspicuous and separated by a distinct palpable groove from the base of the phalanx (Fig. 6.15). This is maximized on reaching full flexion. It is confirmed by palpating whilst alternating between flexion and extension. The **first MCP joint** in the thumb is particularly important. It can be palpated by deep pressure over the medial side of the base of the proximal phalanx in full thumb abduction, whilst alternating flexion and extension of the thumb in this position (Fig. 6.16).

To feel the joint line on **IP joints,** the finger is gripped between the examiner's thumb and middle finger at the level of the joint whilst the examiner uses the index finger tip to locate the base of the phalanx as the subject flexes and extends the distal free part of the finger (Fig. 6.17).

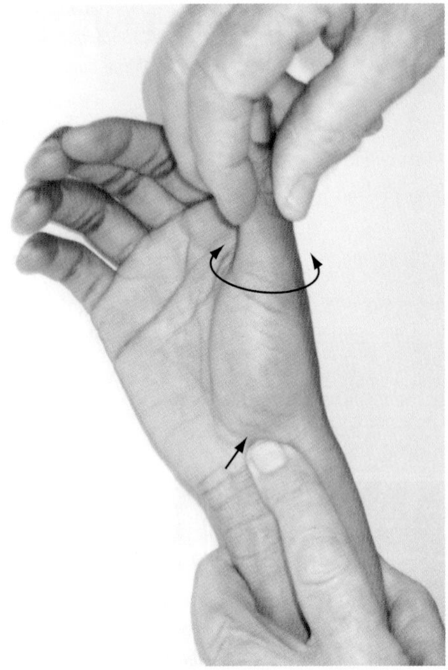

Fig. 6.14 Locating the line of the first carpo-metacarpal joint

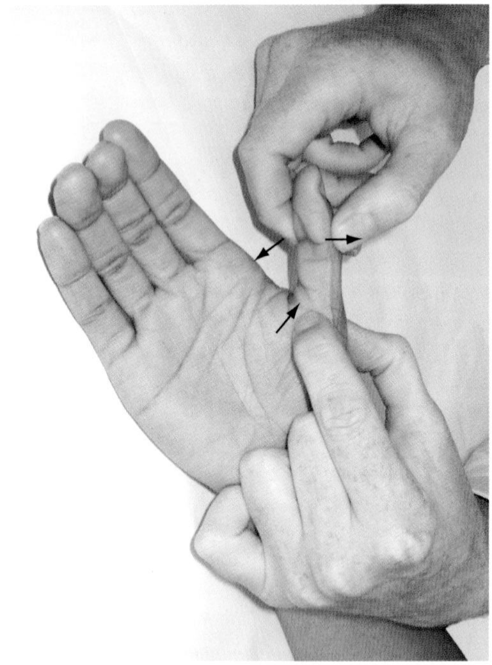

Fig. 6.16 Locating the first metacarpo-phalangeal joint. Palpation is made with the thumb abducted

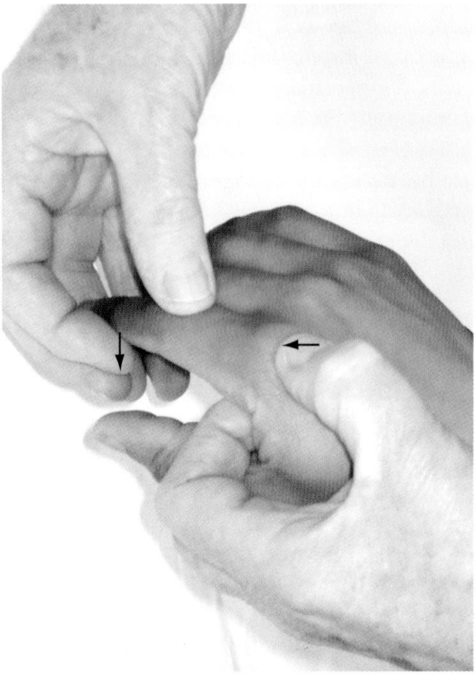

Fig. 6.15 Locating a metacarpo-phalangeal joint line

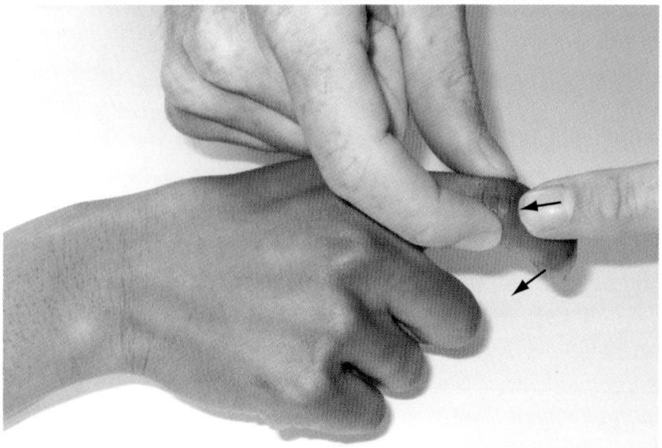

Fig. 6.17 Palpating an interphalangeal joint

# LOCATING SOFT TISSUES

- Tendons:
  Flexor carpi radialis
  Extensor carpi radialis longus and brevis
  Palmaris longus
  Extensor carpi ulnaris
  Flexor carpi ulnaris
  Extensor digitorum
  Flexor digitorum superficialis
  Extensor indicis
  Extensor digiti minimi
  Extensor pollicis longus and brevis
  Abductor pollicis longus
- Muscles:
  Thenar and hypothenar
  Interossei
- Nerves:
  Median, ulnar, radial
- Arteries:
  Radial and ulnar

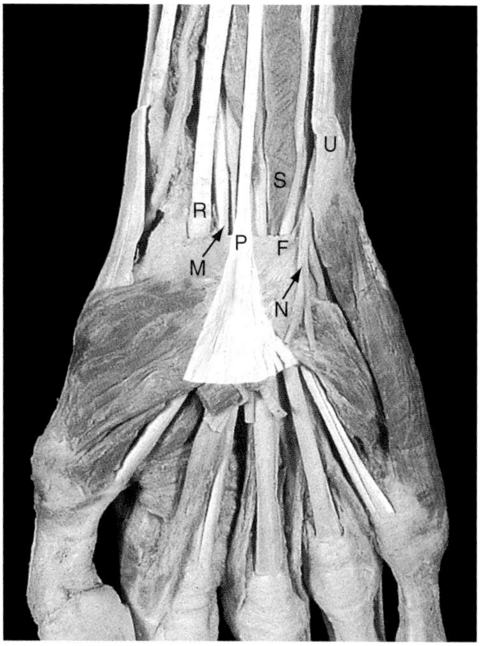


Fig. 6.18 Prosection showing flexor tendons and nerves at the wrist
F = flexor retinaculum, M = median nerve, N = ulnar nerve, P = palmaris longus attaching to palmar aponeurosis, R = flexor carpi radialis, S = flexor digitorum superficialis, U = flexor carpi ulnaris (From Gosling JA, Harris PF, Whitmore I, Willan PLT. 2002 Human Anatomy, 4th edn. London: Mosby)

## FLEXOR TENDONS AT THE WRIST

The tendons are shown in a prosection in Figure 6.18. The subject presents the supinated lower forearm, wrist and hand to the examiner, with the wrist partially flexed and fingers in the position of a power grip. The subject attempts to flex the wrist further against strong resistance applied to the hand and fingers by the examiner (Fig. 6.19).

### FLEXOR CARPI RADIALIS

The tendon is located about two-thirds of the distance along a line passing from the ulnar to the radial border of the wrist. Just beyond the distal skin crease of the wrist the tendon can be traced over the prominence of the scaphoid tubercle near the root of the thumb. Its palpation can be enhanced by moderate flexion and extension of the hand just proximal to the tubercle.

### PALMARIS LONGUS

This muscle lies midway between the radial and ulnar borders of the wrist. When present, it is easily felt and can be confirmed by repeated flexion and extension, whilst applying firm pressure over the distal skin crease.

### FLEXOR CARPI ULNARIS

The tendon lies along the ulnar border and is most easily palpated whilst resisting combined ulnar deviation of the wrist at the same time as flexion. It can be confirmed by tracing the tendon distally on to the firm pisiform bone.

### FLEXOR DIGITORUM SUPERFICIALIS

In the interval between the flexor carpi ulnaris and palmaris longus tendons there is a fullness, made more prominent by extending the wrist. This is due to the underlying tendons of flexor digitorum superficialis. Their presence is confirmed by firm palpation with the index and middle fingers over the fullness whilst the fingers are alternating between flexion and extension.

## EXTENSOR TENDONS AT THE WRIST

The tendons are shown in the prosection in Figure 6.20.

The subject rests the pronated forearm on a table, with the wrist in a neutral position and digits fully extended.

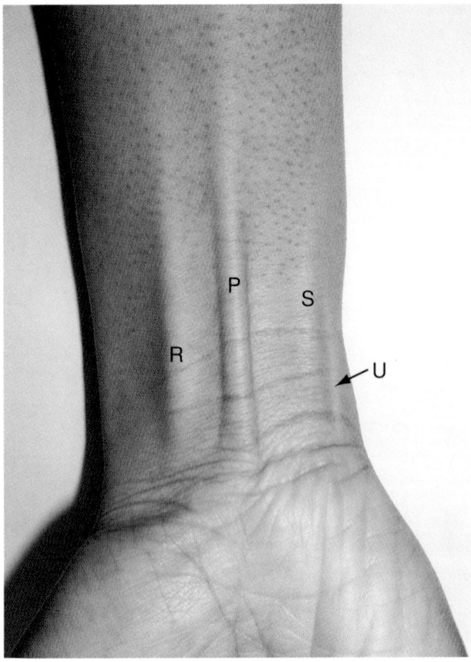


Fig. 6.19 Location of flexor tendons at the wrist
P = palmaris longus, R = flexor carpi radialis, S = flexor digitorum superficialis, U = flexor carpi ulnaris

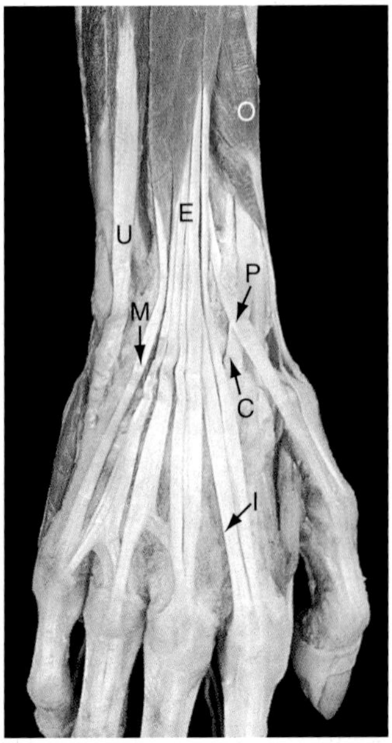


Fig. 6.20 Prosection showing extensor tendons at the wrist
C = extensor carpi radialis brevis, E = extensor digitorum, I = extensor indicis, M = extensor digiti minimi, O = outcropping muscles, P = extensor pollicis longus, U = extensor carpi ulnaris (From Gosling JA, Harris PF, Whitmore I, Willan PLT. 2002 Human Anatomy, 4th edn. London: Mosby)

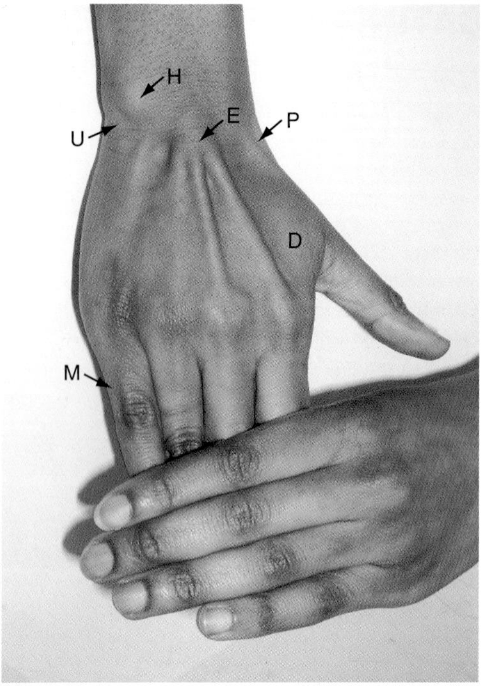


Fig. 6.21 Locating landmarks and extensor tendons at the wrist
D = first dorsal interosseous muscle, E = extensor digitorum (it has emerged from beneath the extensor retinaculum; the tendon to the middle finger crosses the metatarsal head), H = head of ulna, M = extensor digiti minimi, P = extensor pollicis longus, U = extensor carpi ulnaris

Placing the fingers of one hand across the dorsum of the fingers of the subject's hand, the examiner resists attempts to extend the hand at the wrist (Fig. 6.21). The procedure can be enhanced if there is already some dorsiflexion of the subject's hand before the examiner starts to resist it.

## EXTENSOR DIGITORUM (COMMUNIS)

The common tendon is located on the dorsum of the wrist, midway between the ulnar and radial borders. Below this point four tendons can be seen and easily felt as they diverge toward the roots of the fingers. Movement of the common tendon is confirmed by palpation whilst the fingers alternate between extension and flexion.

## EXTENSOR DIGITI MINIMI

The tendon is most easily palpated distal to the head of the ulna where it crosses the distal border of the triquetrum. Using the index finger tip, the examiner rolls it over the slender tendon whilst applying pressure in a radial direction. It is confirmed by alternating strong extension and flexion of the little finger. It should not be confused with the more robust flexor carpi ulnaris tendon.

### EXTENSOR CARPI ULNARIS

The tendon is readily palpable in a deep groove close to the ulnar border of the head of the ulna. It is most easily felt with the wrist in a neutral position whilst palpating on the ulnar border of the wrist immediately below the ulnar head, with the subject producing strong ulnar deviation of the hand at the same time. It can be traced to the base of the fifth metacarpal where it is attached.

### EXTENSOR INDICIS

This tendon is very difficult to define and cannot be detected at the wrist. It may be located on the dorsum of the hand over the shaft of the second metatarsal. Using the long extensor tendon as a guide, the index finger seeks to roll across the indicis tendon lying close by on its ulnar side and activated by extension of the index finger. The impression may be that of a duplicated long extensor tendon.

### EXTENSOR CARPI RADIALIS LONGUS AND BREVIS

With the forearm pronated and wrist in neutral position, the subject clenches the fingers. The examiner locates the base of the third metacarpal in a deep groove separating it from the capitate proximally using the tip of the index finger. The finger tip is then moved laterally toward the thumb and locates a prominent tendon passing to the base of the second metacarpal. This is the extensor carpi radialis longus. It becomes more prominent with further flexion of the wrist whilst maintaining a fist (Fig. 6.22). It also becomes prominent by resisting dorsiflexion of the clenched fist.

## LONG TENDONS OF THE THUMB

There are three tendons, one for each long bone in the thumb. They form the boundaries of the anatomical "snuff box" and are shown in the prosection in Figure 6.23.

The subject presents the hand and wrist in the mid-prone position, with the thumb fully extended. This can be resisted by the examiner applying pressure over the distal phalanx. The tendon of **extensor pollicis longus** is

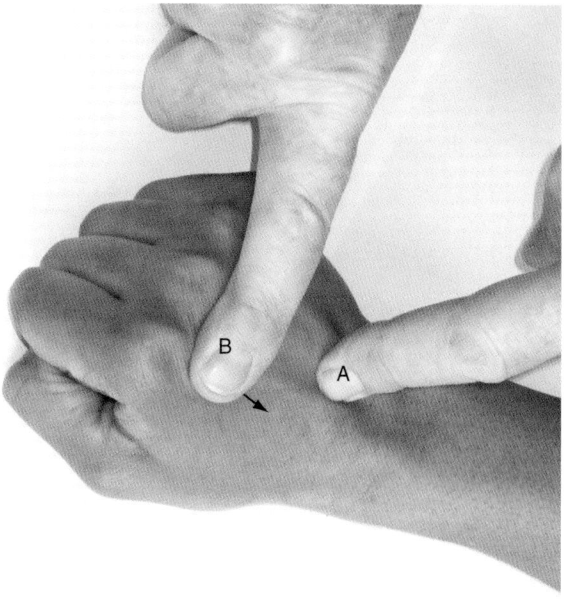


Fig. 6.22 Palpating the tendon of extensor carpi radialis longus
Finger A indicates the base of the third metacarpal. Finger B moves laterally and proximally, seeking the base of the second metacarpal

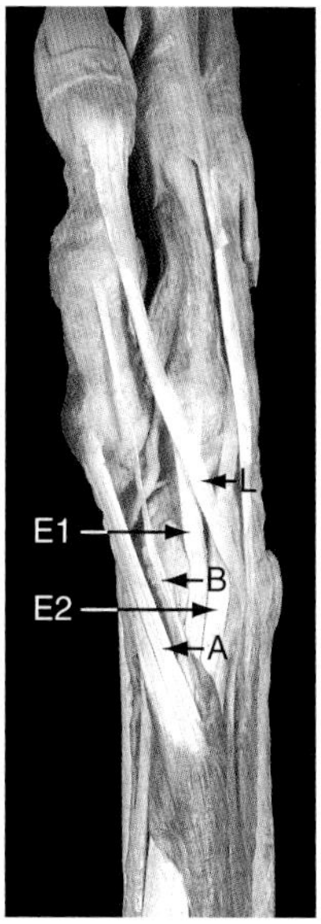


Fig. 6.23 Prosection showing the location of tendons associated with the "snuff box" and thumb
A = abductor pollicis longus, B = extensor pollicis brevis, L = extensor pollicis longus, E1 = extensor carpi radialis longus, E2 = extensor carpi radialis brevis (From Gosling JA, Harris PF, Whitmore I, Willan PLT. 2002 Human Anatomy, 4th edn. London: Mosby)

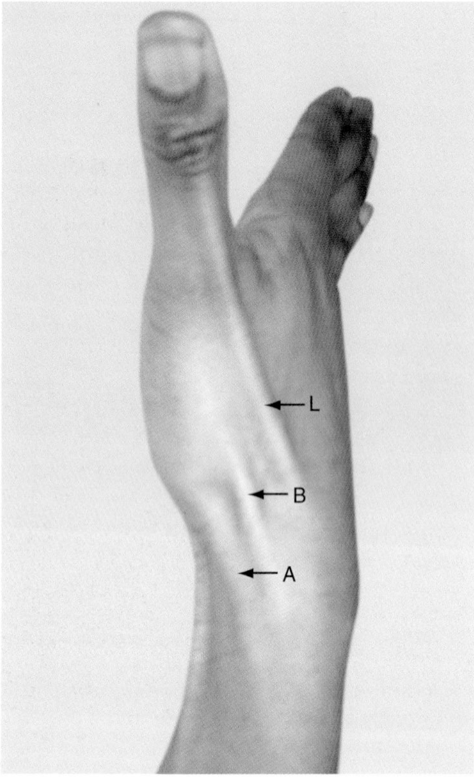


Fig. 6.24 Locating long tendons of the thumb
A = abductor pollicis longus, B = extensor pollicis brevis, L = extensor pollicis longus

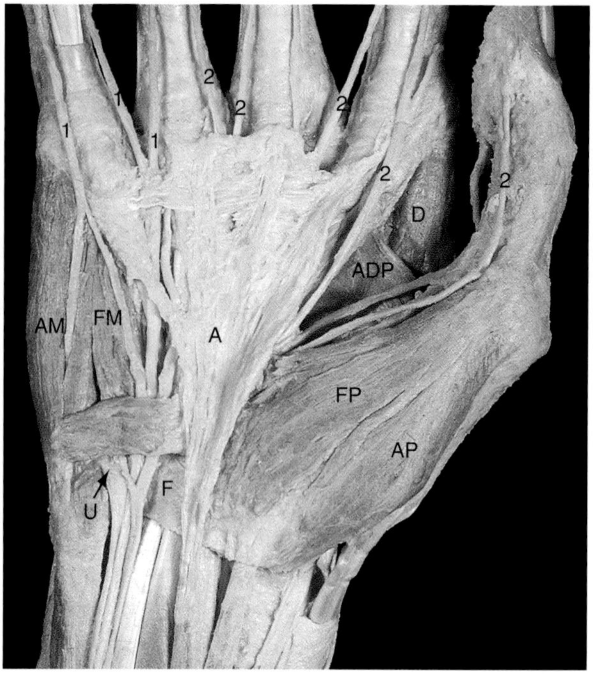


Fig. 6.25 Prosection showing some intrinsic hand muscles and digital nerves
A = palmar aponeurosis, ADP = adductor pollicis, AM = abductor digiti minimi, AP = abductor pollicis brevis, D = first dorsal interosseous, F = flexor retinaculum, FM = flexor digiti minimi, FP = flexor pollicis brevis, U = deep branch of ulnar nerve, 1 = digital branches of ulnar nerve, 2 = digital branches of median nerve (From Gosling JA, Harris PF, Whitmore I, Willan PLT. 2002 Human Anatomy, 4th edn. London: Mosby)

located where it winds round the dorsal radial tubercle and using the tips of the index, middle, and ring fingers traced along the ulnar side of the first metacarpal to its termination at the base of the distal phalanx.

Of the two tendons forming the opposite side of the "snuff box," that of **extensor pollicis brevis** can be easily traced from below the styloid process as far as the base of the proximal phalanx. The **abductor pollicis longus** tendon lies very close by and detailed palpation is required to distinguish them. If the thumb is increasingly abducted at the same time as extended, the distinction becomes clear, a cleft appearing between them as the abductor tendon is traced to its attachment at the base of the first metacarpal (Fig. 6.24).

## THENAR, HYPOTHENAR AND INTEROSSEOUS MUSCLES

A prosection of some of the intrinsic muscles of the hand is shown in Figure 6.25.

Three **thenar** muscles form the thenar eminence. If deep palpation is used on the ulnar side of the distal part of the shaft of the first metacarpal, the short flexor and abductor muscles can be felt to contract when the movements they produce are resisted by pressure over the terminal phalanx. The deepest muscle, the opponens, is palpable at the root of the thenar eminence as the thumb is rotated medially into the palm. The **hypothenar** muscles are smaller and difficult to define. The abductor digiti minimi can be felt contracting on the ulnar border of the hand when resistance is applied as the little finger is abducted. Only the **dorsal interossei** can be located. With the palm facing downward and fingers extended, the examiner uses the tips of the index and middle fingers to palpate in the spaces between the shafts of the metacarpals. The subject is instructed to alternate abduction and adduction of the digits, during which the interossei can be felt to tense and relax. The first dorsal interosseous muscle is particularly prominent.

## MEDIAN, ULNAR, AND RADIAL NERVES

### LOCATION

The **median** nerve is a large nerve. Although impalpable, at the wrist it is very superficial and lies midway between the radial and ulnar borders, immediately deep to the tendon of the palmaris longus. The **ulnar** nerve is also impalpable but is located at the wrist passing lateral to the pisiform and medial to the hook of the hamate. It is deep, but marked pressure with the pad of the thumb lateral to the pisiform may produce pain along the medial side of the palm extending into the little finger. The **radial** nerve at the wrist is very superficial, and at the "snuff box" branches may be palpated by rolling them over the tendon of the extensor pollicis longus as they pass toward the dorsum of the hand.

### MOTOR FUNCTIONS

The ulnar nerve is the major motor nerve, supplying all the intrinsic muscles except the three thenar muscles and the first lumbrical, which are supplied by the median nerve. However, commonly, the opponens pollicis has a dual innervation, with an additional supply from the ulnar nerve. The ulnar nerve is best assessed by asking the subject to adduct and abduct the extended fingers, and the median by opposing the thumb (see "Testing movements"). The radial nerve has no intrinsic motor distribution in the hand, but more proximal damage in the limb can affect the long extensors of the wrist and digits, resulting in wrist drop with impairment of power grip.

### SENSORY CUTANEOUS DISTRIBUTION

This is illustrated in Figure 6.26. The median nerve has the major sensory distribution. On the flexor surface it supplies the lateral $3\frac{1}{2}$ digits and an equivalent area on the palm. Since the palmar branch enters the palm superficial to the retinaculum, sensory disturbances here do not occur with carpal tunnel compression. The remaining $1\frac{1}{2}$ digits and an equivalent area in the palm are supplied by the ulnar nerve. Since the ring finger has a dual nerve supply it should be avoided when testing for sensory disturbance. A small area over the radial border of the thenar eminence is supplied by the radial nerve. Most of the extensor surface is supplied by the radial nerve, except for the nail beds of the lateral $3\frac{1}{2}$ digits which are innervated by the median nerve, and the whole of the medial $1\frac{1}{2}$ digits and equivalent area on the dorsum of the hand which are supplied by the ulnar nerve.

## RADIAL AND ULNAR ARTERIES

**Radial artery** pulsations at the wrist can be easily detected in three locations. With the forearm supinated, the pulse is conventionally taken by compressing the artery with the examiner's finger tip against the expanded distal ventral surface of the radius. It can be followed into the "snuff box," where it is also palpable. Finally, the artery having emerged from the "snuff box" on to the dorsum of the hand, pulsations can be detected proximally in the first intermetacarpal space, where it passes deeply into the palm between the two heads of the first dorsal interosseous muscle. The **ulnar artery** accompanies the ulnar nerve at the wrist, passing from under the flexor carpi ulnaris tendon to lie lateral to the pisiform bone. Exceptionally, pulsations can be felt as the artery emerges from beneath the tendon.

# MOVEMENTS OF THE WRIST, HAND, AND DIGITS

- Wrist and carpus:
  Pronation and supination
  Flexion and extension
  Abduction and adduction
- Thumb:
  Abduction and adduction
  Flexion and extension
  Circumduction
- Fingers:
  Flexion and extension; power grip
  Adduction and abduction; card test

All movements are first tested passively, and then actively against resistance.

## WRIST AND CARPUS

The subject is seated, with the pronated forearm placed on a flat table and the wrist relaxed. Three groups of joints, all synovial, are tested: the wrist joint itself, the distal radio-ulnar, and the mid-carpal. The ellipsoid wrist joint, in particular, allows multi-axial movements. Supination and pronation occur mainly at the distal radio-ulnar joint, although 20–25° can occur at the mid-carpal joint. Other movements of the wrist are not confined to the wrist joint itself, but represent a combination of those at the mid-carpal and wrist joints.

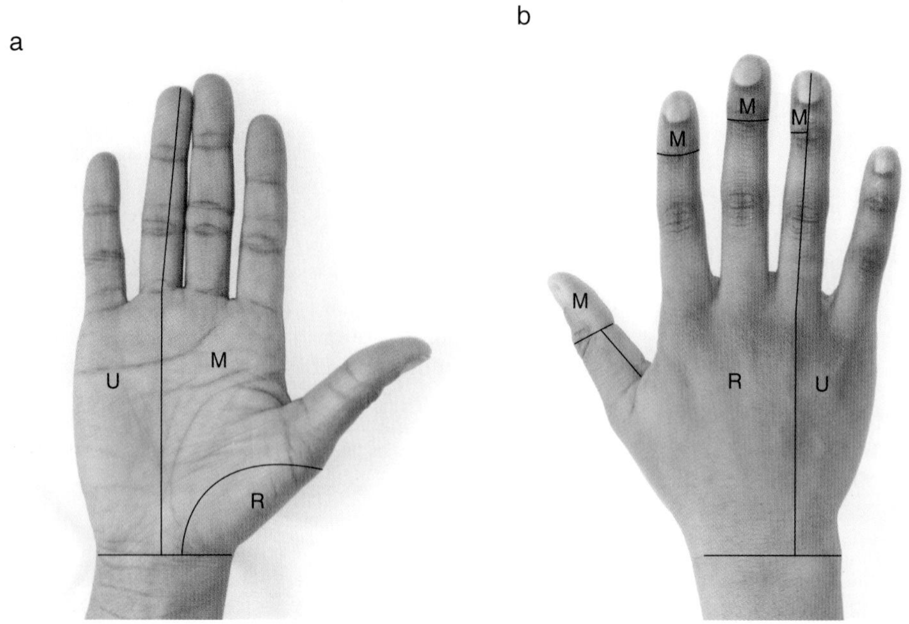


**Fig. 6.26a and b** Sensory nerve distribution on ventral and dorsal surfaces of the hand and fingers
M = median nerve, U = ulnar nerve, R = radial nerve. Note dual supply to ring finger

The range of flexion (palmar flexion) is up to **80°** and extension (dorsiflexion) is **70°** (Fig. 6.27a). Abduction (radial deviation) can reach **20°** and adduction (ulnar deviation) **30°** (Fig. 6.27b).

## PRONATION/SUPINATION

The examiner clasps the subject's extended hand between his or her own two flattened hands applied over the dorsal and ventral surfaces of the subject's hand. Starting with the hand in the neutral mid-supine position, the examiner turns it through 90° so that the palm faces downward on the table. This is repeated in the reverse direction, the hand being turned through 90° so that the dorsum lies flat on the table (Fig. 6.28).

## FLEXION/EXTENSION

The subject's hand is gripped by the examiner's fingers on the dorsum and thumb in the palm, and bent backward into full extension (Fig. 6.29a). Then, with the under-surface of the wrist supported just beneath the joint line by the examiner's extended index finger, the subject's hand is allowed to overhang the finger and assume a flexed position (Fig. 6.29b). Flexion is increased by the examiner exerting pressure over the dorsum of the hand (Fig. 6.29c). It can be seen that palmar flexion appears greater than extension. This is due to the more major contribution of the mid-carpal joint to flexion, whereas the radio-carpal joint has the major role in extension.

## ABDUCTION/ADDUCTION (RADIAL/ULNAR DEVIATION)

With the wrist in neutral position and palm facing downward, the examiner steadies the ulnar border of the subject's forearm between his or her own index finger and thumb. Then, using the other hand, the examiner grips the subject's hand across the dorsum of the metacarpals or fingers and applies traction to pull the hand medially (adduction) (Fig. 6.30a) and then laterally (abduction) (Fig. 6.30b). Of the two movements, it can be seen that adduction is the larger, with most of it occurring at the radio-carpal joint, whereas abduction is more limited and almost all occurs at the mid-carpal joint.

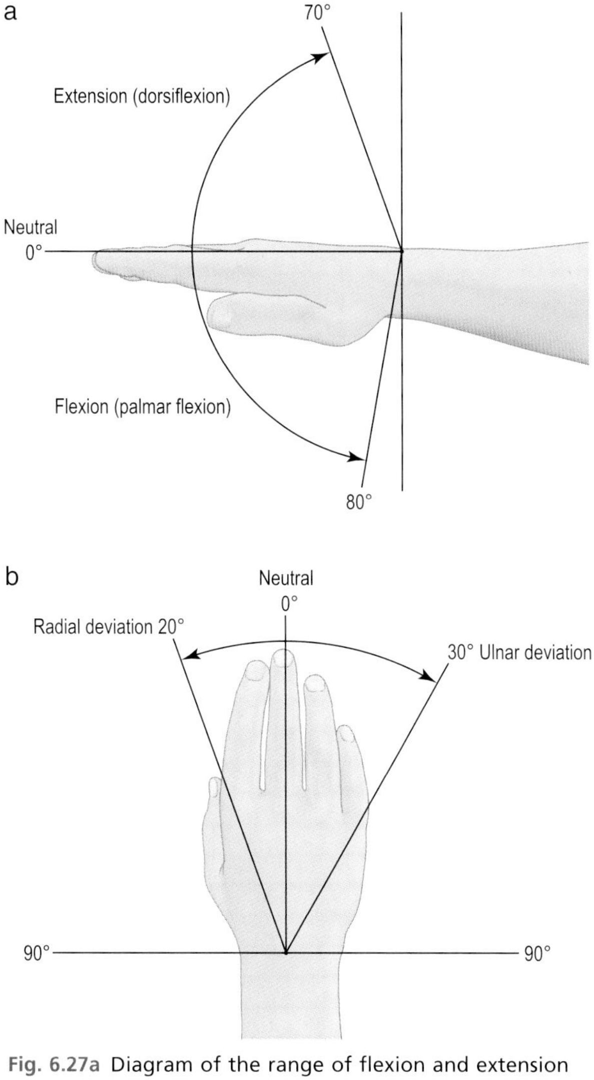


Fig. 6.27a Diagram of the range of flexion and extension at the wrist
Fig. 6.27b Diagram of the range of ulnar deviation (adduction) and radial deviation (abduction) at the wrist
Redrawn from *Joint motion: method of measuring and recording.* Edinburgh: E&S Livingstone, 1965 (with the permission of the American Academy of Orthopedic Surgeons, reprinted with their permission by the British Orthopaedic Association)

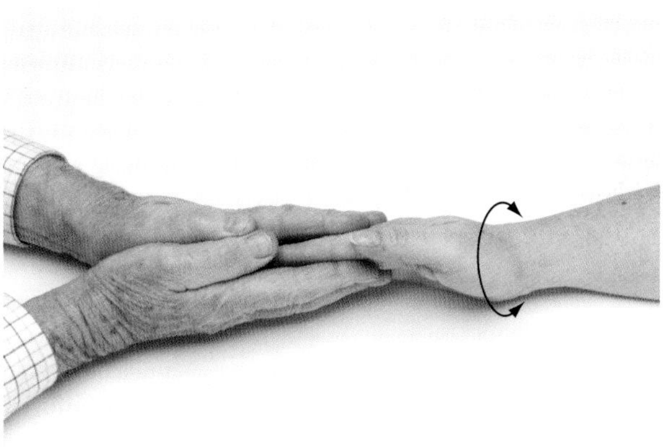

Fig. 6.28 Testing the range of supination and pronation
The subject's hand is in neutral position

## THUMB AND FINGERS

### THUMB

The various movements are shown in Figure 6.31. The subject faces the examiner, with the palm of the hand upward. The thumb is kept straight and is **abducted** by moving it outward (in a plane at right angles) away from the palm and then returned inward in the reverse direction, to lie against the palm and root of the index finger **(adduction).** Then, keeping the thumb against the palm, the subject **flexes** it by bending it toward the ulnar border of the hand and **extends** it by reversing the movement to straighten it. To test movement at the first carpometacarpal joint, passive **circumduction** can be performed by the examiner gripping the terminal segment of the thumb and moving it round in a circular manner. The subject is also asked to perform **opposition** by pressing the pad of the thumb in sequence firmly against the pads of the index, middle, ring, and little finger (Fig. 6.31e).

### FINGERS

The arrangement of the long tendons is shown in the prosections in Figure 6.32. The subject faces the examiner, with palm of the hand outstretched. **Flexion** is tested by asking the subject to make a **power grip,** and **extension** by straightening out the fingers from the position of the power grip (Fig. 6.33a and b). The strength of these movements can also be assessed by the examiner actively resisting attempts to flex and extend individual fingers (Fig. 6.33c).

The **card test** assesses movement at the MP joint produced by the interosseous muscles, and also tests their innervation by the deep branch of the ulnar nerve. To test **adduction,** the subject extends and spreads the fingers apart whilst the examiner introduces a small piece of card or slip of paper between two adjacent fingers, the subject

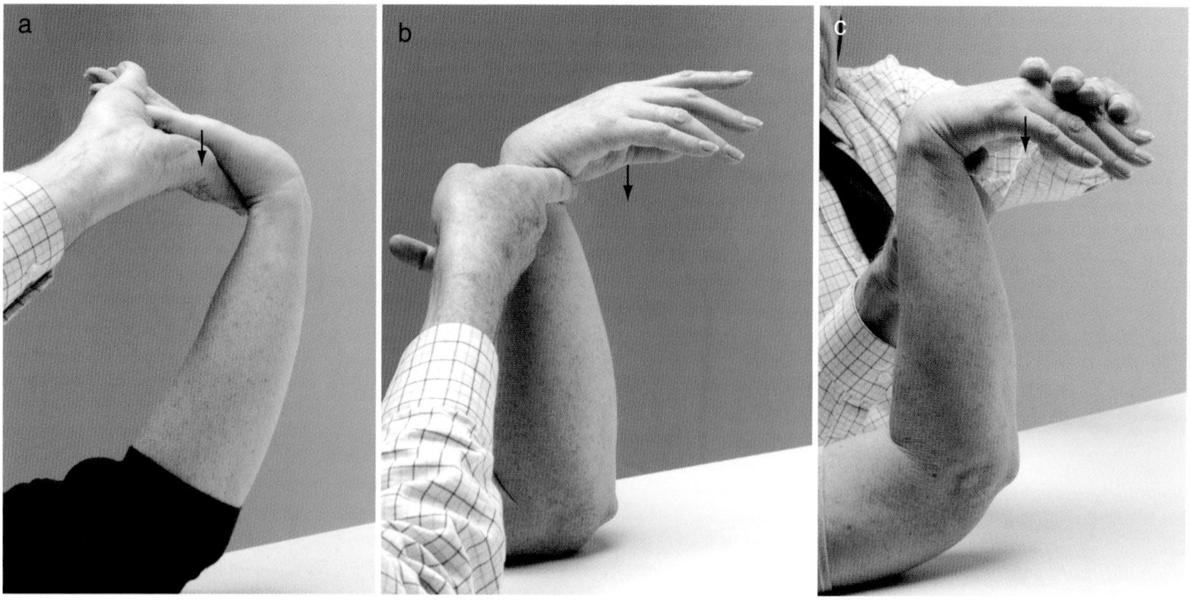


**Fig. 6.29a** Testing the range of extension at the wrist
Most of the movement occurs at the wrist joint
**Fig. 6.29b and c** Testing the range of flexion at the wrist
Appropriate pressure may be applied **(c)**. The mid-carpal joint makes an important contribution to flexion

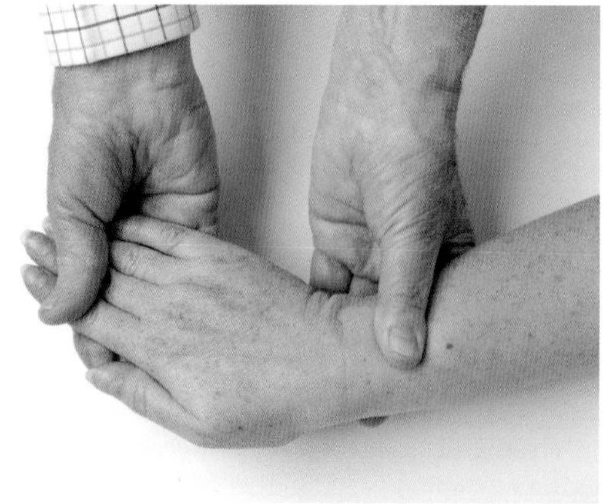

**Fig. 6.30a** Testing the range of adduction (ulnar deviation) at the wrist

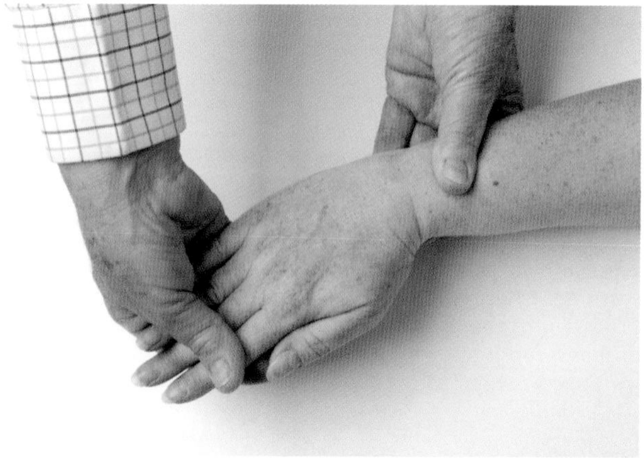

**Fig. 6.30b** Testing the range of abduction (radial deviation) at the wrist

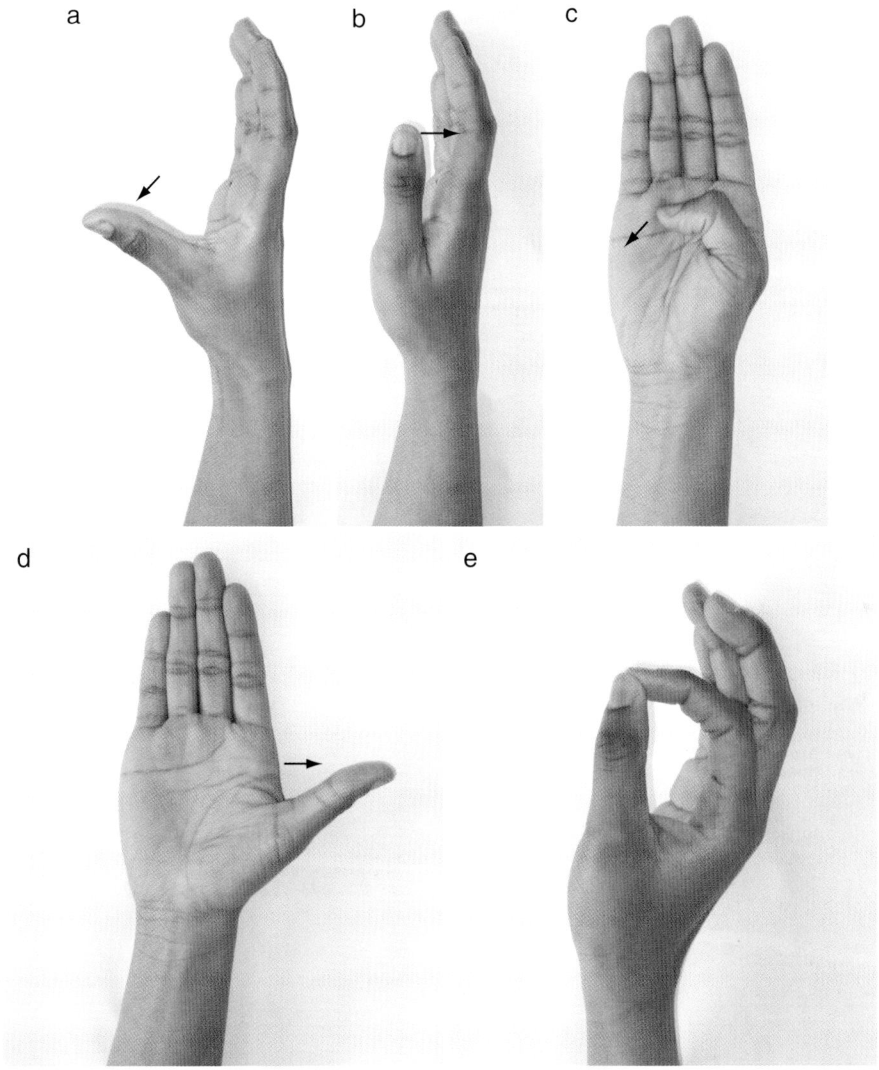


Figs. 6.31a–e Movements of the thumb
**a** Abduction. **b** Adduction. **c** Flexion. **d** Extension. **e** Precision ("pinch") grip

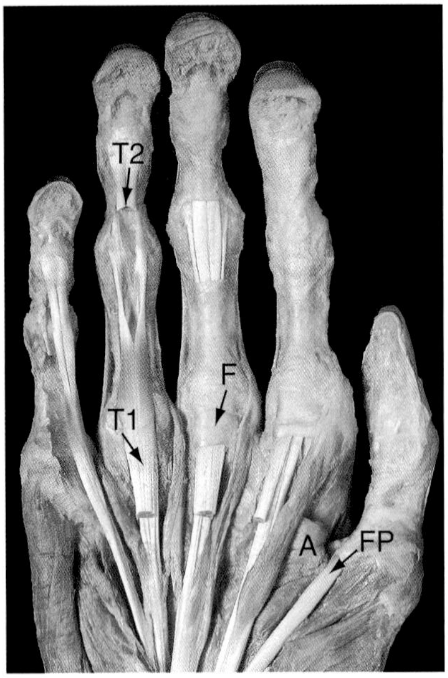


Fig. 6.32a Prosection showing the long flexor tendons of fingers and thumb
A = adductor pollicis, F = fibrous flexor sheath (pulley), FP = flexor pollicis longus tendon, T1 = flexor digitorum superficialis tendon attaching to sides of middle phalanx, T2 = flexor digitorum profundus tendon attaching to base of terminal phalanx (From Gosling JA, Harris PF, Whitmore I, Willan PLT. 2002 Human Anatomy, 4th edn. London: Mosby)

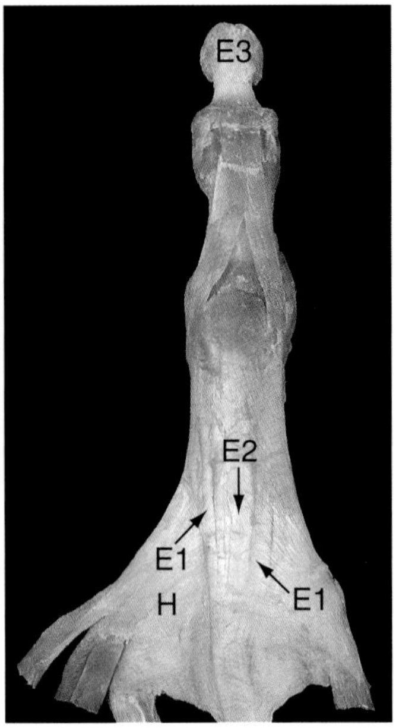


Fig. 6.32b Prosection showing attachments of the long extensor tendon in the finger
E1 = lateral slips converging distally to insert (E3) on to the base of the terminal phalanx, E2 = middle slip inserts on to the base of the middle phalanx, H = extensor hood covering metacarpal head (From Gosling JA, Harris PF, Whitmore I, Willan PLT. 2002 Human Anatomy, 4th edn. London: Mosby)

then being asked to close the fingers tightly together to prevent the examiner withdrawing it (Fig. 6.34a). To test **abduction,** the subject presents the dorsum of the hand to the examiner with extended fingers held firmly together. The examiner uses his or her own hands to press against the ulnar and radial borders of opposed adjacent fingers, resisting attempts to spread them apart (Fig. 6.34b).

## DERMATOMES OF THE UPPER LIMB

The dermatome arrangement in the upper limb is shown in Figure 6.35. The cord segments involved are C4–T1. There is an orderly numerical progression from C4 down the pre-axial border to the thumb, and then up the post-axial border to the axilla, ending at T1. Note that the C7 segment is confined to the hand and middle fingers.

## SPECIAL TESTS

- Grip strength
- Luno-triquetral instability
- Scaphoid fracture
- Wrist joint synovitis
- Extensor tendon tenosynovitis
- Scaphoid-lunate instability
- Distal radio-ulnar joint (DRUJ) instability
- Finkelstein's test
- Phalen's test
- Stress test for collateral ligaments: first MCP, PIP, DIP joints
- Tendon tears: long flexors and extensors

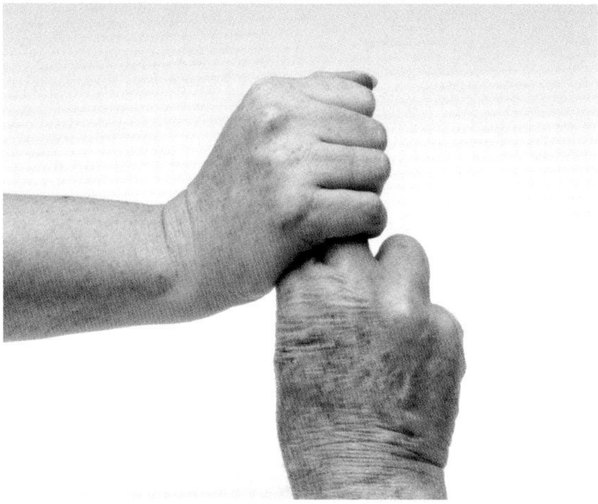

Fig. 6.33a Testing flexion power of the fingers with the power grip
Note some dorsiflexion at subject's wrist

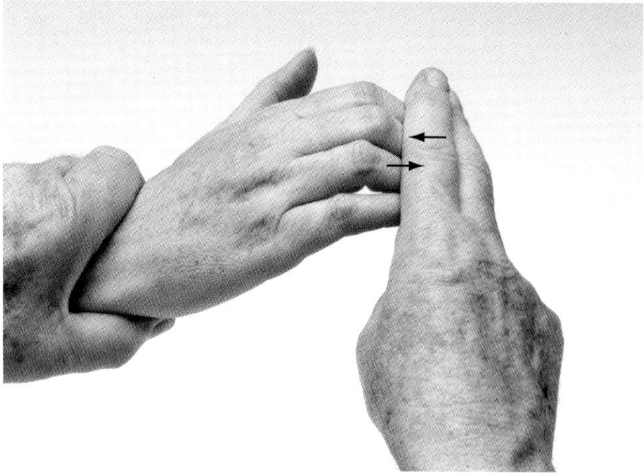

Fig. 6.33b Testing extension power of the fingers

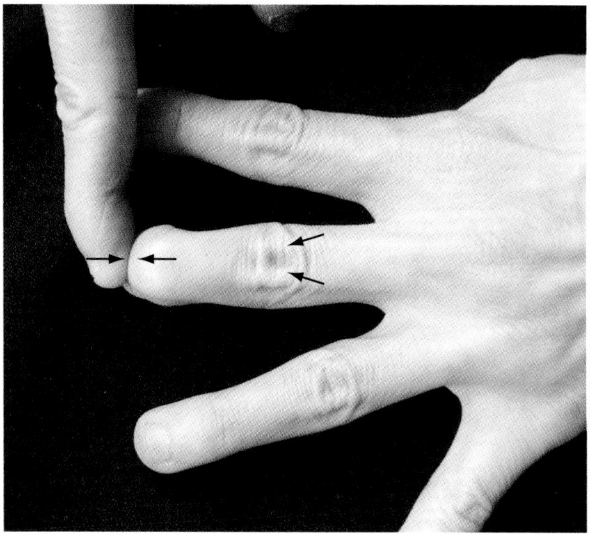

Fig. 6.33c Testing a long extensor finger tendon
The two tendon slips (small arrows) are clearly visible. Compare with Figure 6.32b

## GRIP STRENGTH

Since wrist and carpal injuries may affect grip, it is important to test the **power grip** if wrist or carpal disturbances are suspected. Using his or her own hand and with the fingers held closely together, the examiner presents the extended middle and index fingers to the subject, who is asked to grip the fingers tightly, the subject's wrist being slightly dorsiflexed to maximize the power grip. Power can be assessed by the examiner seeing how much force is needed to withdraw the fingers from the subject's grip (Fig. 6.33a).

## LUNO-TRIQUETRAL INSTABILITY

The subject's forearm and hand are positioned in pronation (palm facing down). The examiner fixes the lunate by gripping it between thumb and index finger, thus locking the wrist (Fig. 6.36). The pisiform and tubercle of the triquetrum are gripped between the other index finger and thumb, and ballotted in an anterior and posterior direction. Excessive mobility may indicate luno-triquetral instability.

## SCAPHOID FRACTURE

The wrist is placed in ulnar deviation and slight flexion. The waist of the scaphoid is palpated in the anatomical "snuff box" formed by the extensor pollicis longus and extensor pollicis brevis tendons over the dorso-radial wrist (Fig. 6.37). Acute tenderness may indicate scaphoid fracture.

## SYNOVITIS OF THE WRIST JOINT

### FINGER EXTENSION TEST

The subject rests the elbow on the table with the forearm vertical. The wrist and MCP joints are held in flexion. The

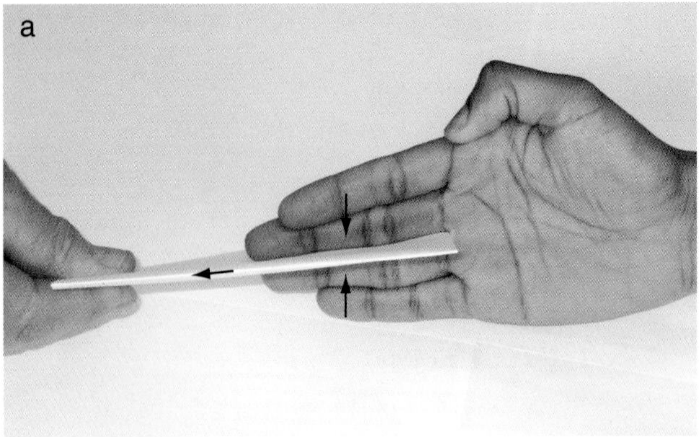


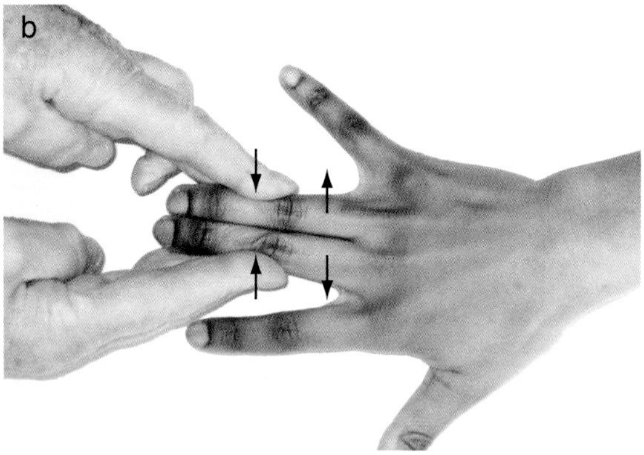


Fig. 6.34a and b Testing palmar and dorsal interossei muscles
The palmar adduct and the dorsal abduct the fingers

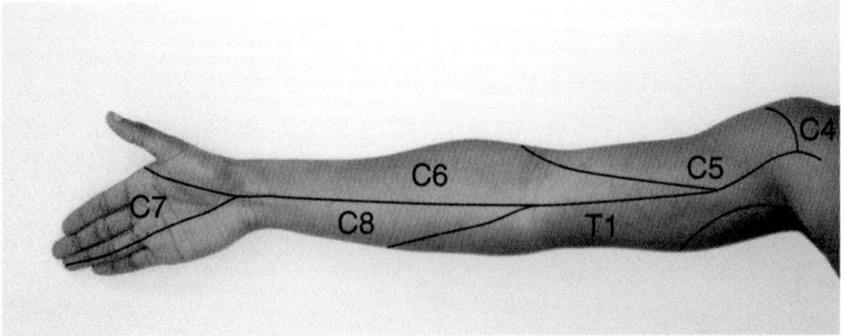


Fig. 6.35 Dermatome distribution in the upper limb

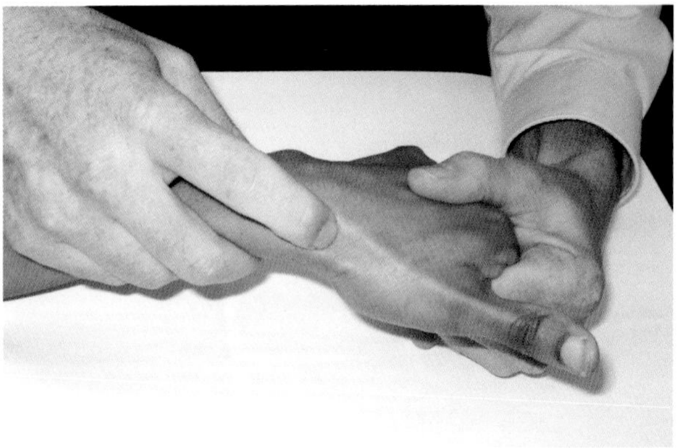

Fig. 6.37 Testing for scaphoid fracture by palpating in the anatomical "snuff box"

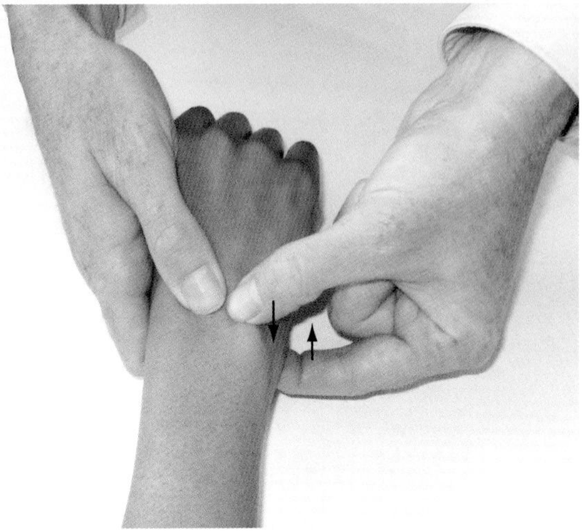

Fig. 6.36 Testing for luno-triquetral instability

examiner resists active extension of the fingers with his or her own fingers over the dorsum of the subject's proximal phalanges (Fig. 6.38). This is a sensitive but non-specific test for synovitis of the wrist/carpal articulations.

## EXTENSOR TENDON TENOSYNOVITIS

With the subject's palm facing downward and the wrist in neutral position, the examiner grips the wrist so that his or her own fingers lie across the dorsum. The subject repeats active full-range wrist flexion and extension whilst the examiner feels for crepitation in the extensor tendons (Fig. 6.39), which may indicate tenosynovitis.

## SCAPHOID-LUNATE INSTABILITY

### WATSON'S TEST

The subject rests the elbow on the table with the forearm vertical. For this test, the wrist and fingers are initially in a neutral position. The examiner supports the dorsum of the wrist with his or her own fingers, whilst palpating the (palmar) tubercle of the scaphoid with the thumb (Fig. 6.40). The examiner moves the wrist from ulnar deviation to radial deviation applying a dorsally directed force on the scaphoid with his or her own thumb. If the scapholunate joint is stable, the scaphoid will be felt to push in a palmar direction under the examiner's thumb as the wrist is moved into radial deviation. Scapho-lunate instability is suspected if the scaphoid is displaced dorsally in radial deviation, or suddenly "pops" into its normal position with this maneuver.

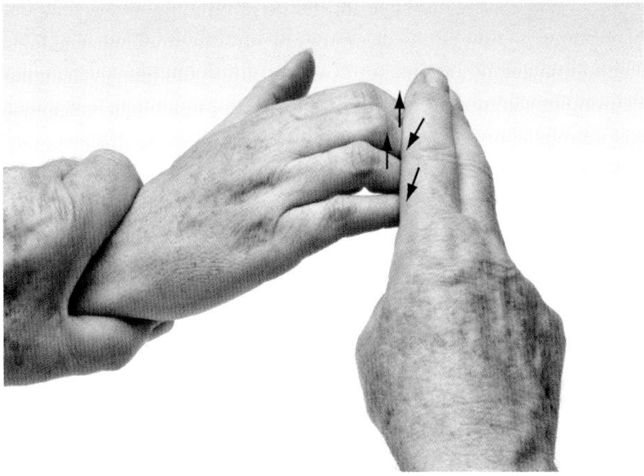

Fig. 6.38 Finger extension test for synovitis of wrist joint

## INSTABILITY OF THE DISTAL RADIO-ULNAR JOINT (DRUJ) DUE TO TEAR OF THE TRIANGULAR FIBRO-CARTILAGE COMPLEX (TFCC)

### DRUJ BALLOTTEMENT

The subject sits with the upper arm supported on a table with the forearm vertical. The examiner holds the patient's hand and wrist in ulnar deviation, and with the thumb and forefinger of the other hand, performs an antero-posterior glide of the distal ulna (Fig. 6.41). The same maneuver is performed with the hand and wrist in radial deviation. If the TFCC is intact, there should be considerably less antero-posterior play in the DRUJ when tested in radial deviation.

## DE QUERVAIN'S SYNDROME

This is stenosing tenosynovitis of the tendon sheath of extensor pollicis brevis and abductor pollicis longus as they approach the thumb.

### FINKELSTEIN'S TEST

The subject makes a modified fist with the thumb placed in the palm of the hand and the fingers flexed over it, or alternatively, with fingers extended, the flexed thumb is

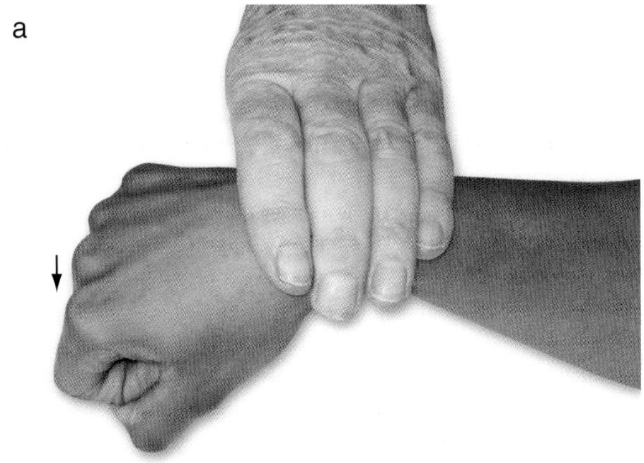


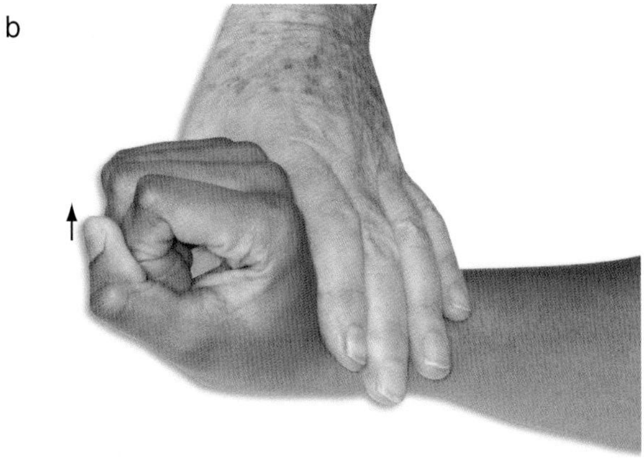


Fig. 6.39a and b Testing for extensor tendon tenosynovitis

a

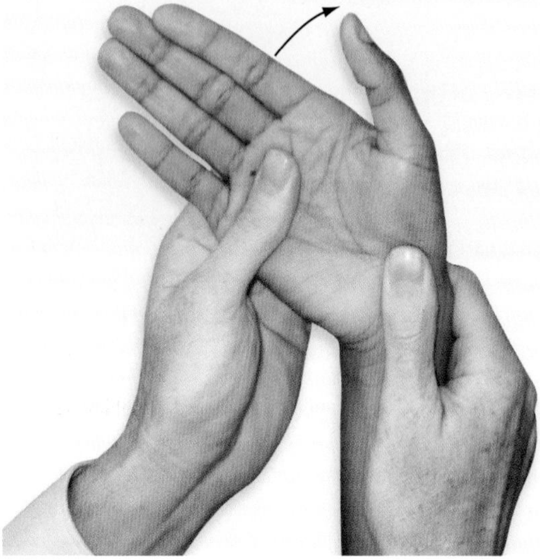

b

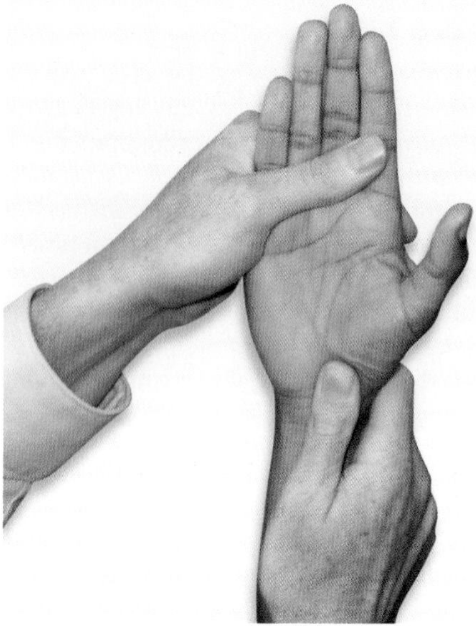

**Fig. 6.40a and b** Watson's test for scaphoid-lunate instability

a

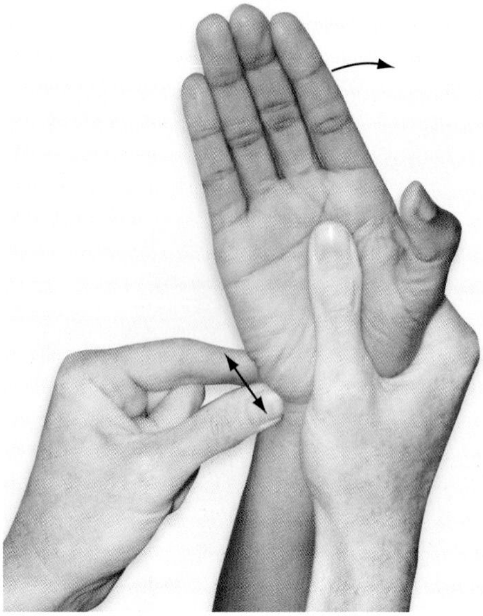

b

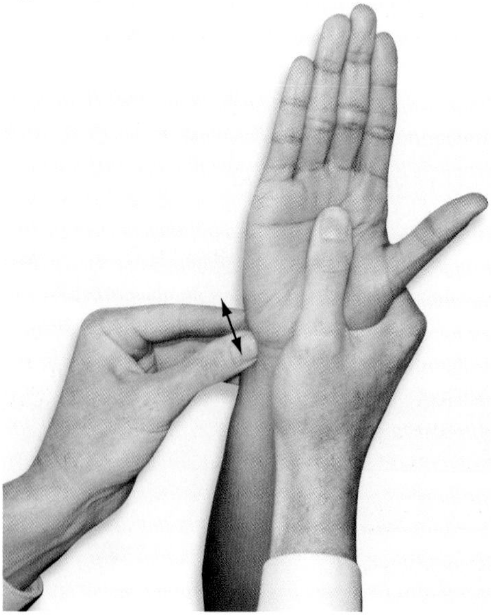

**Fig. 6.41a and b** Ballottement test for distal radio-ulnar instability

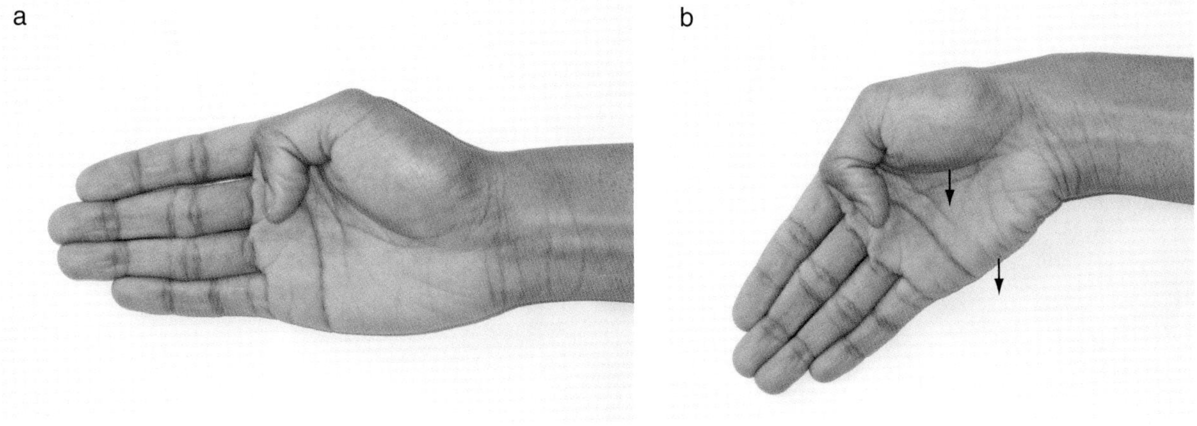

Fig. 6.42a and b Finkelstein's test for stenosing tenosynovitis of extensor pollicis brevis and abductor pollicis longus

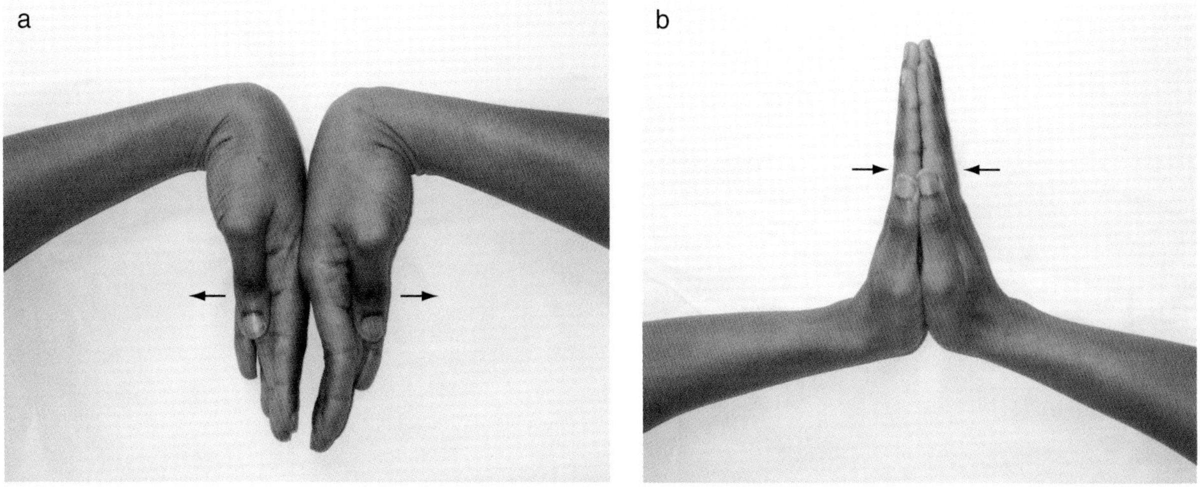

Fig. 6.43a and b Phalen's test for carpal tunnel compression

placed across the palm; with the thumb in position, the hand is then actively ulnar-deviated (Fig. 6.42). If positive, this maneuver causes pain at the base of the thumb.

## CARPAL TUNNEL SYNDROME

**PHALEN'S TEST** (Fig. 6.43)

The subject puts both hands into extreme palmar flexion and then strongly opposes the dorsum of each hand; conversely, the subject brings the palms face together in extreme dorsiflexion, as in praying, and strongly opposes them. The position is maintained for at least 30 seconds. Numbness in the area of distribution of the median nerve indicates tunnel compression.

## STRESS TEST OF THE ULNAR COLLATERAL LIGAMENT OF THE FIRST MCP JOINT

The examiner uses the thumb and forefinger of each hand to grip the proximal phalanx and the metacarpal either side of the first MCP joint respectively. To test the true ulnar collateral ligament, the MCP joint is flexed and a gapping force applied to the ulnar side of the joint (Fig. 6.44). Performing this test with the MCP joint in

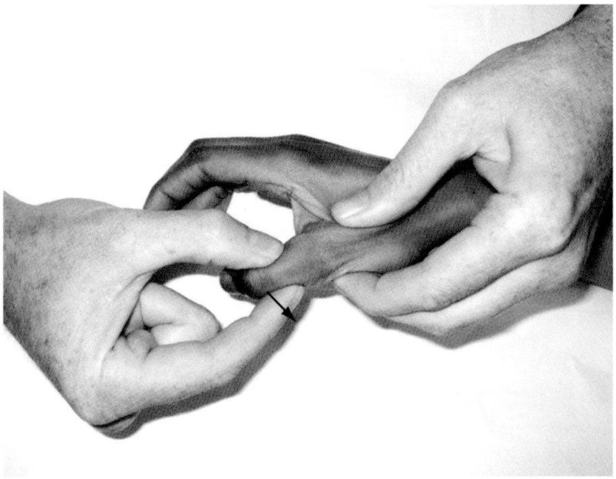

Fig. 6.44 Stress test of the ulnar collateral ligament of the first MCP joint

extension tests the stability of the accessory ulnar collateral ligament. Instability and pain indicate disruption of the ligament.

## STRESS TEST OF THE ULNAR AND RADIAL COLLATERAL LIGAMENTS OF THE PROXIMAL (PIP) AND DISTAL (DIP) INTERPHALANGEAL JOINTS

The collateral ligaments of the IP joints are frequently sprained during sporting activities, especially those involving catching a ball. Damage to the volar plate of the IP joints often occurs in conjunction with IP joint collateral ligament sprains. The integrity of the IP joint collateral ligaments is assessed by the examiner gripping the lateral aspect of the phalanges either side of the joint to be tested (PIP or DIP), with the thumb and forefinger of each hand (Fig. 6.45). A gapping force is then applied to the ulnar

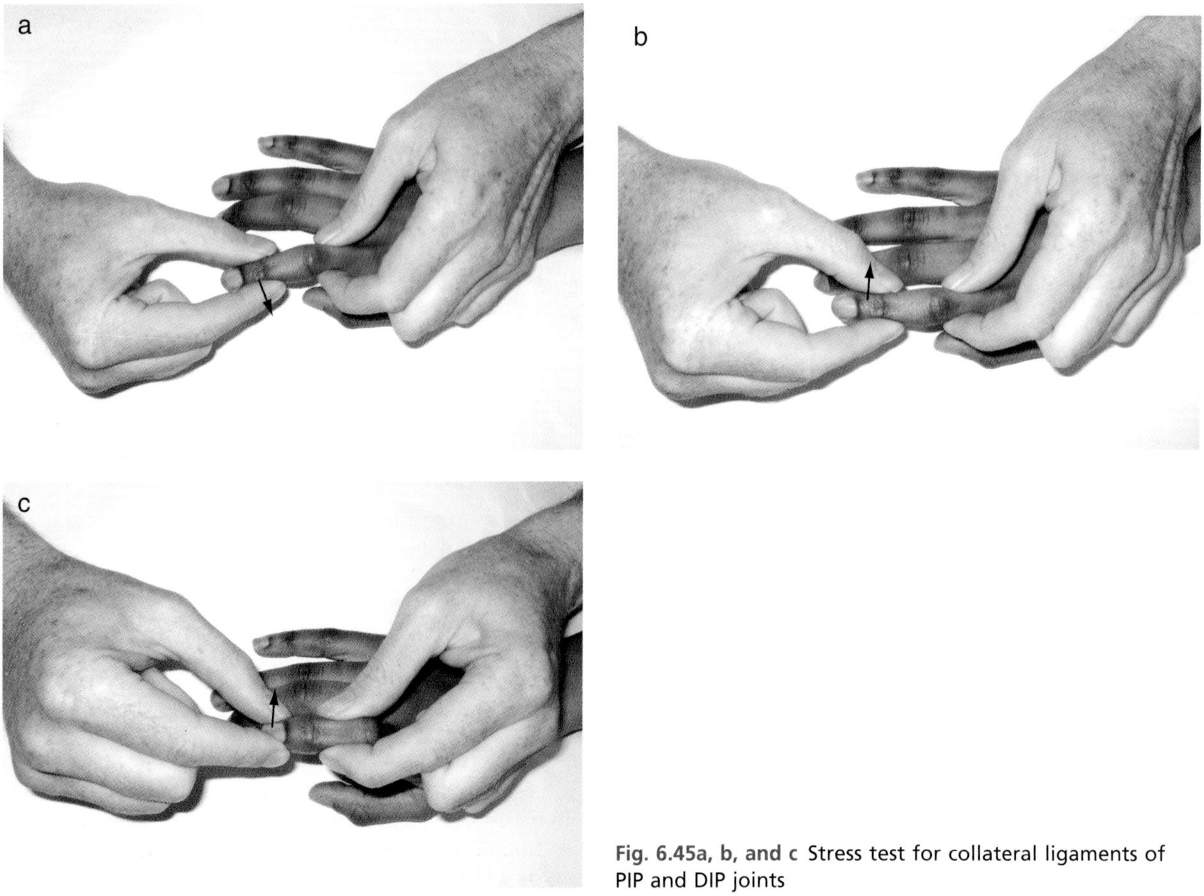

Fig. 6.45a, b, and c Stress test for collateral ligaments of PIP and DIP joints

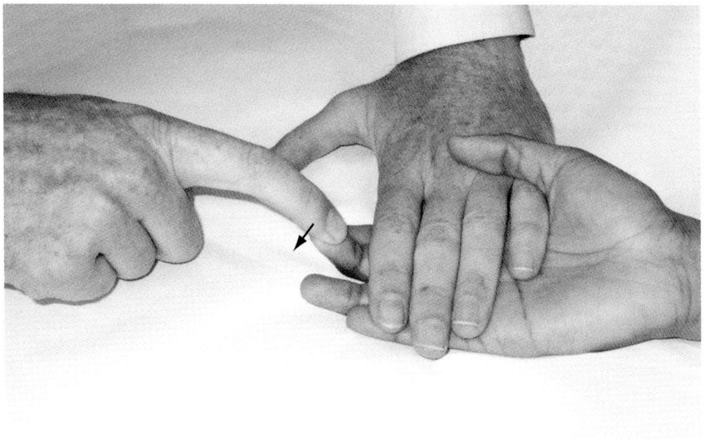

Fig. 6.46a Testing for tear of tendon of flexor digitorum profundus

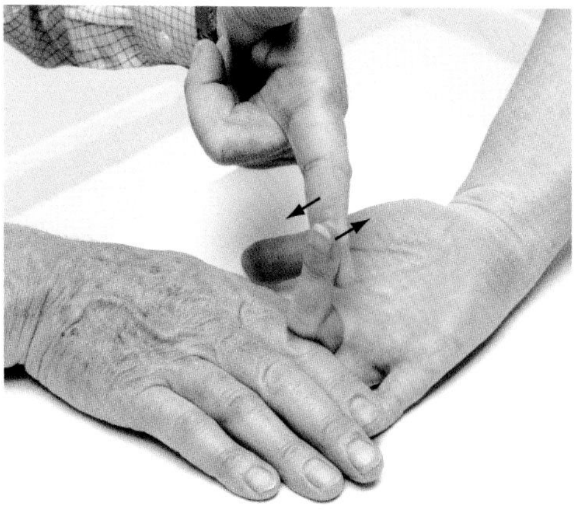

Fig. 6.46b Testing for tear of tendon of flexor digitorum superficialis

and radial side of the joint, with it both in approximately 20° of flexion and in the extended position. Laxity of the joint when tested in the extended position may indicate a fracture into the IP joint. If the joint is stable in the extended position but lax when assessed in flexion, the degree of movement and presence or absence of an "end fee" to the maneuver can be used to determine the extent of sprain of the collateral ligament.

## TEARS OF LONG FLEXOR TENDONS OF THE FINGERS

The subject rests the hand on a table, palm upward, with fingers extended (Fig. 6.46). The examiner places his or her own hand firmly across the subject's fingers, restraining them in extension. Inability to flex a terminal phalanx, especially against resistance, indicates damage to the **flexor digitorum profundus.** To test for damage to a **flexor digitorum superficialis** tendon, the examiner's own fingers are used to keep in full extension those digits of the subject which are not being tested. The subject is then asked to flex against resistance the finger that requires testing, whilst keeping its DIP joint extended.

## TEARS OF LONG EXTENSOR TENDON

The subject presents the hand with the palm facing downward (Fig. 6.47). The examiner uses a finger and thumb to grip the sides of the PIP joint of a finger, with the finger tip flexed. The subject is asked to straighten the finger, whilst the examiner resists by applying pressure over the dorsum of the terminal phalanx.

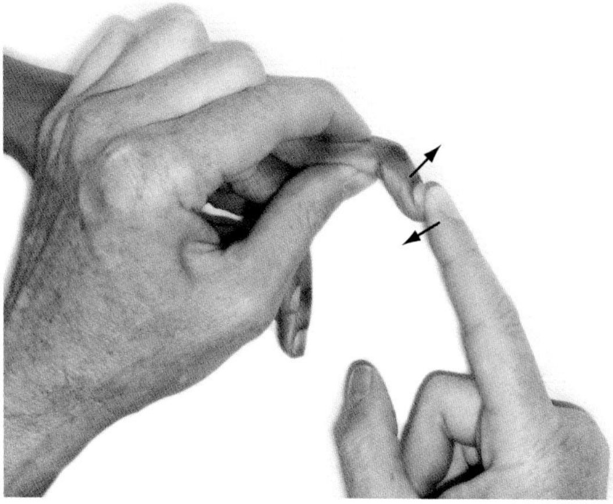

Fig. 6.47 Testing for tear of long extensor tendon of finger

### FURTHER READING

Galati G, Cosenza UM, Sammartino F et al. True aneurysm of the ulnar artery in a soccer goalkeeper. American Journal of Sports Medicine 2003; 31:457–458.

Hsu W-C, Chen W-H, Oware A. A distal ulnar neuropathy in a golf player. Clinical Journal of Sport Medicine 2005; 15:189–191.

Logan AJ, Makwana N, Mason G et al. Acute hand and wrist injuries in experienced rock climbers. British Journal of Sports Medicine 2004; 38:545–548.

Patterson JMM, Jaggars MM, Boyer MI. Ulnar and median nerve palsy in long-distance cyclists. American Journal of Sports Medicine 2003; 31:585–589.

Rettig AC. Athletic injuries of the wrist and hand. Part II: overuse injuries of the wrist and traumatic injuries to the hand. American Journal of Sports Medicine 2004; 32:262–273.

Rossi C, Cellococo P, Margaritondo E et al. De Quervain disease in volleyball players. American Journal of Sports Medicine 2005; 33:424–427.

Wang C, Gill TJ, Zarins B et al. Extensor carpi ulnaris tendon rupture in an ice-hockey player. American Journal of Sports Medicine 2003; 31:459–461.

## CASE STUDY 6 • CLINICAL PROBLEMS

**Problem 1.** *A professional baseball player feels a tearing sensation in the ulnar side of his left wrist whilst performing triceps dips in the gym. Subsequently he experiences ulnar side wrist pain and reduced grip strength whilst batting.*

a) What is the likely diagnosis?
b) Which clinical tests should be performed?
c) What are three possible differential diagnoses?

**Problem 2.** *A mountain bike rider falls on to an outstretched hand and experiences radial sided wrist pain with mild wrist swelling.*

a) What are four possible diagnoses?
b) What clinical test should be conducted to exclude scaphoid fracture? Initial radiography does not reveal a fracture. What is your working diagnosis and how should the injury be managed?
c) What are two common complications associated with scaphoid fracture?

**Problem 3.** *An American football player is struck on the tip of the index finger whilst receiving a pass. He suffers an avulsion fracture of the extensor digitorum tendon at the base of the distal phalanx.*

a) What is the name of the deformity that commonly results from this injury?
b) What clinical test should be performed?
c) How should this injury be managed?

**Problem 4.** *A rock climber experiences palmar forearm and hand pain toward the end of long climbs. His doctor makes a diagnosis of carpal tunnel syndrome.*

a) What other symptoms might the climber experience?
b) What clinical tests could be performed to aid diagnosis?
c) What are three possible differential diagnoses?

**Problem 5.** *A Tour de France cyclist who fell onto his outstretched hand two days ago now complains of paresthesia in his little and ring finger when resting his hands on the top of the handle bars of his bicycle.*

a) What nerve is likely to have been affected?
b) What is the name of the canal in the wrist that this nerve passes through?
c) What other symptoms might the cyclist experience?

**Problem 6.** *A basketball player injures his little finger when attempting to catch a hard thrown pass. He is unable to play on and a radiograph of the finger (Fig. 6.48) is obtained.*

a) What is the likely mechanism of injury?
b) What abnormalities are shown on the X-ray film?
c) What soft-tissue structures overlying the anterior surface of the affected joint could be damaged with this type of injury?
d) What treatment is likely to be required?

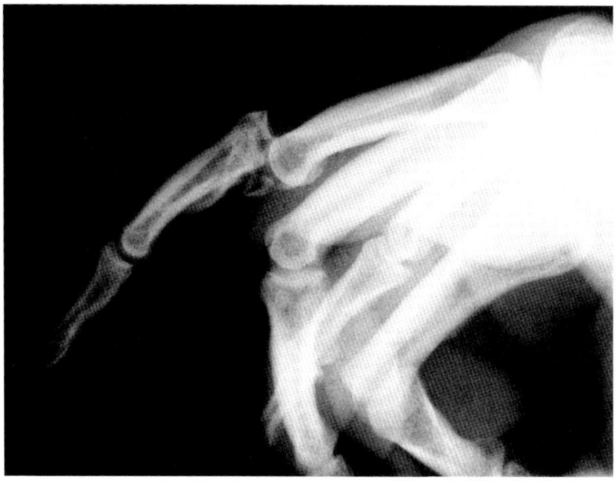

Fig. 6.48 Radiograph of hand injury

CHAPTER 7

# Hip, gluteal region, and thigh

## INTRODUCTION

The hip and gluteal region form the root of the lower limb where it joins the postero-inferior part of the trunk below the rim of the iliac crest. Much of the gluteal prominence (buttock) consists of subcutaneous fat covering the considerable mass of the gluteus maximus. Two smaller gluteal muscles, the medius and minimus, lie under the maximus and contribute to the size of the buttock, but to a much lesser extent. They are important hip abductors and stabilizers, preventing pelvic tilt during gait. Deep-seated beneath the gluteus maximus is the stable, ball-and-socket, multi-axial hip joint. The gluteal tuberosity, to which the hamstring muscles are attached, lies below it.

Entering the region through the greater sciatic foramen, the large sciatic nerve descends through the buttock behind the hip joint (where it is vulnerable to posterior dislocation), to reach the posterior compartment of the thigh. It is the major nerve supply to the lower limb, supplying the hamstring muscles and all parts of the limb below the knee.

The thigh lies distal to the buttock and extends as far as the knee. It forms the proximal segment in the lever system of the lower limb. It has three compartments, which surround the shaft of the femur. The anterior compartment contains the quadriceps group supplied by the femoral nerve, the medial contains the adductor group supplied by the obturator nerve, and the posterior contains the hamstrings supplied by the sciatic nerve. Muscles in all three compartments are vulnerable to injury. The compartments are enveloped by the stocking-like investing layer of deep fascia, which is particularly thick laterally where it forms the ilio-tibial tract.

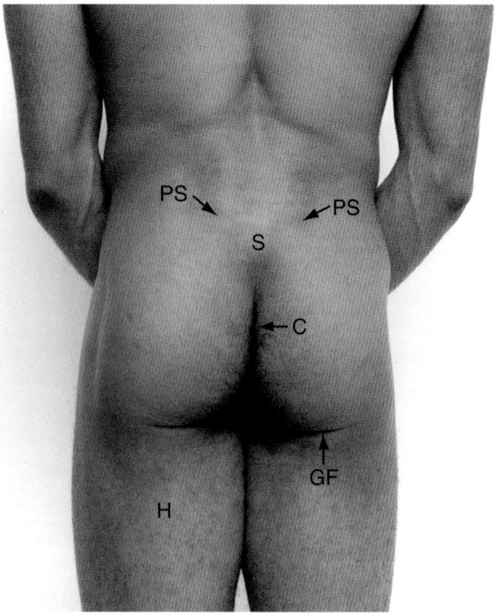


Fig. 7.1 Gluteal region and thigh from posterior aspect C = location of coccyx in depth of upper end of gluteal cleft, GF = gluteal fold, H = hamstrings, PS = posterior superior iliac spine, S = dorsum of sacrum

## INSPECTION OF NORMAL CONTOURS

- Gluteal fold
- Posterior superior iliac spine
- Gluteal depression
- Hamstrings

The subject stands upright, facing away from the examiner. From posteriorly, although the overall shape of the human buttock is the same, it varies considerably in size and shape from person to person, for reasons that include race, sex, age, and the amount of subcutaneous fat. In a muscular subject, it is firm and its contours are well defined, descending from the level of the iliac crest to its typical rounded prominence and then diminishing inferiorly to reach the crease of the **gluteal fold** (Fig. 7.1) at its junction with the thigh. Note that the fold does not correspond with the lower margin of the gluteus maximus, which crosses it obliquely.

If the superior margin of the buttock is followed downward and medially, it is seen to lie close to the dimple marking the **posterior superior iliac spine (PSIS)**; it then continues medially along the edge of the sacrum, to converge with the opposite side at the upper end of the natal (gluteal) cleft. From the upper part of the hip, the lateral contour of the buttock forms a smooth convex profile passing downward to be continuous with the lateral margin of the thigh, which tapers to the level of the knee. Often in the female the lateral contour of the buttock is

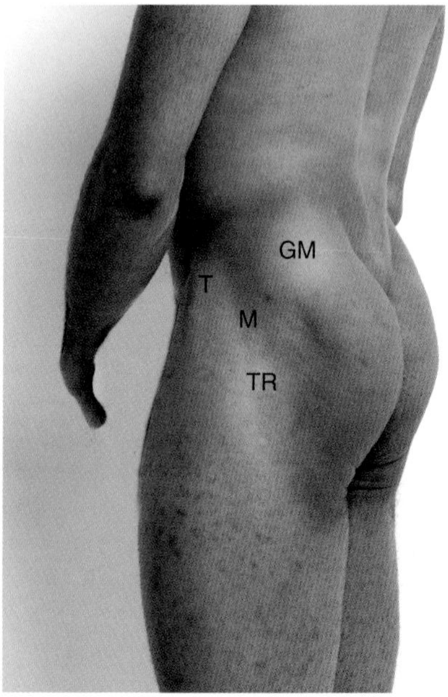


Fig. 7.2 Gluteal region and thigh from lateral aspect Gluteal muscles are tensed; GM = gluteus maximus, M = gluteus medius, T = tensor fasciae latae, TR = greater trochanter

accentuated by the wider pelvis and more subcutaneous fat. On the lateral surface of the buttock there is a marked **gluteal depression** (Fig. 7.2) located behind the fullness of the greater trochanter and below the middle of the iliac crest. It is emphasized if the subject is asked to tense the buttock.

The thigh lies distal to the buttock and extends as far as the knee. It is cylindrical in shape, tapering toward the knee and flattening on its posterior surface as the **hamstring muscles** give way to their tendons, which approach the upper part of the popliteal fossa where they form its boundaries on each side. The medial side of the thigh continues distally, initially in line with the gluteal cleft but with a distinct curve laterally as it approaches the knee. The lateral contour of the buttock curves smoothly downward in continuity with the lateral margin of the thigh, which converges toward the knee.

## LOCATING BONY LANDMARKS

- Anterior superior iliac spine
- Iliac tubercle
- Adductor tubercle
- Greater trochanter
- Ischial tuberosity
- Sacrum and coccyx

Bony landmarks are shown on the skeleton in Figure 7.3a and b and in the radiograph in Figure 7.3c.

### ANTERIOR SUPERIOR ILIAC SPINE, ILIAC TUBERCLE, AND ADDUCTOR TUBERCLE

The subject lies supine on the examination couch, with the extended thigh available for examination. Palpation of the iliac crest and its anterior landmarks is described in Chapter 3. The landmarks include the **anterior superior iliac spine,** close to which the lateral cutaneous nerve of the thigh may become entrapped, and more posteriorly the **tubercle.** Moving to the medial border of the thigh about its midpoint, and with the limb relaxed, the examiner applies firm pressure, guiding the fingers distally over the underlying soft tissues toward the knee until a conspicuous bony point is reached. This is the **adductor tubercle,** which marks the distal attachment of the adductor magnus and where the femoral vessels leave the adductor canal to enter the popliteal fossa behind the knee.

### GREATER TROCHANTER

To locate the greater trochanter (Fig. 7.4), the palmar surfaces of the fingers on one hand palpate the lateral side of the buttock about a hand's breadth or more below the tubercle of the iliac crest. The broad lateral subcutaneous surface of the trochanter is easily felt using a massaging type of palpation. By passively flexing the thigh to 90°, and then using the index and middle finger tips, the examiner can readily palpate the posterior, upper, and anterior borders of the greater trochanter. This part of the examination may be facilitated if subjects lie on their side.

### ISCHIAL TUBEROSITY

The subject now turns face down (prone) on the examination couch. Grasping the leg below the knee, the examiner passively flexes the knee, keeping the thigh flat on the couch so that the hamstrings and gluteus maximus are relaxed. The pads of several fingers are used to locate the ischial tuberosity, using a massaging motion about 5 cm above and medial to the midpoint of the gluteal fold. Since it lies under the lower part of gluteus maximus, it is not easily located and requires careful deep palpation. It is essential that gluteus maximus and the hamstrings are relaxed. Once it has been located, confirmation is given by making the hamstrings attached to it contract.

### SACRUM AND COCCYX

Finally, the bony features of the sacrum and coccyx, as described in Chapter 2, can be revisited, as they lie at the medial boundary of the buttock.

## LOCATING JOINT LINES

- Hip
- Sacro-iliac

### HIP JOINT

In the stable hip, a line (Nelaton's line) joining the anterior superior iliac spine to the ischial tuberosity just crosses the top of the greater trochanter. This intersection point marks the center of the hip joint. The joint itself is deeply placed in the floor of the femoral triangle beneath the inguinal ligament, about its midpoint, where it is crossed by the tendon of the iliopsoas muscle.

Although the head of the femur is impalpable, its movement in the acetabulum can be detected. The subject lies supine, with the knee and also the hip flexed. With the

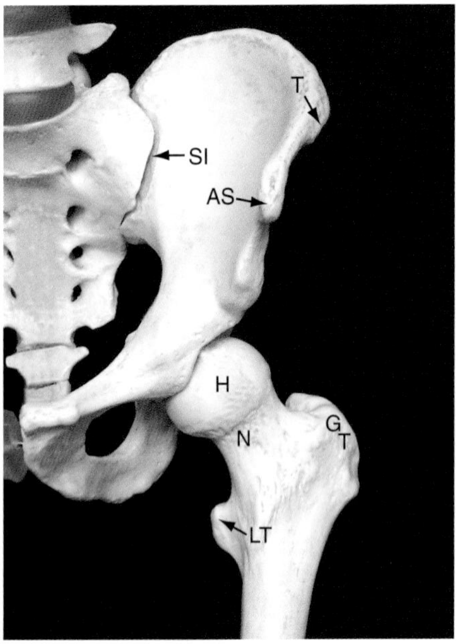


Fig. 7.3a Bony skeleton of hip and thigh from anterior
AS = anterior superior iliac spine, GT = greater trochanter, H = femoral head, LT = lesser trochanter, N = femoral neck, SI = sacro-iliac joint, T = tubercle of iliac crest

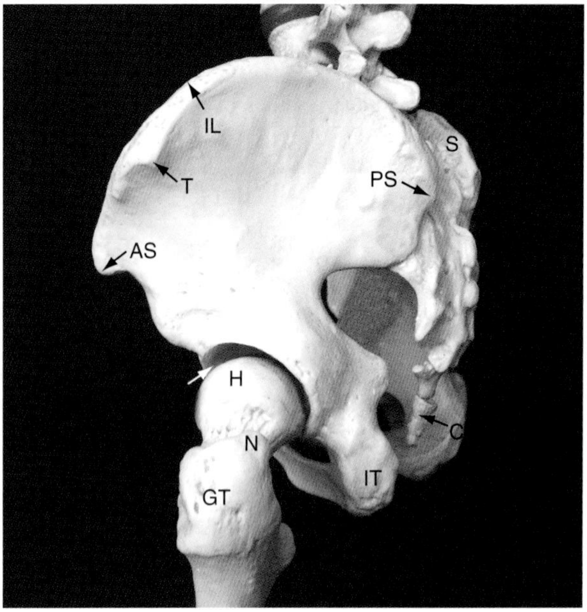


Fig. 7.3b Bony skeleton of hip and thigh from postero-lateral
AS = anterior superior iliac spine, C = coccyx, GT = greater trochanter, H = femoral head, IL = iliac crest, IT = ischial tuberosity, N = femoral neck, PS = posterior superior iliac spine, S = dorsum of sacrum, T = tubercle of iliac crest

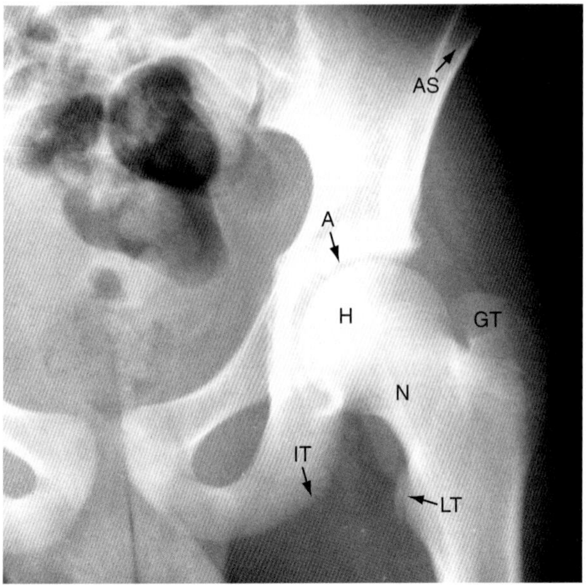


Fig. 7.3c Frontal radiograph of hip
A = acetabulum, AS = anterior superior iliac spine, GT = greater trochanter, H = femoral head, IT = ischial tuberosity, LT = lesser tuberosity, N = femoral neck

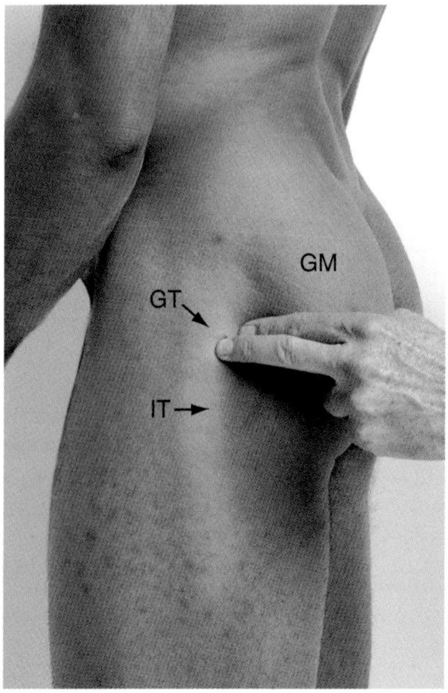


Fig. 7.4 Locating the greater trochanter
GM = gluteus maximus, GT = greater trochanter, IT = ilio-tibial band

subject's thigh muscles relaxed, the examiner grips the knee and alternates the position of the hip between abduction and adduction, allowing the limb to pivot on the heel of the foot as it lies on the couch. By applying deep pressure with the finger tips of one hand immediately below the midpoint of the inguinal groove, movement in the hip can be detected.

### SACRO-ILIAC JOINT

This joint is also considered in Chapter 2. It is normally very stable, with minimal movement, having strong interosseous and posterior sacro-iliac ligaments. It is inaccessible anteriorly, where it forms part of the pelvic brim. However, it is accessible posteriorly in the floor of the skin dimple close to the posterior superior iliac spine (Fig. 7.1). Deep palpation with a finger tip in the dimple reveals a bony edge where the PSIS overhangs the joint line, covered by posterior sacro-iliac ligaments.

## LOCATING SOFT TISSUES

- Piriformis
- Sciatic nerve

Prosections showing gluteal structures and the hamstrings are provided in Figure 7.5.

### PIRIFORMIS

The subject lies face down on the examination couch. The gluteal muscles must be relaxed. The line of the piriformis beneath the gluteus maximus is traced by first locating the midpoint of a line from the dimple marking the PSIS to the tip of the coccyx in the lower part of the gluteal cleft. From this midpoint, another line is taken across the buttock to the upper border of the greater trochanter. This locates the piriformis. With the subject's knee flexed, the examiner supports and grasps the leg so that the thigh can be alternated between resisted medial and lateral rotation. During this maneuver, the other hand is used to palpate along the line of the piriformis (Fig. 7.6), which can be felt to tense through the gluteus maximus during lateral rotation. The lateral (peroneal) division of the sciatic nerve may traverse the muscle and become entrapped.

### SCIATIC NERVE

The subject lies prone on the couch, with the gluteal muscles relaxed. Three bony landmarks must be palpated

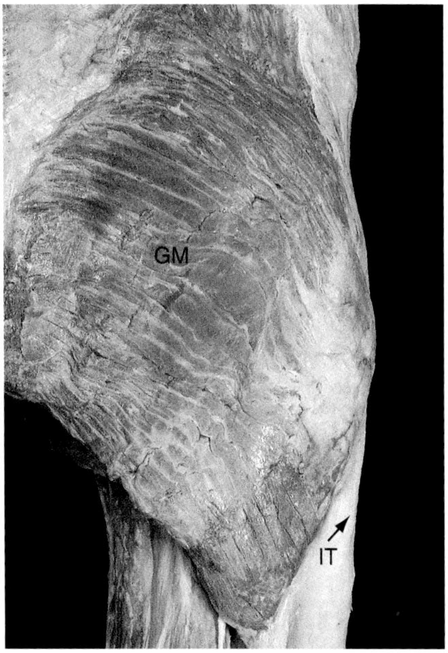


Fig. 7.5a Prosection to show gluteus maximus
GM = gluteus maximus, IT = ilio-tibial band (From Gosling JA, Harris PF, Whitmore I, Willan PLT. 2002 Human Anatomy, 4th edn. London: Mosby)

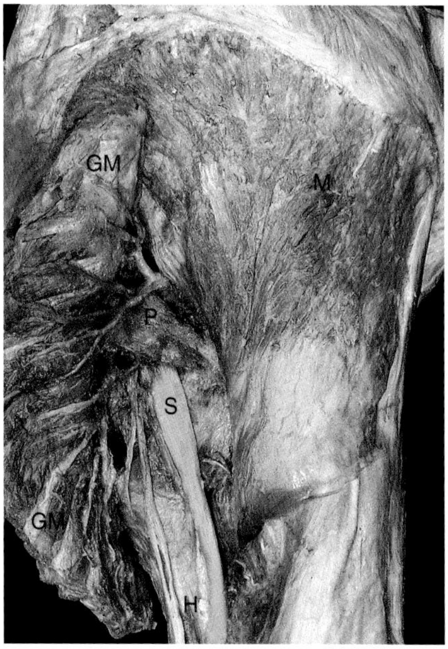


Fig. 7.5b Prosection to show deep gluteal structures
GM = gluteus maximus (reflected), H = hamstrings, M = gluteus medius, P = piriformis, S = sciatic nerve (From Gosling JA, Harris PF, Whitmore I, Willan PLT. 2002 Human Anatomy, 4th edn. London: Mosby)

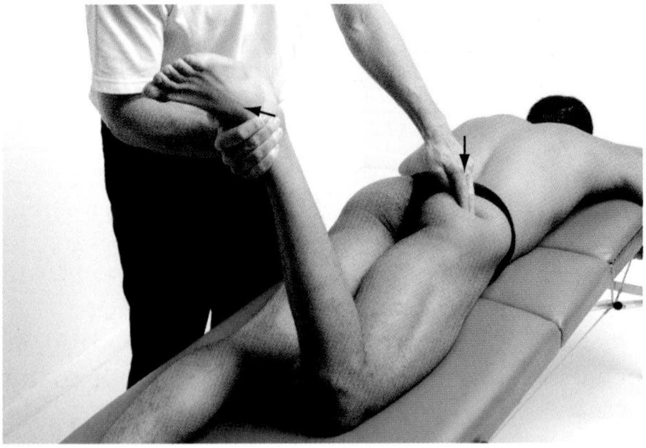

Fig. 7.6 Locating piriformis
The hip is laterally rotated whilst the muscle is palpated

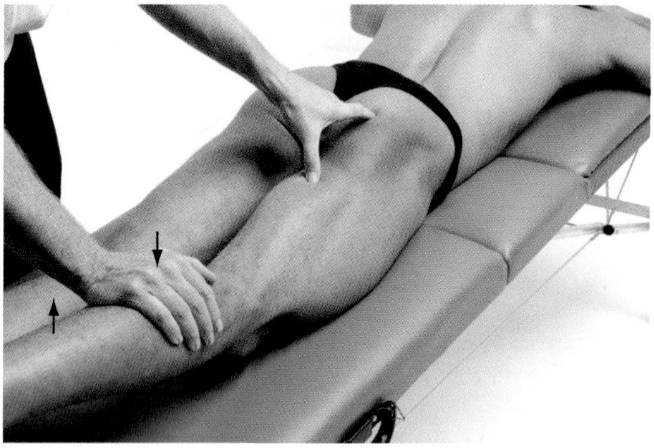

Fig. 7.7 Demonstrating and testing the hamstrings

in order to trace the course of the nerve. The first point is marked by the junction between the upper and middle third of a line between the PSIS and the ischial tuberosity. The second point lies midway between a line connecting the ischial tuberosity and the upper border of the greater trochanter. The sciatic nerve is located by following a gently convex line inclining laterally and joining the two predetermined points. It continues vertically and distally midway between the medial and lateral borders of the thigh to the junction between the lower and middle thirds of the thigh, where it usually terminates as the tibial and common peroneal nerves.

# TESTING MUSCLES

- Quadriceps femoris
- Adductors
- Hamstrings
- Gluteus maximus
- Gluteus medius and minimus
- Tensor fasciae latae
- Hip rotators

## QUADRICEPS FEMORIS

As the quadriceps group acts principally on the knee, it is considered and examined in Chapter 8.

## ADDUCTORS

The adductor group is considered in the groin section of Chapter 3.

## HAMSTRINGS

These anti-gravity muscles extend the hip and flex the knee (see Ch. 8). To test the ability of the hamstrings to extend the hip, the subject lies prone on the examination couch, with both lower limbs fully extended. Keeping the limb straight, the subject is asked to raise the thigh off the couch by extending the hip. At the same time, the examiner applies downward pressure over the proximal leg, resisting the movement. The contracting hamstrings can be palpated and cause a visible bulge on the back of the thigh (Fig. 7.7). The method of defining the individual hamstring tendons in the distal thigh is described in Chapter 8.

## GLUTEUS MAXIMUS

This is the most powerful anti-gravity extensor muscle of the hip. To test its power, the subject lies prone with the hip in neutral and the knee flexed 90° so that the hamstrings are relaxed. The subject is asked to lift the thigh off the couch against resistance provided by the examiner's hand, which is placed over the distal posterior thigh. Contraction is confirmed by palpating tension in the buttock during the maneuver (Fig. 7.8).

## GLUTEUS MINIMUS, GLUTEUS MEDIUS, AND TENSOR FASCIAE LATAE

The hip abductors, gluteus minimus, gluteus medius, and tensor fasciae latae, can all be tested if subjects lie on their side on the couch, with both lower limbs fully extended. To isolate the **gluteus minimus,** the subject abducts the uppermost limb, raising it upward away from the couch, whilst the examiner resists the movement by downward pressure on the thigh. Repeating this maneuver with the subject rolled slightly toward prone biases the **gluteus medius** (Fig. 7.9a), whilst resisting hip abduction with the subject rolled slightly toward supine tests the **tensor fasciae latae** (Fig. 7.9b).

The two muscles also have an important role in gait. They act from their distal (trochanteric) to their proximal (iliac) attachment, contracting on the side of the supporting limb to prevent downward tilting of the pelvis and trunk on the unsupported side. To test this function, the subject stands upright, with the examiner standing behind. The subject is asked to stand on one leg. A drop in the level of the iliac crest on the unsupported side (Trendelenburg sign) indicates weakness in the hip abductors of the stance limb.

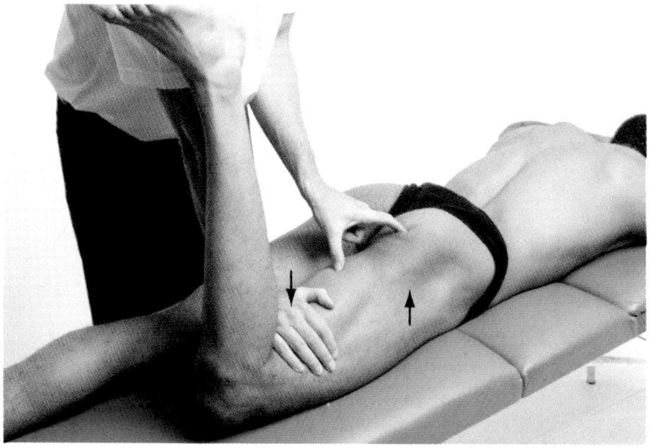

Fig. 7.8 Demonstrating and testing gluteus maximus

## HIP ROTATORS

These require brief attention. To test the passive ROM in extension, the subject lies face downward on the couch and flexes the knee to 90°. Using the leg and foot as a lever, the examiner grips the foot and pivots the leg, first inward and then outward. Active resistance to these movements is also tested.

# RANGE OF MOVEMENTS

- Hip
- Flexion/extension
- Abduction/adduction
- Rotation: medial/lateral

The hip joint is a synovial multi-axial joint. Testing its range of motion is illustrated in Figure 7.10. Hip **flexion** may reach **120°** but **extension** is restricted to **30°**. In the movement of **abduction, 45°** is possible and **up to 60°** when attempted with the hip flexed to 90°. However, only **30°** can be attained in **adduction. Rotation** movements are more variable in range, but on average **up to 45°** can be reached in each direction with the hip flexed, particularly in passive movement.

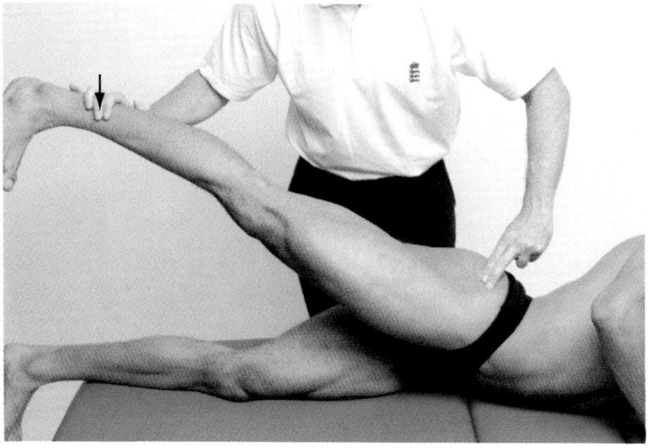

Fig. 7.9a Testing and palpating the gluteus medius

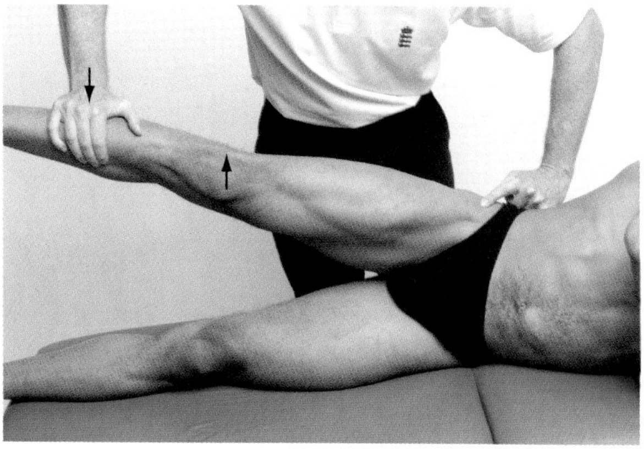

Fig. 7.9b Locating and demonstrating tensor fasciae latae during thigh abduction
The examiner has a finger tip on the muscle and the ilio-tibial band is visible on the lateral side of the knee (see ↑)

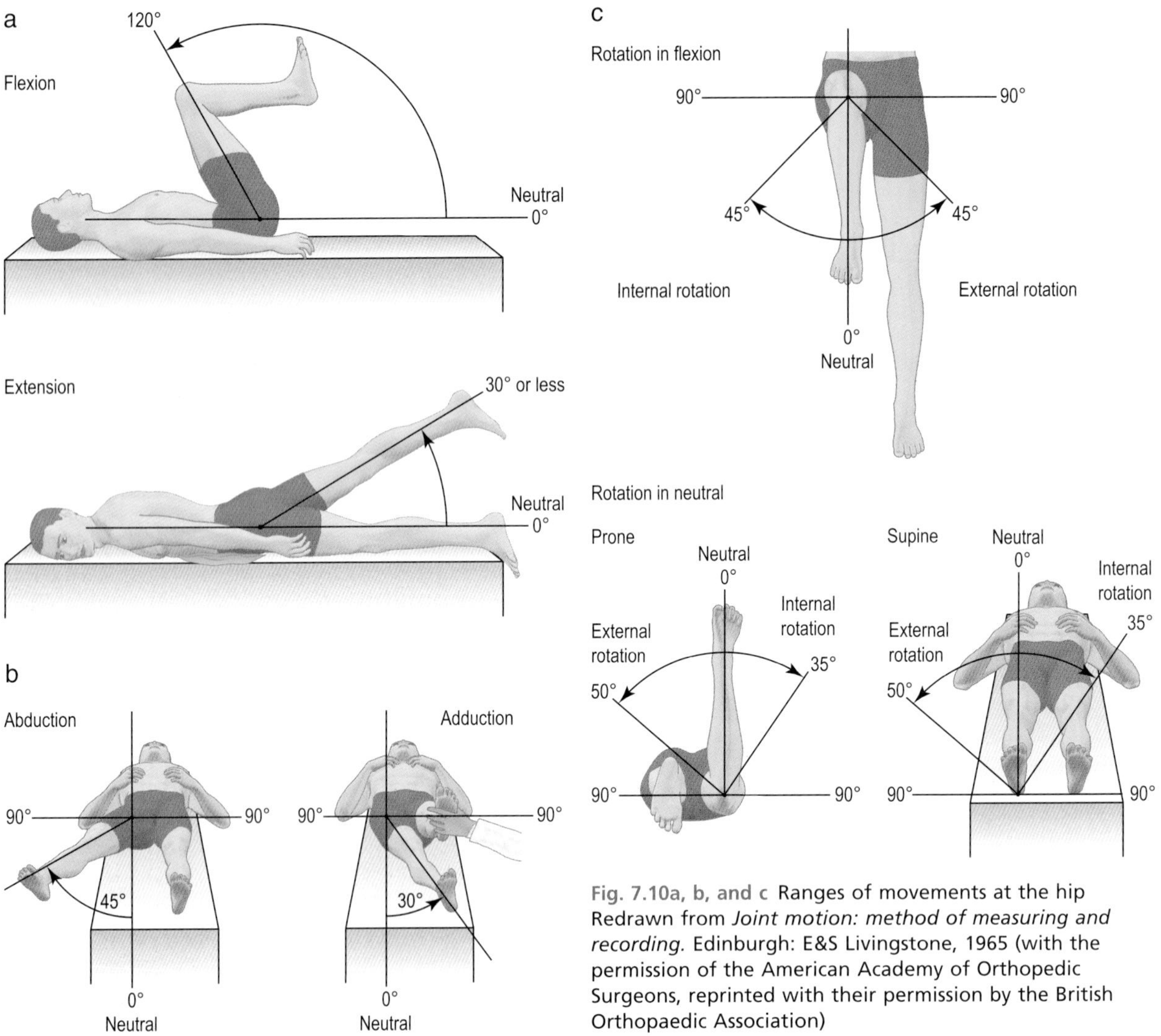


**Fig. 7.10a, b, and c** Ranges of movements at the hip Redrawn from *Joint motion: method of measuring and recording.* Edinburgh: E&S Livingstone, 1965 (with the permission of the American Academy of Orthopedic Surgeons, reprinted with their permission by the British Orthopaedic Association)

# TESTS FOR HIP DERANGEMENTS AND MUSCLE STRAINS

- Thomas test
- Ober's test
- Faber test

## THOMAS TEST

The modified Thomas test can be used to assess for tightness of the hip flexors: rectus femoris, the ilio-psoas and the tensor fasciae latae. The subject, sitting on the end of the couch, is asked to hold one knee to the chest and roll on to the back. The limb is then released, allowing the foot to be supported on the examiner's hip and keeping the lumbar spine in a flat position against the couch. Tightness of the hip flexors is indicated when the hip on the unsupported, relaxed side exhibits an element of flexion (Fig. 7.11a). Tightness of the ilio-psoas can be differentiated from that of the rectus femoris by the examiner attempting to flex the unsupported knee (Fig. 7.11b). If the knee cannot be flexed further, then the rectus femoris is probably limiting hip extension.

Assessment for strains or avulsion of the ilio-psoas and the rectus femoris can also be conducted in the modified Thomas test position. Applying resistance to hip flexion

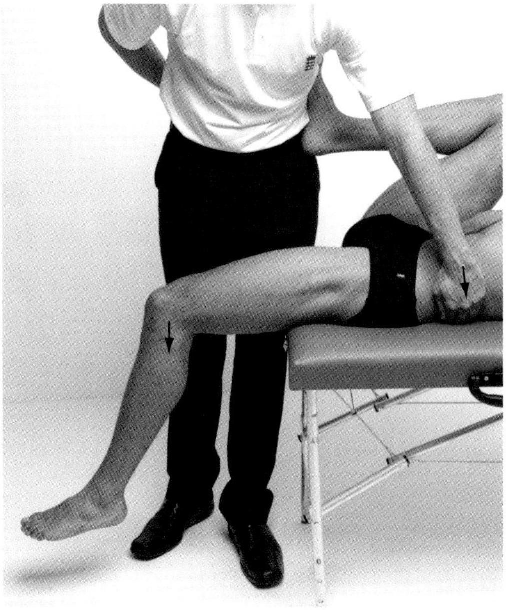

Fig. 7.11a Modified Thomas test for tightness in the hip flexors

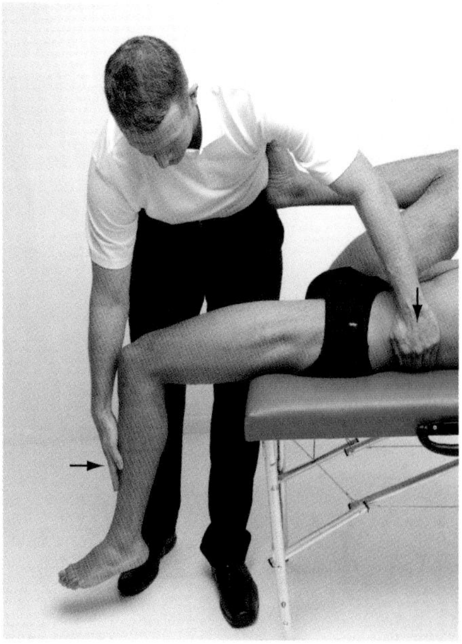

Fig. 7.11b Differentiating rectus femoris and ilio-psoas tightness

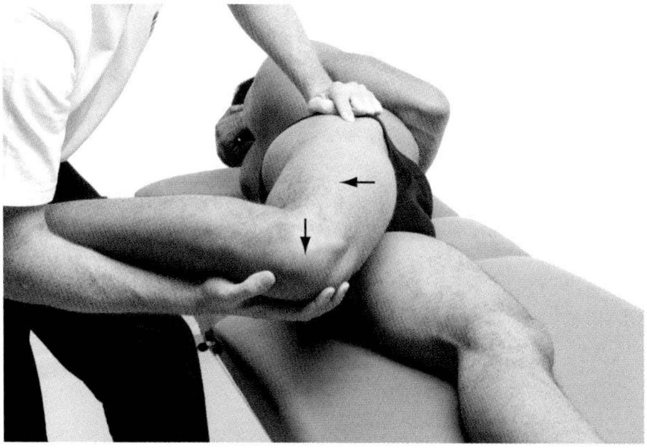

Fig. 7.11c Testing for tensor fasciae latae length and tightness

over the distal anterior thigh tests the iliopsoas (Fig. 7.12a). To test the rectus femoris, the examiner maintains this resistance whilst asking the subject to "kick out" the leg isometrically against the examiner's thigh (Fig. 7.12b).

## OBER'S TEST

Tightness of the tensor fasciae latae and ilio-tibial band can be detected by Ober's test. The subject turns to lie on one side and the examiner applies firm downward pressure over the ilium. The subject's uppermost leg is flexed at the knee and cradled firmly along the examiner's forearm, with the hand holding the knee. This gives control over the hip, which is then passively extended so that the ilio-tibial band lies directly over the greater trochanter. With the limb in this position, the examiner allows it to drop toward the couch. If the limb remains in an abducted position, this indicates tightness in the ilio-tibial band, and the tension can be palpated with a finger on the band as it passes over the trochanter (Fig. 7.11c).

## HIP JOINT TEST

The Faber test (described in Ch. 2), or limitation of hip internal rotation (Fig. 7.13a and b) or external rotation ROM (Fig. 7.13c and d), and groin discomfort when overpressure is applied in **combined hip flexion and adduction** (Fig. 7.14), are all non-specific indicators of possible hip derangements such as osteochondral defects, labral tears, capsulitis, and hip impingement. Readers are directed to a special edition of *Clinics in Sports Medicine,* Volume

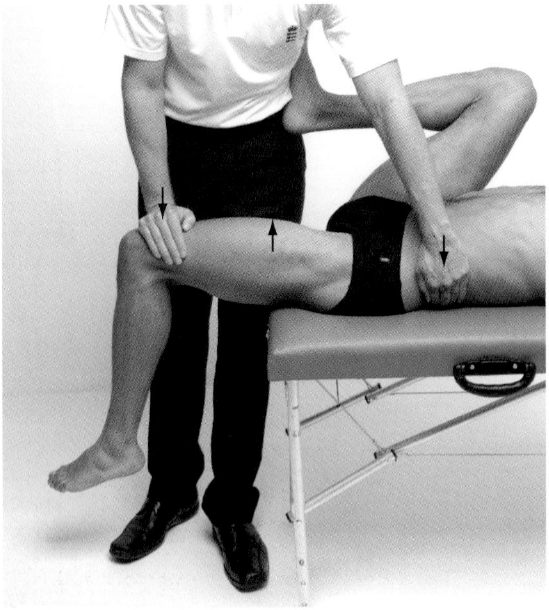

Fig. 7.12a Testing iliopsoas strength

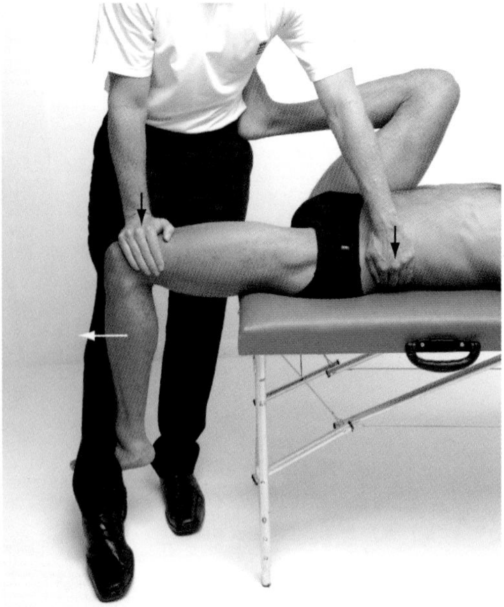

Fig. 7.12b Testing rectus femoris strength

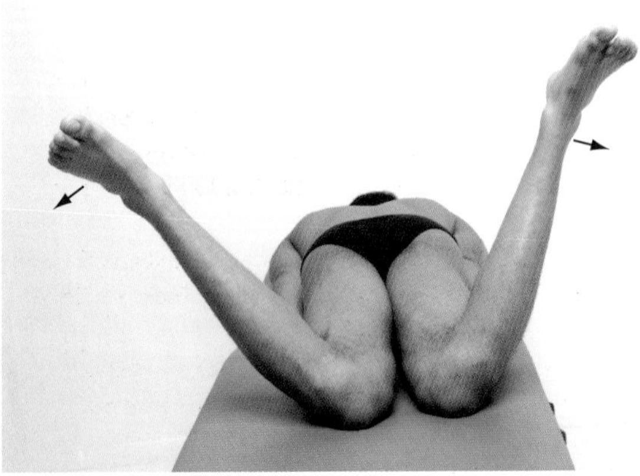

Fig. 7.13a Demonstrating hip internal rotation ROM

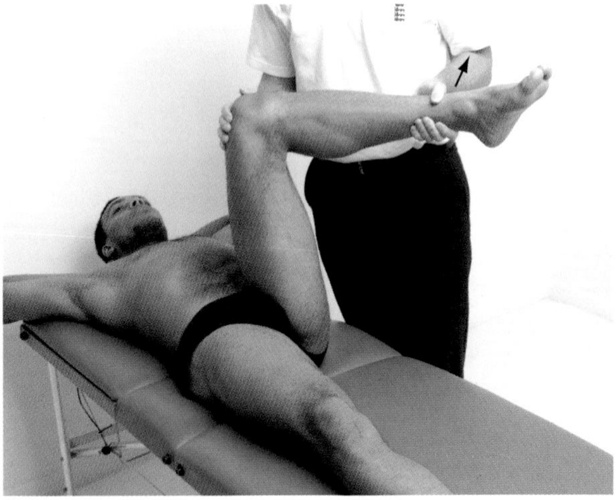

Fig. 7.13b Demonstrating passive hip internal rotation ROM

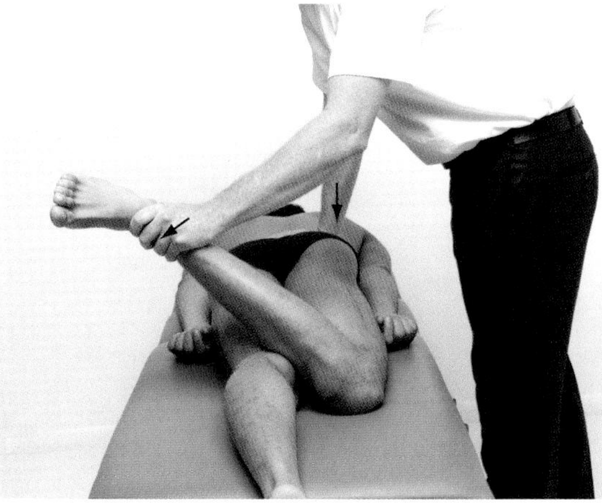

Fig. 7.13c Demonstrating passive hip external rotation ROM

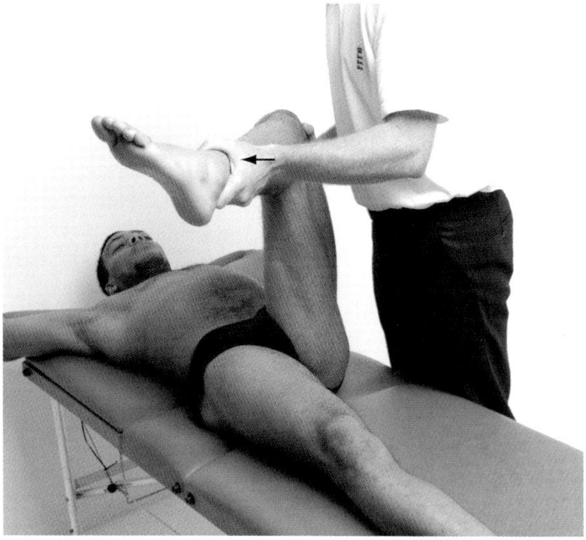

Fig. 7.13d Demonstrating passive hip external rotation ROM in hip flexion

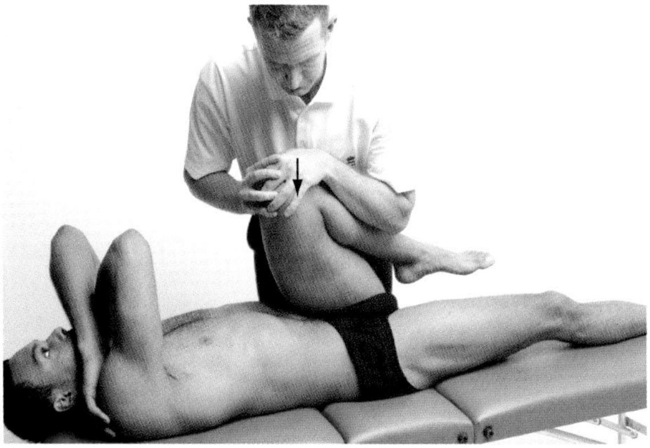

Fig. 7.14 Applying over-pressure in combined hip flexion and adduction

25 (2006), for a comprehensive review of the diagnosis, investigation, surgical management, and rehabilitation of sporting hip derangements.

## FURTHER READING

Diaz JA, Fischer DA, Rettig AC et al. Severe quadriceps muscle contusions in athletes: a report of three cases. American Journal of Sports Medicine 2003; 31:289–293.

Fredericson M, Cookingham CL, Chaudhari AM et al. Hip abductor weakness in distance runners with ilio-tibial band syndrome. Clinical Journal of Sport Medicine 2000; 10:169–175.

Hernesman SC, Hoch AZ, Vetter CS et al. Foot drop in a marathon runner from chronic complete hamstring tear 2003; 13:365–368.

Hsu JC, Fischer DA, Wright RW. Proximal rectus femoris avulsions in National Football league kickers: a report of two cases. American Journal of Sports Medicine 2005; 33:1085–1087.

Mitchell B, McCrory P, Brukner P et al. Hip joint pathology: clinical presentation and correlation between magnetic resonance arthrography, ultrasound, and arthroscopic findings in 25 consecutive cases. Clinical Journal of Sport Medicine 2003; 15:152–156.

Moazzaz P, Chang CJ. Two unusual cases of acetabular fractures sustained during sports. Clinical Journal of Sport Medicine 2002; 12:127–129.

Ulkar B, Yildiz Y, Kunduracioglu B. Meralgia paresthetica. A long-standing performance-limiting cause of anterior thigh pain in a soccer player. American Journal of Sports Medicine 2003; 31:787–789.

Wahl CJ, Warren RF, Adler RS et al. Internal coxa saltans (snapping hip) as a result of overtraining: a report of three cases in professional athletes with a review of causes and the role of ultrasound in early diagnosis and management. American Journal of Sports Medicine 2004; 32:1302–1309.

Willick SE, Lazarus M, Press JM. Quadratus femoris strain. Clinical Journal of Sport Medicine 2002; 12:130–131.

## CASE STUDY 7 • CLINICAL PROBLEMS

**Problem 1.** *A 14-year-old soccer goalkeeper reports experiencing a sharp pain and a popping sensation in the front of his right hip when attempting to kick a waterlogged ball with that leg. It is now uncomfortable for him to lift his right leg.*

a) What are at least two possible diagnoses?
b) Which test can be used to test the length of the long and the short hip flexors?
c) How can the strength of the long and the short hip flexors be differentiated?

**Problem 2.** *A 25-year-old American football wide receiver suddenly experiences a sharp pain in his posterior thigh when sprinting for a touchdown.*

a) Which muscle group is likely to have been affected?
b) The player's trainer concludes that weakness of the gluteus maximus is a contributing factor to the injury. How can the relative hip extension strength of the gluteus maximus and the hamstrings be assessed?

**Problem 3.** *After about 30 mins of each training session in the boat, a 20-year-old female rower experiences a toothache-like pain in her left buttock that radiates to the posterior thigh.*

a) Compression of the sciatic nerve by which buttock muscle might be a cause of these symptoms?
b) What is the surface marking of this muscle?
c) Name three other possible causes of sciatic nerve irritation in this situation.
d) Which test could be used to assess for adverse mechanical tension of the sciatic nerve?

**Problem 4.** *A 30-year-old male Thai boxing exponent is kicked in the lateral thigh. An hour later he is unable to flex his knee beyond 45°.*

a) What is the most likely cause of the restricted ROM?
b) In what position should the knee be immobilized and why?
c) What are possible short- and long-term complications of this injury?

**Problem 5.** *An ice hockey player in the National Hockey League (NHL) complains of a painful click that radiates along his left groin when skating fast. The sports physician orders an MRI hip scan.*

a) Which structure in the hip joint, indicated by the arrow in Figure 7.15, is likely to be implicated? Note: F = head of femur; A = acetabulum.
b) Derangements of what other structures might be causing these symptoms? Name at least three.
c) Which tests might indicate hip joint pathology?

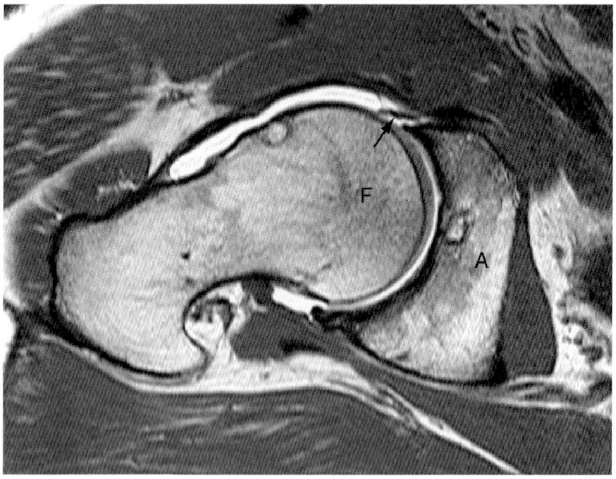


Fig. 7.15 Axial MRI of the hip joint
A = acetabulum, F = femoral head

8

CHAPTER

# Knee

## INTRODUCTION

As the knee joint and adjacent structures are relatively superficial, they are readily palpated and are accessible anteriorly, medially and laterally. Posteriorly, the joint is not accessible since it lies deep in the floor of the popliteal fossa, through which passes the main vascular and nerve supply to the leg and foot. The joint has two components, patello-femoral and tibio-femoral, which share a common synovial cavity.

CHAPTER

# INSPECTION OF NORMAL CONTOURS

- Patella
- Quadriceps
- Patellar ligament
- Tibial tuberosity and tibia
- Ilio-tibial tract
- Vastus medialis
- Lateral tibial condyle
- Head of fibula
- Hamstring tendons

Wearing shorts, the subject is examined either sitting, or lying supine and then prone on the examination couch.

Visible contours depend upon the position of the knee, the amount of subcutaneous fat, and the development of the musculature, especially the quadriceps femoris.

Viewed from anteriorly, with the knee extended, a central feature is the prominence of the **patella,** broader above and narrower below. Continuing from its upper border, the fullness of the thigh is due to the underlying **quadriceps** tendon and the muscles comprising the quadriceps femoris, the three vasti and the rectus femoris.

Inferiorly, the patellar profile narrows, continuing to the prominence of the underlying **patellar ligament,** and below this, the **tibial tuberosity** and anterior border of the **tibia.** On each side of the patella is a distinct depression, more evident laterally than medially. On the lateral side, if the knee is tensed, fullness appears in the upper part, which is due to the vastus lateralis. Behind this, extending the length of the depression, is a ridge formed by the anterior border of the **ilio-tibial tract** (Fig. 8.1). Much of the upper part of the medial depression is encroached upon by a distinctive bulge due to the lower fibers of the **vastus medialis** passing to their attachment on the medial border of the patella. The depression is therefore most evident in its lower part.

Viewing from the lateral side, with the subject's knee flexed at 90°, there is a fullness formed by the distal part of vastus lateralis, and below this a small groove followed by a slight prominence caused by the underlying lateral femoral condyle. Below this is a shallow groove marking the line of the knee joint. Immediately distal is a flat area overlying the **lateral tibial condyle.** Just below this and more posterior is a distinct prominence caused by the underlying **head of the fibula.** Two ridges passing down the lateral side of the knee may be visible. The more anterior marks the posterior border of the ilio-tibial tract, whilst the posterior is due to the underlying tendon of the biceps femoris leading down to the head of the fibula (Fig. 8.2).

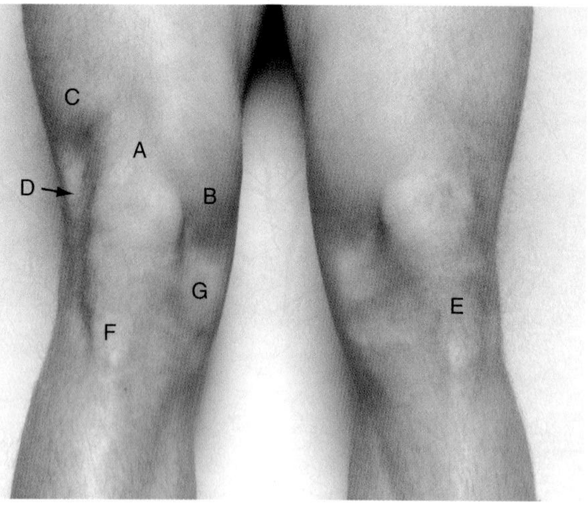


Fig. 8.1 Surface features of the knee from anterior A = quadriceps femoris tendon, B = vastus medialis, C = vastus lateralis, D = ilio-tibial tract, E = patellar ligament, F = tibial tuberosity, G = insertions of sartorius, gracilis, and semi-tendinosus (pes anserinus)

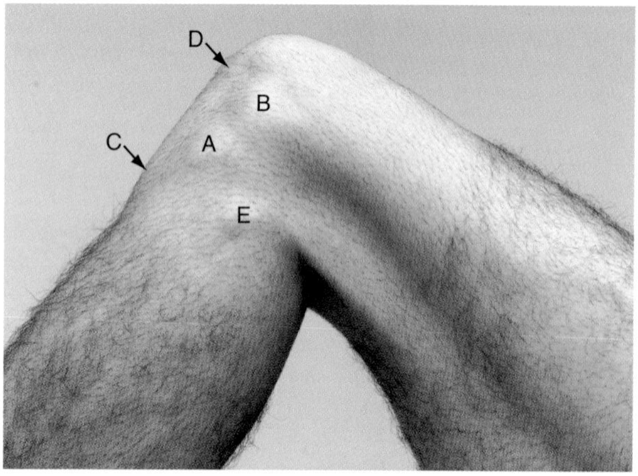


Fig. 8.2 Surface features of the knee from lateral side A = tibial condyle, B = femoral condyle, C = tibial tuberosity, D = apex of patella, E = head of fibula with biceps tendon. The well-defined groove between A and B marks the line of the knee joint

Viewed from medially, the bulge of the vastus medialis is very conspicuous; below this a shallow groove separates

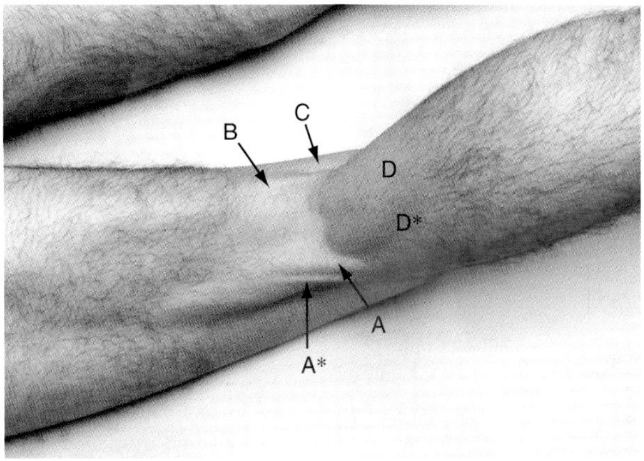


Fig. 8.3 Surface features of the knee from posterior A = biceps femoris: short head, A* = biceps femoris: long head, B = semi-tendinosus, C = semi-membranosus, D = medial head of gastrocnemius, D* = lateral head of gastrocnemius

it from a prominence overlying the medial femoral condyle, whose distal margin may be visible. A sulcus can be clearly seen medial to the patellar ligament, and this overlies the medial tibial condyle. Posteriorly, a small bulge descending to the medial tibial condyle marks the underlying sartorius, gracilis, and semi-tendinosus tendons (Fig. 8.1).

From posteriorly, with the knee extended, the upper boundaries of the popliteal fossa are marked by two grooves commencing on each side of the joint, which converge superiorly in the lower part of the thigh. They mark the underlying **hamstring tendons.** These tendons are biceps femoris laterally, with semi-tendinosus and semi-membranosus medially. With the subject lying prone, they are easily palpable and form well-defined ridges when the knee is flexed to 90° against resistance on the part of the examiner (Fig. 8.3). In the lower part of the fossa, the infero-lateral and infero-medial boundaries may be visible as diffuse elevations caused by the underlying medial and lateral heads of gastrocnemius. They become more prominent if the subject attempts plantar flexion of the foot against resistance and with the leg extended. The two heads of the gastrocnemius blend into the fullness of the upper calf, where they join with the underlying soleus muscle, these three muscles contributing to the rounded contour of the calf. The roof of the diamond-shaped fossa bulges distinctly when the leg is fully extended due to the underlying fat and fascia.

# LOCATING BONY LANDMARKS

- Patella: apex, base, borders, anterior surface
- Tibial condyles and tuberosity
- Femoral condyles, adductor tubercle
- Fibular head

## PATELLA

The bony features that may be palpated around the knee are illustrated on the skeleton in Figure 8.4. With the subject lying supine, the knee extended and the quadriceps relaxed, the borders of the patella can be defined and its medio-lateral mobility tested (Fig. 8.5) by gripping it between the fingers and thumb. Continuing the grip on the patella and asking the subject to tense the quadriceps allow lateral tracking of the patella, to be assessed as it stabilizes. With the quadriceps relaxed, the following structures can be palpated, working distally in the midline: **base of patella, anterior subcutaneous surface, apex**, and **tibial tuberosity** (Fig. 8.1). Palpation of the **patellar apex** is facilitated by diverging the thumb and index finger and spreading them across the base of the patella, pressing it firmly backward. This displaces the patella and tilts the apex forward (Fig. 8.6).

## TIBIAL CONDYLES/TUBEROSITY AND FEMORAL CONDYLES

From the tibial tuberosity, using firm palpation and moving the finger tip upward and medially (or laterally) for 2 cm will locate the **anterior border of the tibial condyle.**

With the knee flexed to about 90° and the finger tips pointing firmly backward in the recess either side of the patellar ligament, the **distal surface of the femoral condyles** (Fig. 8.7) can be palpated. Repeating this maneuver but pointing the fingers downward either side of the patellar ligament locates the **upper surface of the tibial condyles** with the overlying menisci (Fig. 8.8).

## HEAD OF THE FIBULA

To palpate the head of the fibula, the pads of the index and middle fingers are moved firmly upward along the lateral border of the leg toward the knee. Near the knee, the soft tissues give way to the bony head of the fibula (Fig. 8.9). Its characteristic rounded shape is confirmed by rolling the finger tips over it.

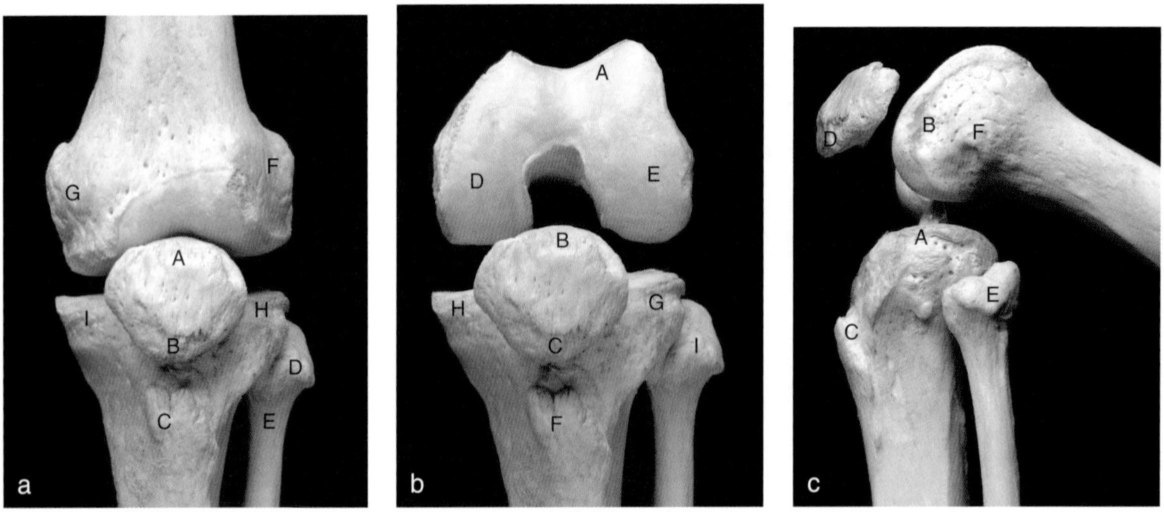


Fig. 8.4a Bony points of the extended knee skeleton from anterior
A = base of patella, B = patellar apex, C = tibial tuberosity, D = head of fibula, E = neck of fibula, F = lateral femoral condyle, G = medial femoral condyle, H = lateral tibial condyle, I = medial tibial condyle
Fig. 8.4b Bony points of the flexed knee skeleton from anterior
A = trochlear surface of femur, B = patellar base, C = patellar apex, D = medial femoral condyle, E = lateral femoral condyle, F = tibial tuberosity, G = lateral tibial condyle, H = medial tibial condyle, I = head of fibula
Fig. 8.4c Bony points of the flexed knee skeleton from lateral
A = lateral tibial condyle, B = lateral femoral condyle, C = tibial tubercle, D = apex of patella, E = head of fibula, F = lateral epicondyle

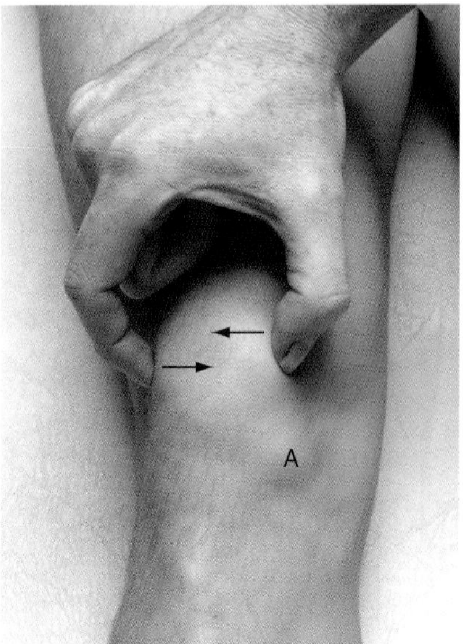


Fig. 8.5 Testing medio-lateral mobility of the patella
A = bulge of infra-patellar fat pad

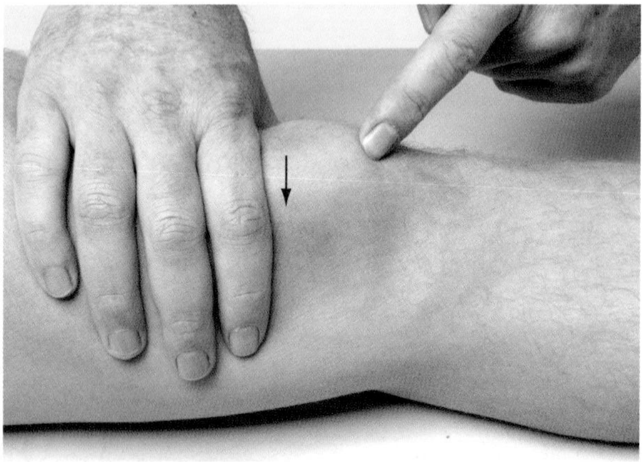

Fig. 8.6 Palpating the apex of the patella

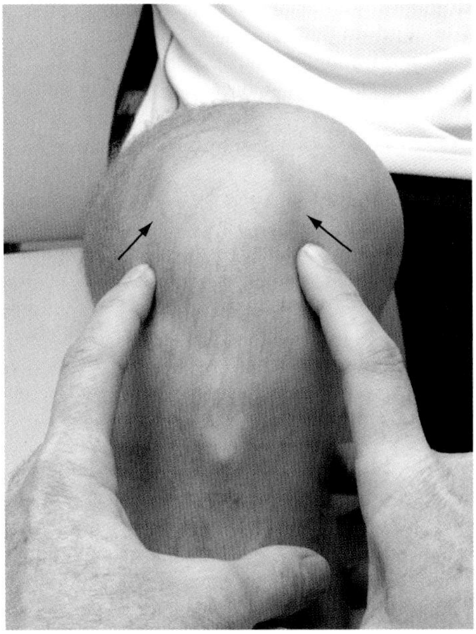

Fig. 8.7 Palpating the distal articular surface of the femoral condyles with the knee flexed

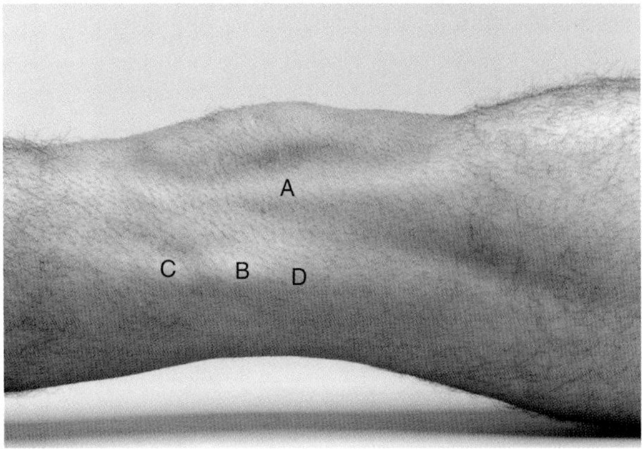


Fig. 8.9 Surface features of the knee and upper leg from the lateral side
A = ilio-tibial tract, B = head of fibula, C = fibula neck, D = location of lateral collateral ligament

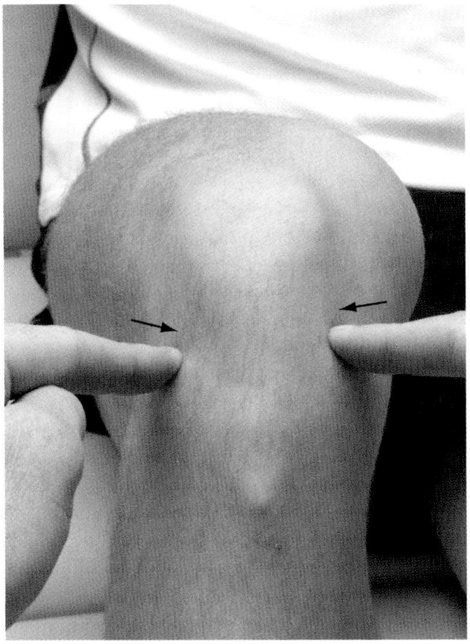

Fig. 8.8 Palpating the tibial condyles and menisci with the knee flexed

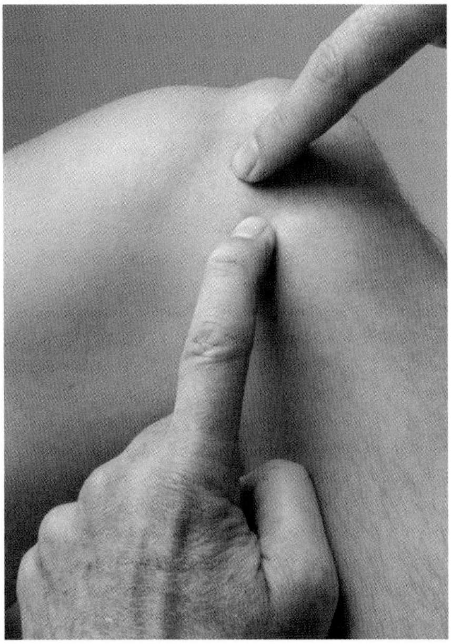

Fig. 8.10 Palpating the knee from the medial side
The lower finger lies in the groove of the joint line and the upper palpates the medial femoral condyle

Palpating progressively down the medial side of the lower thigh toward the knee, the first conspicuous bony point located is the **adductor tubercle**, which lies immediately above a large bony prominence, the **medial femoral condyle**, the full extent of which can be gauged by the fingers using a massaging motion over it (Fig. 8.10). Below the condyle lies a palpable groove which marks the joint line, and below this the fingers can palpate a large triangular bony area which is the **medial tibial condyle** (Fig. 8.10).

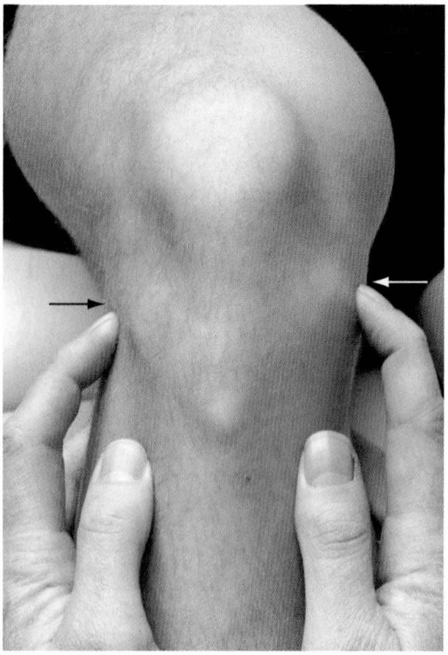

Fig. 8.11 Palpating the joint line

## LOCATING THE KNEE JOINT LINE

The joint line passes horizontally between the femoral and tibial condyles. It is best located with the knee flexed to 90°. Starting below the knee and working upward along the medial or lateral side whilst using firm palpation, the fingers are moved across the tibial condyle until a distinct groove is located between the femoral and tibial condyles (Fig. 8.11). Keeping the fingers in the groove whilst grasping the leg and passively flexing and extending the knee confirms that the groove is the joint line.

## LOCATING SOFT TISSUES

- Quadriceps tendon
- Patellar ligament
- Patellar retinacula
- Quadriceps femoris
- Ilio-tibial tract
- Collateral ligaments
- Infra-patellar fat pad
- Popliteal artery
- Supra-patellar bursa

### QUADRICEPS TENDON

The subject lies supine with legs extended and muscles relaxed. The palpating finger is placed horizontally across the thigh immediately above the base of the patella and the subject asked to tense the quadriceps. The quadriceps tendon (Fig. 8.1) can be felt to tighten. Whilst the **quadriceps femoris** is contracting, continued palpation proximally along the line of the quadriceps tendon leads to the prominence of the **rectus femoris.** The **vastus medialis** and **lateralis** are also easily palpable and form distinctive swellings on the respective sides of the lower thigh, the medialis appearing characteristically lower as it pulls on the medial border of the patella (Fig. 8.1).

### PATELLAR RETINACULA AND LIGAMENT

By using firm palpation with the flattened fingers along the infero-medial and infero-lateral borders of the patella, whilst asking the subject to tense the quadriceps, the **patellar retinacula** can be felt to tighten. Relocating the palpating finger across the leg below the apex of the patella and asking the subject to contract the quadriceps allow the tensed **patellar ligament** (Fig. 8.1) to be palpated. Keeping the leg fully extended, the subject is asked to raise the limb to approximately 45°.

### ILIO-TIBIAL TRACT

The anterior border of the ilio-tibial tract (Fig. 8.1) is clearly visible, and can be easily palpated approximately three finger-breadths postero-lateral to the lateral border of the patella, as it passes distally to attach to the lateral tibial condyle.

With the knee flexed to approximately 90°, the mid-point of the joint line is palpated exactly halfway around the knee, first on the medial and then on the lateral border (Fig. 8.11). To feel the collateral ligaments, the leg is grasped above the ankle, and whilst the joint is palpated, is passively extended to 180°. The **lateral collateral ligament** is the most easily located, and is felt as a strong rounded cord-like band (Fig. 8.12) over which the finger tip can be easily rolled, extending upward from the head of the fibula toward the femoral condyle. The **medial collateral ligament** is a much broader structure (Fig. 8.13) and less easily defined. It can be felt as a general tightening over the medial side of the joint line, as the movement of passive extension moves toward completion.

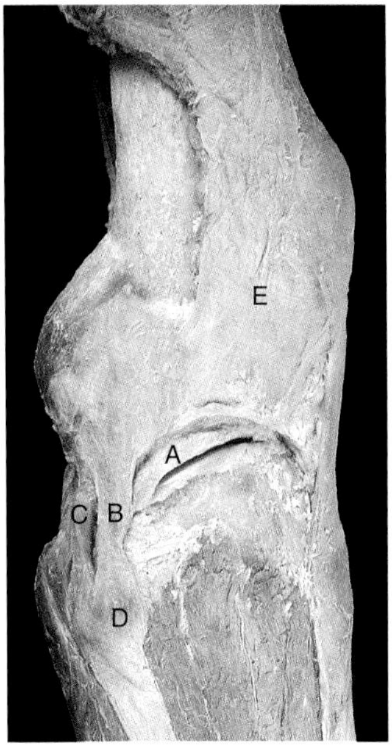


Fig. 8.12 Prosection of the knee joint from the lateral side A = meniscus, B = lateral collateral ligament, C = biceps femoris, D = head of fibula, E = retinaculum (From Gosling JA, Harris PF, Whitmore I, Willan PLT. 2002 Human Anatomy, 4th edn. London: Mosby)

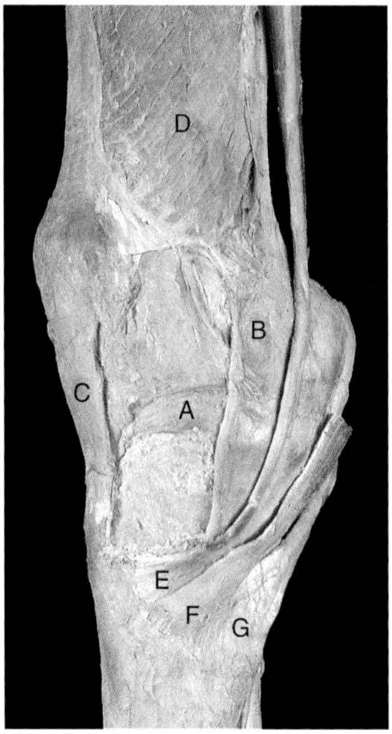


Fig. 8.13 Prosection of the knee joint from the medial side A = meniscus, B = medial collateral ligament, C = patellar ligament, D = vastus medialis, E = sartorius, F = gracilis, G = semitendinosus (From Gosling JA, Harris PF, Whitmore I, Willan PLT. 2002 Human Anatomy, 4th edn. London: Mosby)

## INFRA-PATELLAR FAT PAD

To locate the position of the infra-patellar fat pad (Fig. 8.14), the subject lies supine, with the knee flexed to approximately 90° and the foot flat on the couch. The examiner locates the patellar ligament, and with a finger tip on either the medial or lateral side of the ligament, applies firm pressure horizontally behind it (Fig. 8.15). The fat cannot normally be felt but, when damaged, is tender to palpation. Its presence may also be indicated by a soft tissue fullness on one or both sides of the patellar ligament.

## POPLITEAL ARTERY

Because the popliteal artery lies deeply in the popliteal fossa, it is not easily palpated. If the subject sits cross-legged on a couch or chair, with the point of the lower knee impinging into the back of the overlying knee, slight rhythmical forward movement of the overlying leg may be visible which synchronizes with the pulse. Alternatively, the subject lies prone on the couch and the leg is passively supported at 90° by the examiner. With the fingers of one or both hands, firm pressure is applied deeply over the lower part of the popliteal fossa in an attempt to compress the artery against the upper part of the tibia, where the artery lies on the popliteus muscle.

## SUPRA-PATELLAR BURSA

With the subject lying supine and the leg fully extended, the examiner places all the outstretched fingers of the examining hand across the front of the subject's thigh, immediately above the base of the patella. The upper limit of the suprapatellar bursa (pouch) is marked by the upper border of the hand. At the level of the upper border of the patella, the bursa is continuous behind the patella with the main synovial cavity of the knee joint (Fig. 8.14a).

# TESTING JOINT MOVEMENTS

- Flexion
- Extension

The knee is essentially a hinge joint, whose principal movements are **flexion** and **extension** over a range of 135° (Fig. 8.16). Passive movement can be tested with

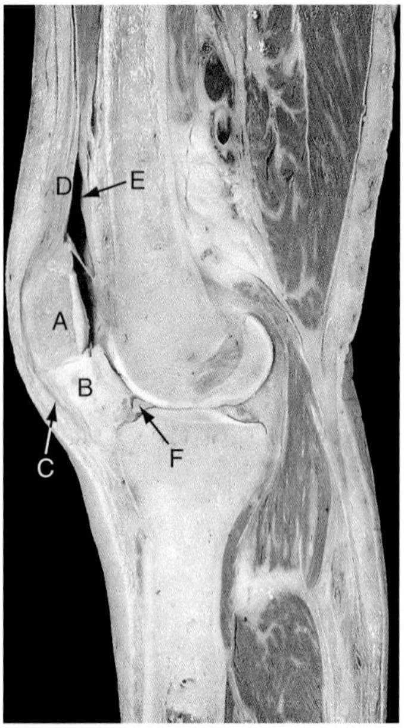


Fig. 8.14a Sagittal section through a prosection of the knee joint
A = patella, B = infra-patellar fat pad, C = patellar ligament, D = quadriceps tendon, E = suprapatellar pouch, F = meniscus (From Gosling JA, Harris PF, Whitmore I, Willan PLT. 2002 Human Anatomy, 4th edn. London: Mosby)

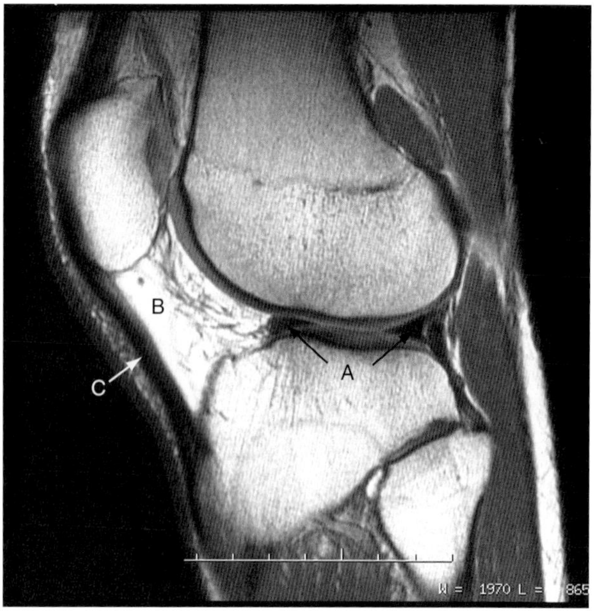


Fig. 8.14b MRI sagittal scan of knee joint
A = meniscus, B = infra-patellar fat pad, C = patellar ligament

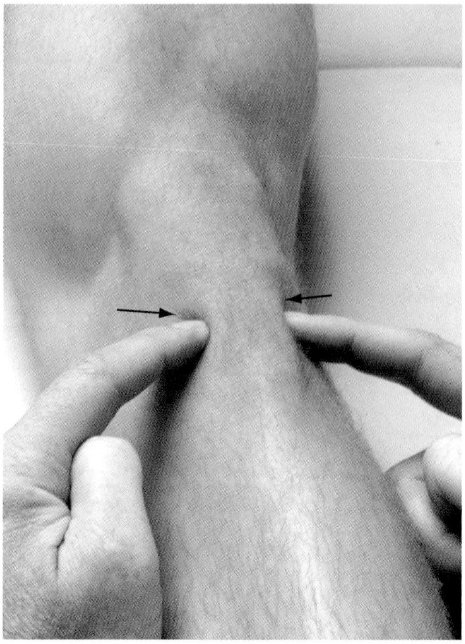

Fig. 8.15 Palpating the infra-patellar fat pad

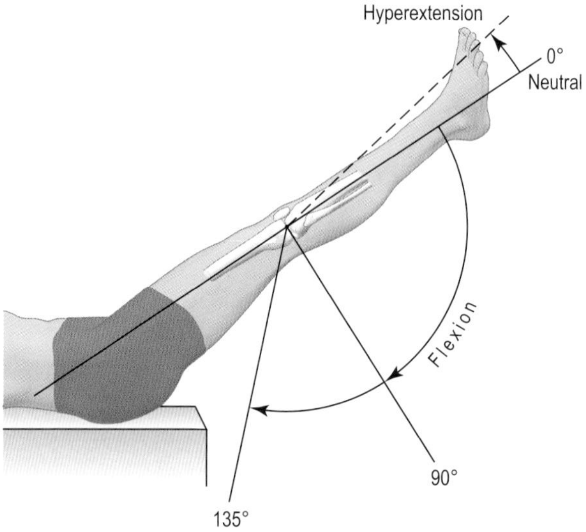


Fig. 8.16 Diagram showing the range of movement in the knee joint
Redrawn from *Joint motion: method of measuring and recording.* Edinburgh: E&S Livingstone, 1965 (with the permission of the American Academy of Orthopedic Surgeons, reprinted with their permission by the British Orthopaedic Association)

the subject lying supine, by grasping the leg above the ankle and flexing and extending it on the thigh. During termination of extension, a small amount of medial rotation of the femur on the tibia may be observed. Conversely, as flexion commences, this is accompanied by a limited amount of lateral rotation. If the subject is seated with the knee flexed over the edge of the couch and leg dependent, the examiner can test rotation by grasping the foot firmly and passively rotating it medially or laterally.

# TESTING MUSCLES

- Quadriceps femoris
- Hamstrings

## QUADRICEPS FEMORIS

The quadriceps femoris is the principal extensor of the knee. The subject sits with the knees bent to 90° over the edge of the couch or chair. The examiner applies firm pressure over the front of the distal part of the leg, resisting attempts to extend it. At the same time, a hand placed across the front of the mid-thigh palpates the tightening quadriceps.

## HAMSTRINGS

The hamstrings are the principal flexors of the knee. The subject lies prone on the couch, with the leg flexed to about 30°. The examiner firmly grips the posterior aspect of the leg just above the ankle and resists attempts to flex the joint further. The tightened hamstring tendons can be seen outlining the upper part of the popliteal fossa (Fig. 8.3), and a hand placed across the mid-thigh confirms contraction of the hamstrings as the joint is flexed.

# TESTING REFLEXES

## QUADRICEPS REFLEX (KNEE JERK)

Cord segments and nerve roots involved are L3 and L4. The subject is seated on a chair, thighs crossed, with one knee flexed to 90° and lying in front of the supporting knee. The examiner locates the patellar ligament and percusses it directly with a tendon hammer. Alternatively, the subject sits on the examination couch with knees projecting over the edge and legs lying dependent at 90°. The patellar ligament is located and percussed with the tendon hammer.

# SPECIAL TESTS

- Effusion:
  Wipe test
  Patellar tap
- Patellar tracking
- Infra-patellar fat pad
- Cruciate ligaments:
  Anterior cruciate ligament: Lachman's test
  Posterior cruciate ligament: 90/90 sag test
- Collateral ligaments:
  Medial collateral ligament: valgus stress
  Lateral collateral ligament: varus stress
- Menisci:
  Palpation
  McMurray test

## EFFUSION

Two tests are available, depending on the size of the effusion.

### WIPE TEST

This can be used to detect small effusions. The subject lies supine, with the knee fully extended and the muscles relaxed. The palmar surfaces of the examiner's fingers are placed on the lower antero-medial surface of the knee and moved firmly and progressively upward along the medial border of the patella (Fig. 8.17a). Any intra-articular fluid will be flushed into the supra-patellar pouch. The fluid in the supra-patellar pouch can then be returned to the knee joint by brushing the dorsal surface of the fingers distally along the lateral side of the knee down to the level of the joint line (Fig. 8.17b). The presence of an effusion will be confirmed by visible refilling of the fossa medial to the patella.

### PATELLAR TAP

This can be used to detect medium or larger effusions. The subject lies supine, with the knee fully extended and the muscles relaxed. The thumb and fingers of one hand are arched across the front of the thigh about a hand's breadth above the base of the patella. Whilst applying firm back-

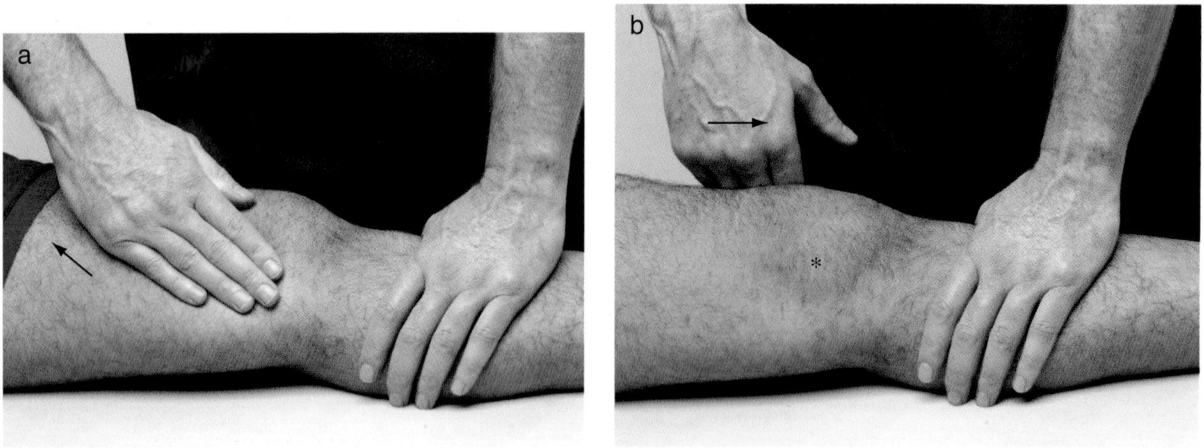


Fig. 8.17a and b Wipe test for knee joint effusion
* = effusion

ward pressure against the thigh, the hand slides slowly down the thigh to reach the patella. Observation is made for fullness appearing on either side of the patella. The index finger or thumb of the free hand is placed on the anterior surface of the patella, which is then pushed firmly backward on to the femur (Fig. 8.18). If excessive fluid is present, the "floating" patella is felt to move backward and suddenly impact against the femur.

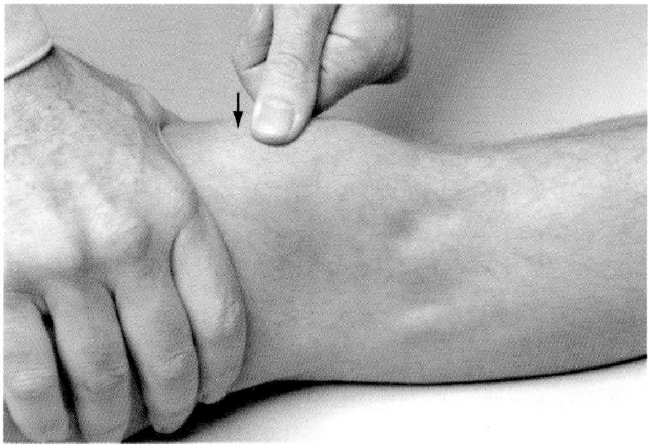

Fig. 8.18 Patellar tap test for knee joint effusion

## ABNORMAL PATELLAR TRACKING

### APPREHENSION TEST

The subject lies supine with the knee fully extended and relaxed. The examiner uses a thumb to glide and hold the patella in a lateral position (Fig. 8.19). The subject is then told to flex the knee; if the patella is abnormal, it tries to sublux laterally, causing discomfort and apprehension.

## INFRA-PATELLAR FAT PAD

The subject lies supine, with the knee flexed between 70 and 90°, thigh relaxed and foot flat on the couch. Using the tip of the index finger, the examiner directs palpation postero-medially or postero-laterally either side of the patellar ligament, inclining the finger toward the deep aspect of the ligament (Fig. 8.15).

## KNEE LIGAMENT TESTING

There are two groups of ligaments: cruciate (Fig. 8.20) and collateral (Figs 8.12 and 8.13).

### CRUCIATE LIGAMENTS

The cruciate ligaments lie deeply within the capsule, being invested by a posterior invagination of synovial membrane into the joint cavity. Their relative positions are shown in the MRI scan in Figure 8.20.

#### *Anterior cruciate ligament (ACL)*

For **Lachman's test for the integrity of the ACL,** the subject lies supine, with the examiner's knee over the edge of the couch supporting the back of the subject's knee in approximately 20° of flexion. The examiner's palm is used to stabilize the distal femur above the patella. If possible, the thumb and forefinger are used to palpate the lateral and medial joint line throughout the maneuver. The

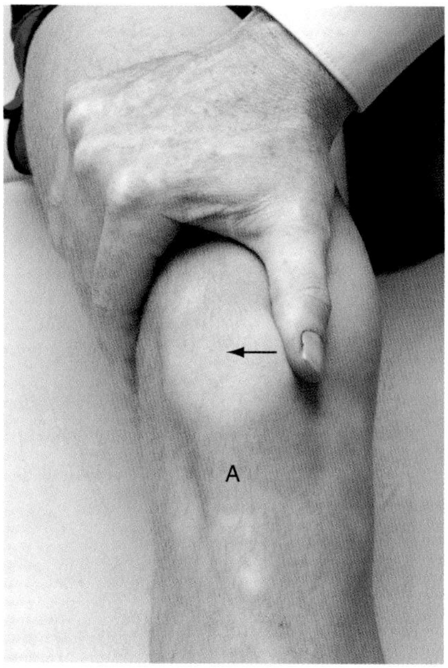


Fig. 8.19 Patellar apprehension test
A = patellar ligament

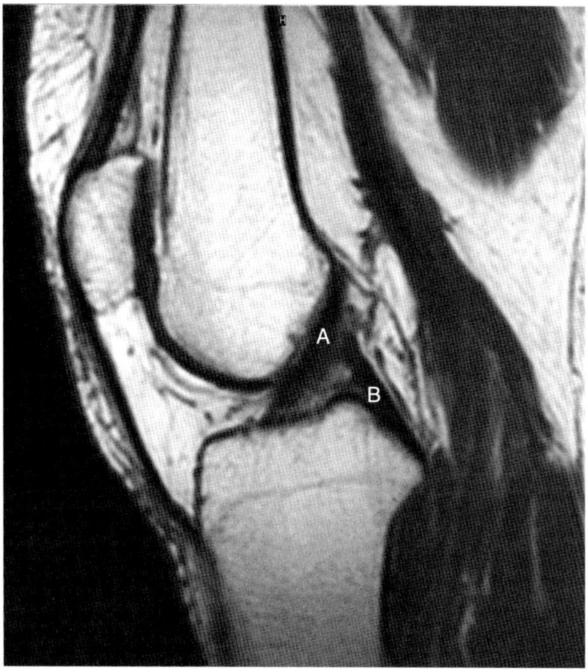


Fig. 8.20 MRI scan of the knee joint showing the location of the cruciate ligaments
A = anterior cruciate ligament, B = posterior cruciate ligament

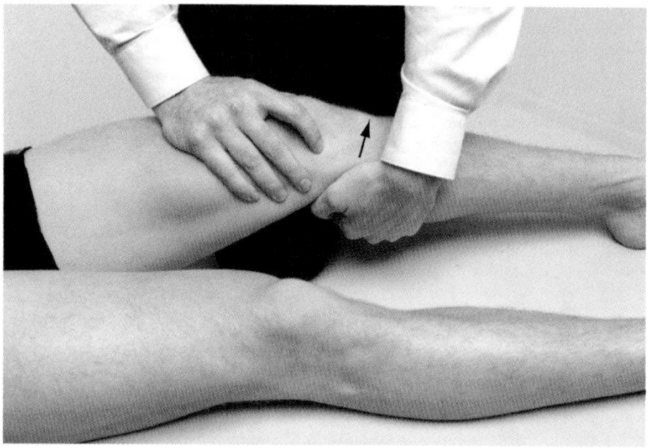

Fig. 8.21 Lachman's test for a tear of the anterior cruciate ligament

opposite hand grips the proximal end of the tibia from behind. Maintaining an extended elbow, the examiner attempts to pull the proximal end of the tibia forward on the distal end of the femur (Fig. 8.21). The degree of anterior translation of the tibia can be visualized and palpated by the thumb and forefinger of the other hand, and is compared to the uninjured knee. The lack of an "end feel," or a soft "end point" with a large anterior tibial translation, indicates rupture of the ACL.

Additionally, the **pivot-shift** and **anterior drawer** tests may be used to test the integrity of the ACL. These are demonstrated on the accompanying DVD.

### *Posterior cruciate ligament (PCL)*

For the **90/90 sag test,** the subject lies supine, with both hips and knees flexed to 90° and supported in this position by the examiner's forearm, which is placed under both legs. The examiner views the knees in profile, side-on (Fig. 8.22). Rupture or a significant tear of the PCL is indicated by the posterior displacement (sag sign) of the tibial tuberosity of the affected leg.

The **posterior drawer test** may also be used to assess the PCL. This is demonstrated on the accompanying DVD.

## COLLATERAL LIGAMENTS

### *Medial collateral ligament (MCL)*

For the **valgus stress test,** the subject lies supine. Placed over the edge of the couch, the examiner's knee supports the subject's knee in 20° flexion. The examiner cradles the leg with a forearm placed along its medial side, and palpates the medial joint line with the forefinger of that hand.

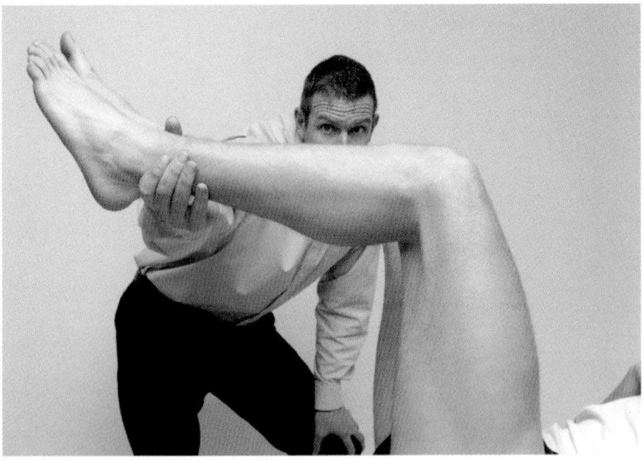

Fig. 8.22 90/90 Sag test for a tear of the posterior cruciate ligament

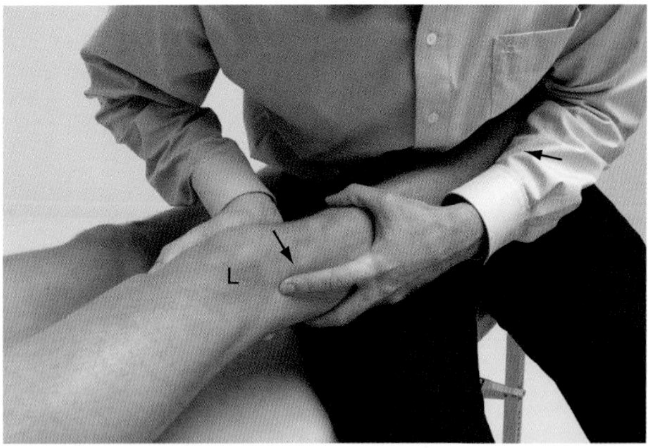


Fig. 8.24 Varus stress test for a tear of the lateral collateral ligament with the knee in 20° of flexion
L = vastus lateralis

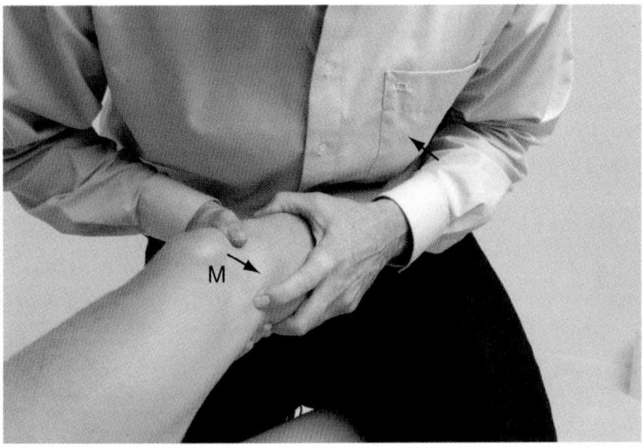


Fig. 8.23 Valgus stress test for a tear of the medial collateral ligament
M = vastus medialis

The examiner's other hand is used to apply a valgus force at right angles to the lateral side of the knee (Fig. 8.23). The degree of laxity and the presence or absence of an "end feel" to the MCL can be appreciated by palpating the degree of abnormal widening of the joint line on the medial side.

### *Lateral collateral ligament (LCL)*

The **varus stress test** is conducted in a similar manner to that for the MCL, except that the examiner's hand positions are reversed. A varus force is applied at right angles to the subject's knee, with the forefinger of the examiner's other hand palpating to detect any abnormal widening of the joint line on the lateral side (Fig. 8.24).

## MENISCI

### PALPATION

Direct palpation over the joint line at its midpoint on the medial side of the knee may reveal tenderness, since the medial meniscus is attached to the medial collateral ligament. With the subject supine, knee flexed to 70–90°, and foot flat on the couch, firm backward pressure with the tip of a finger or thumb directed toward the tibial condyles either side of the patellar ligament may elicit tenderness (Fig. 8.8).

### MCMURRAY'S TEST

To test for a tear of the medial meniscus, the examiner grips the leg above the ankle, flexing the hip and knee and applying a slight varus force on the knee in the fully flexed position (Fig. 8.25a). Examiners with small hands may prefer to grip the heel of the subject's foot, with the sole of the foot lying along their own forearm. Using the other hand to steady the knee and palpate the joint line, the examiner slowly extends the knee whilst laterally rotating the leg (Fig. 8.25b). A click in the knee that may be associated with pain indicates a positive test. The lateral meniscus is tested via a similar maneuver, except that the knee is first flexed with a slight valgus stress (Fig. 8.25c) and then extended as the leg is medially rotated (Fig. 8.25d).

Additionally, **Apley's test (anvil)** may be used to detect meniscal tears. This is demonstrated in the accompanying DVD.

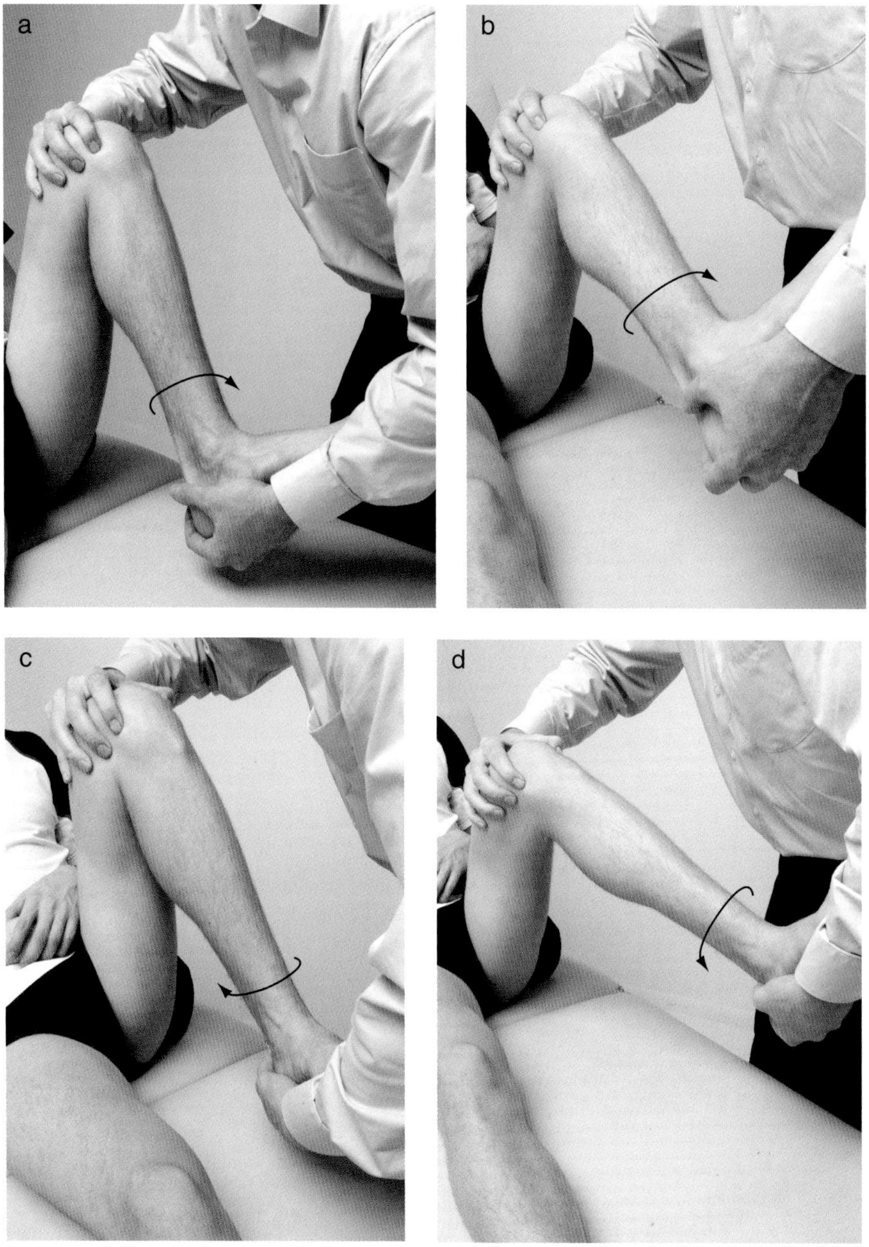


Fig. 8.25 McMurray test for a meniscal tear; **a and b** Medial meniscus, **c and d** Lateral meniscus

## FURTHER READING

Beynnon BD, Johnson RJ, Fleming BC. The science of anterior cruciate ligament rehabilitation. Clinical Orthopaedics and Related Research 2002; 402:9–20.

Boyd CR, Eakin C, Matheson GO. Infrapatellar plica as a cause of anterior knee pain. Clinical Journal of Sport Medicine 2005; 15:98–102.

Fulkerson J. Diagnosis and treatment of patients with patellofemoral pain. American Journal of Sports Medicine 2002; 30:447–456.

Kocabey Y, Tetic O, Isbell WM et al. The value of clinical examination versus magnetic resonance imaging in the diagnosis of meniscal tears and anterior cruciate ligament damage. Journal of Arthroscopic and Related Surgery 2004; 20:696–700.

Radhakrishna M, Macdonald P, Davidson M et al. Isolated popliteus injury in a professional football player. Clinical Journal of Sport Medicine 2004; 14:365–367.

Sims WF, Jacobson K. The posteromedial corner of the knee. American Journal of Sports Medicine 2004; 32:337–345.

## CASE STUDY 8 • CLINICAL PROBLEMS

**Problem 1.** *Three days ago, a 20-year-old female basketball player was attempting to avoid an opponent whilst dribbling the ball. As she was pushing off from the right leg, she felt a "popping" sensation in her knee. It was not particularly painful at the time but she was unable to carry on, as she felt the knee would "give way" if she tried to run. Within an hour the knee was very swollen.*

a) What is the most likely diagnosis?
b) Which is the most important manual test that should be performed on the structure labeled "A" in Figure 8.20?
c) What associated structures could also be damaged?
d) What manual tests are most appropriate for these structures?

**Problem 2.** *A 15-year-old male high jumper complains of 6 months of intermittent, superficial, anterior knee pain when running and jumping. It is relieved with ice and rest. The knee does not swell. A Doppler ultrasound scan is performed* (Fig. 8.26a and b).

a) What are three possible diagnoses?
b) What structures should be palpated?
c) Which muscle group should be tested?

**Problem 3.** *A 30-year-old soccer player is tackled from the side. His opponent's boot strikes the upper lateral tibia, forcing the knee into a valgus position. The player feels a tearing sensation in the medial knee.*

a) What is the most likely structure to have been damaged?
b) What other structures could have been damaged with this mechanism of injury?
c) A small knee effusion develops gradually over the 12 hours following the injury. What test should be used to identify this sign and what is the significance of this finding?

**Problem 4.** *A handball player notices a large ball-shaped swelling on the top of his kneecap following a match. He recalls falling heavily on to that knee during the match.*

a) What could cause this type of swelling?
b) Housemaid's knee is the common name given to which knee condition?

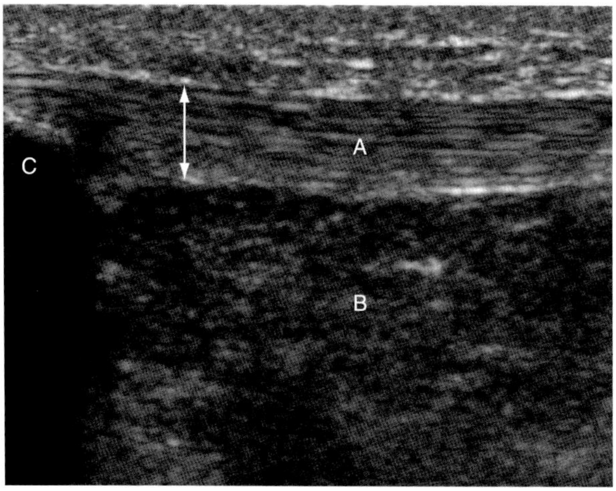


Fig. 8.26a Doppler ultrasound scan of the knee: normal
A = patellar ligament, B = fat pad, C = patella

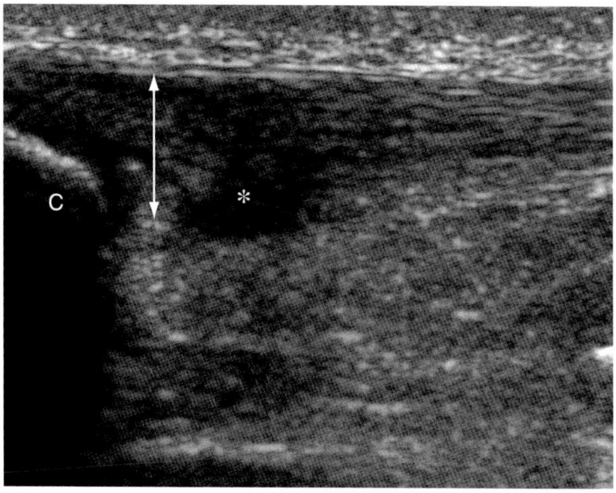


Fig. 8.26b Doppler ultrasound scan of the knee: tendinosis (*)
C = patella

## CASE STUDY 8 • CLINICAL PROBLEMS—cont'd

**Problem 5.** *A 19-year-old female volleyball player complains of a deep ache in the anterior knee that is aggravated by sitting in the car when returning from matches and training. She also has difficulty climbing steps. There is no knee effusion.*

a) What is a likely cause of this athlete's anterior knee pain?
b) What manual test should be performed?

**Problem 6.** *A 37-year-old rugby forward twists his knee whilst pushing in a scrum. He complains of a painful clicking in the lateral knee after the injury, and a day later, wakes up with a moderate knee effusion.*

a) What structure is most likely to have been damaged?
b) During performance of the McMurray's test, in which direction should the tibia be rotated in order to test the lateral meniscus?
c) What treatment is this player likely to require?

**Problem 7.**

a) Which muscles underlie the operation scar shown in Figure 8.27?

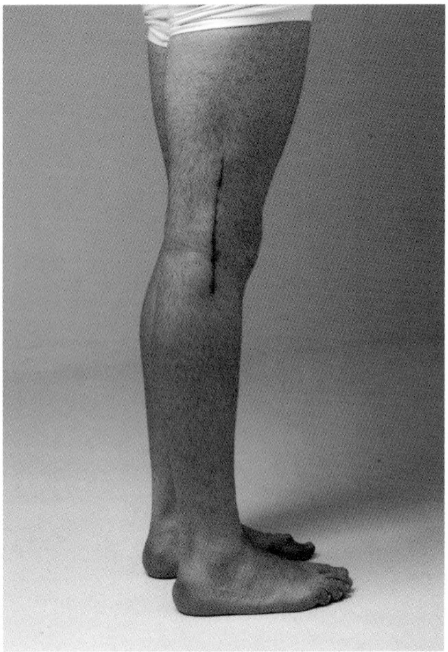

Fig. 8.27 Operation wound on the leg

CHAPTER 9

# Leg and ankle

## INTRODUCTION

The leg is the middle segment in the lever system of the lower limb. Connected by the interosseous membrane, two long bones, the tibia medially and the fibula laterally, together form its core. The tibia is the more significant, being larger, and has the major role in terms of muscle attachments and taking stresses and forces acting on the leg during weight-bearing and locomotion. It is also more superficial for much of its length. For these reasons, it is more vulnerable to injury.

The leg has three muscle compartments enclosed by thick, unyielding deep fascia. The anterior compartment contains the dorsiflexors, which raise the foot during locomotion. The lateral compartment is the smallest and encloses the evertors of the foot. The posterior compartment is much the largest, and includes the substantial gastrocnemius–soleus group, which are strong anti-gravity muscles and are important in stepping, running, and jumping. They also play a big part in the pump mechanism of venous return from the lower limb.

Distally, the ankle lies in a crucial position in the lever system of the lower limb, providing both stability and support for the leg, as well as allowing movement of the foot in its basic roles of weight-bearing and locomotion. Both sides of the ankle are superficial, making this part of the joint accessible for examination but also vulnerable. The front and back of the ankle are less accessible, being crossed by long tendons entering the dorsal and plantar aspects of the foot.

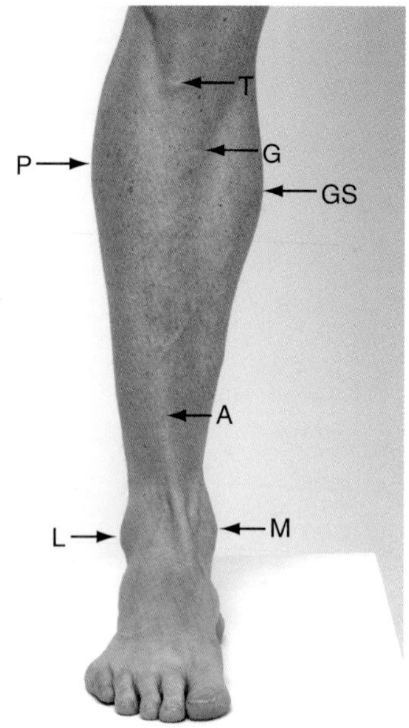


**Fig. 9.1** Frontal view of the leg, ankle, and foot
Note the relative levels of the malleoli. A = anterior subcutaneous border of tibia, G = groove marking anteromedial border of tibia, GS = gastrocnemius–soleus muscles, L = lateral malleolus, M = medial malleolus, P = peroneal muscles, T = tibial tubercle

## INSPECTION OF NORMAL CONTOURS

- Tibia
- Peroneal muscles
- Calf muscles:
  Gastrocnemius
  Soleus
- Malleoli
- Long saphenous vein
- Foot: long tendons
- Achilles tendon
- Calcaneum
- Heel pad

Viewed from anteriorly, an indistinct ridge, the anterior subcutaneous border of the **tibia,** may be seen extending from the tibial tuberosity downward in the midline. If visible, it is evident only in the upper two-thirds of the leg. The lateral profile forms a slight outward curve, especially in the proximal part of the leg, and this is due to the underlying **peroneal muscles.** The medial profile is more obvious, especially in the upper half of the leg, appearing as a distinct convex bulge, which is due to the underlying bulk of the **calf muscles.** The profiles converge into the lower, narrower part of the leg, where the muscles give way to their tendons descending toward the ankle.

On each side of the ankle, the characteristic bony prominences of the **malleoli** are clearly visible, the lateral being more distal and posterior compared with the more proximal and anterior medial malleolus (Fig. 9.1). The **long saphenous vein** may be visible as it passes subcutaneously immediately in front of the medial malleolus. With the foot in a neutral position or only slightly dorsiflexed, the **long tendons** crossing the joint may be visible as longitudinal ridges, the most medial being the inner border of the tibialis anterior tendon, and the most lateral the outer border of the extensor digitorum longus tendon.

Viewed from posteriorly in the upper part of the leg, the two heads of the **gastrocnemius** form indistinct bulges continuing from the infero-lateral and infero-medial borders of the popliteal fossa, as the bulging roof gives way to a slight depression between the two heads. Below the fossa, the prominent fullness of the **calf** indicates the union of the two heads of gastrocnemius with the underlying **soleus.**

The convex curvature of the calf occupies the upper half of the leg and is slightly asymmetrical, since the medial head of the gastrocnemius is somewhat larger than the lateral and extends more distally. This is particularly shown when standing on tip-toes (Fig. 9.2).

The leg tapers considerably toward the ankle, as the calf muscles give way to the well-defined midline **Achilles tendon,** which is several centimeters in length. On each side of the tendon are hollows, one lying behind each malleolus; their asymmetry in respect to the profile of the

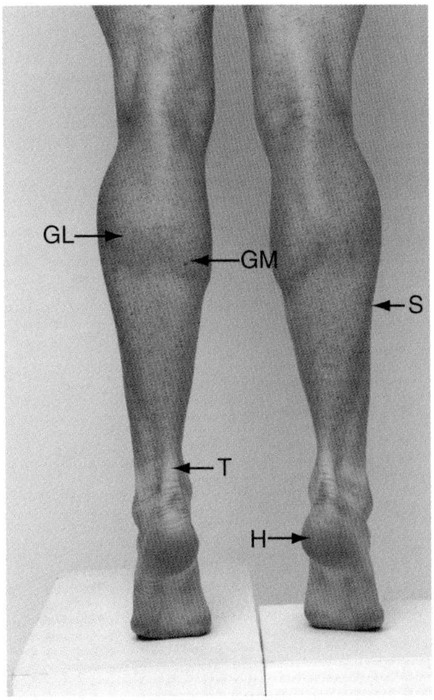


Fig. 9.2 Posterior view of the superficial calf muscles with the subject standing on tip-toes
GL = lateral head of gastrocnemius, GM = medial head of gastrocnemius, H = heel fat pad, S = soleus, T = Achilles tendon

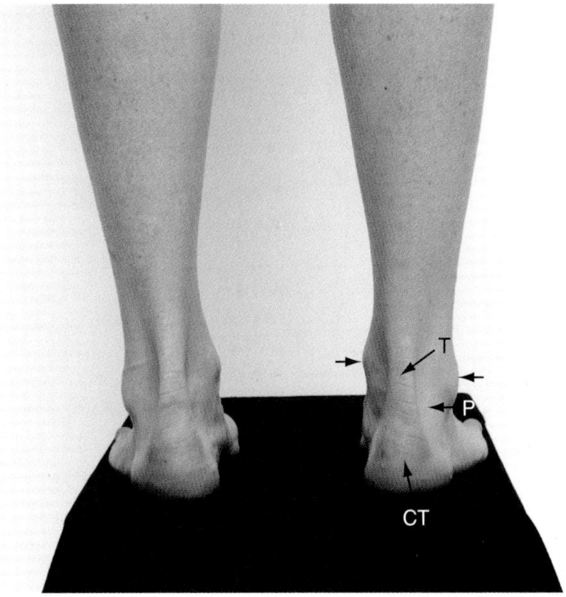


Fig. 9.3 Posterior standing view to show alignment of the ankles, heels, and feet
Note the relative levels of the malleoli (small arrows)
CT = calcaneal tuberosity, P = location of tendons of peronei, T = Achilles tendon

ankle is clearly visible, as already described. Following the Achilles tendon toward the back of the heel, the profile broadens to the skin overlying the **calcaneum** and finally the weight-bearing **heel pad.** This is an important region to inspect from posteriorly. The subject stands with the feet slightly apart, facing away from the examiner (Fig. 9.3). Observation is made for any broadening of the heel, obliteration of the hollows below the malleoli, relative levels of the medial and lateral borders of the foot, and misalignment of the Achilles tendons indicating abnormal positioning of the feet.

## LOCATING BONY LANDMARKS

- Tibia:
  Tubercle
  Anterior border
  Antero-medial surface
  Medial border
  Medial malleolus
- Fibula:
  Head and styloid process
  Neck
  Distal lateral surface
  Lateral malleolus
- Talus:
  Posterior tubercle
  Superior/anterior surface
- Calcaneum:
  Posterior surface

The main features of the skeleton of the leg and ankle are shown in Figure 9.4.

### TIBIA

From anteriorly, the tibia is palpable along its entire length. Starting just below the knee in the midline of the leg, the **tibial tubercle** is easily located. With the tip of the index finger held close to that of the middle finger, the groove formed between them glides downward along the sharp **anterior border** of the tibia, inclining medially. In the lower third of the leg, the border becomes obscured

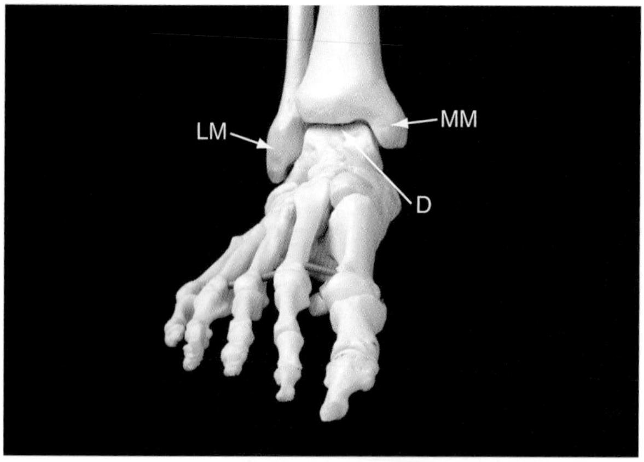


Fig. 9.4a–d Skeleton of the ankle and foot
a Frontal view. D = dome of talus, LM = lateral malleolus, MM = medial malleolus

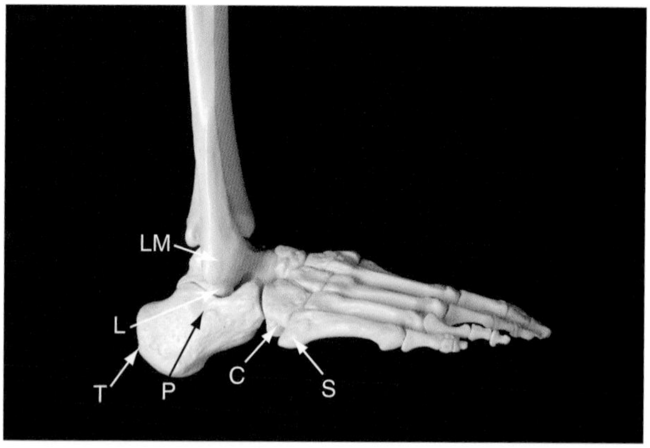


Fig. 9.4b Lateral view
C = cuboid, L = lateral process of talus, LM = lateral malleolus, P = peroneal tubercle, S = styloid process (base) of fifth metatarsal, T = calcaneal tuberosity

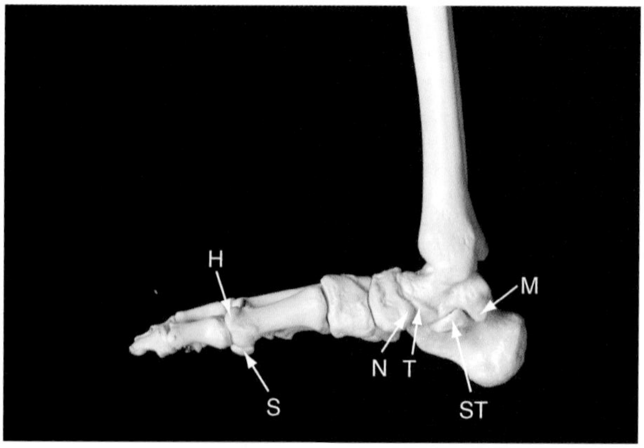


Fig. 9.4c Medial view
H = head of first metatarsal, M = medial process of talus, N = navicular tuberosity, S = sesamoid bone, ST = sustentaculum tali, T = head of talus

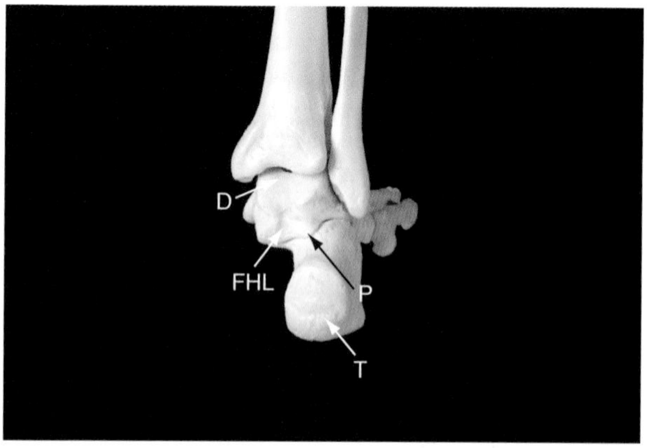


Fig. 9.4d Posterior view
D = dome of talus, FHL = groove for tendon of flexor hallucis longus, P = posterior tubercle of talus, T = calcaneal tuberosity

by the long tendons, as they descend to cross the ankle joint. The tips of the index, middle and ring fingers can be used to locate the diffuse subcutaneous anterior surface of the medial **tibial condyle** immediately below the joint line and, using firm palpation, guided distally along the wide subcutaneous **antero-medial surface** of the shaft (Fig. 9.5), terminating over the subcutaneous medial surface of the **malleolus.** The anterior border and tip of the medial malleolus are easily palpable, as is its posterior surface, which lies immediately in front of the hollow adjacent to the prominent Achilles tendon. Finally, returning to the upper part of the shaft, the **medial border** of the tibia (the site of pain and tenderness in conditions associated with medial tibial stress syndrome) can be palpated easily in the upper two-thirds of the leg by drawing the pad of the forefinger firmly down the groove marking the junction of the hard bone with the soft edge of the calf muscles.

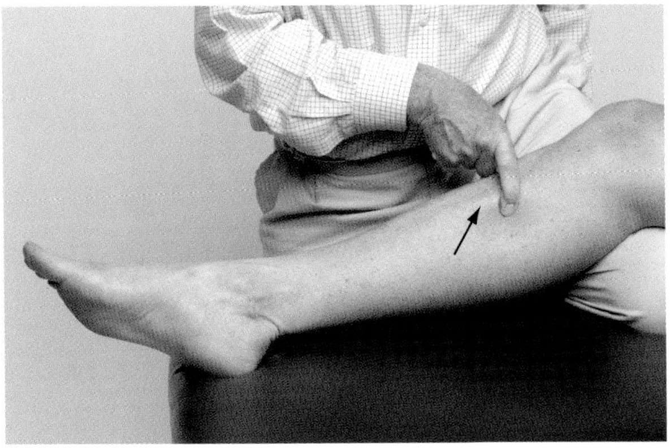

Fig. 9.5 Palpation of the antero-medial border of the tibia
The edge of the border is indicated by the small arrow

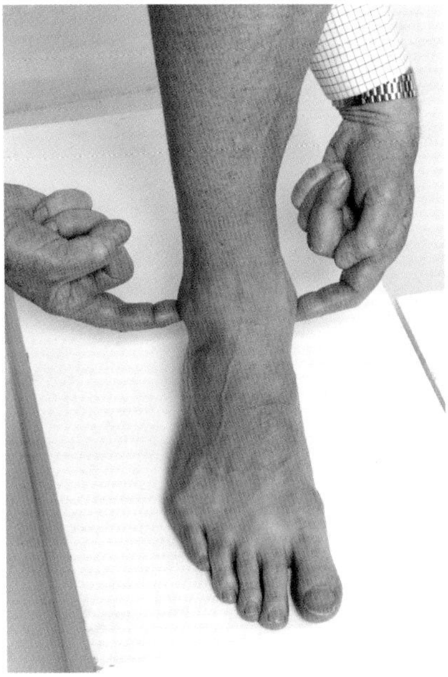

Fig. 9.6 Locating the tips of the malleoli

## FIBULA

Unlike the tibia, the fibula is not accessible for its whole length; only its upper and lower ends may be palpated. Starting distally, the outer subcutaneous surface of the **lateral malleolus,** smaller but more prominent than the medial, can be readily defined, as can its anterior border, tip, and posterior surface too. Using palpation to confirm their differences, the level of the tips of the malleoli should be compared, along with the relative positions of their anterior borders (Fig. 9.6). These differences have already been described. Maintaining palpation, the finger tips are moved firmly in a proximal direction off the malleolus and on to the small triangular subcutaneous surface of the lower end of the shaft of the fibula; the latter disappears, however, as palpation continues upward along the lateral border of the leg over the tendons and, more proximally, the softer muscle bellies of the peroneus longus and brevis. Palpation continuing upward and using firm, deep pressure as the knee is approached, the hard round prominence of the **head of the fibula** (Fig. 9.7) suddenly presents and can be gripped between finger and thumb. It tapers superiorly into the styloid process, marking the attachment of the lateral collateral ligament of the knee. If palpation is retraced downward from the head, a distinct depression can be felt below the head marking the position of the fibular neck and where the common peroneal nerve passes round it. Deep palpation here may cause pain, indicating that the nerve has been located.

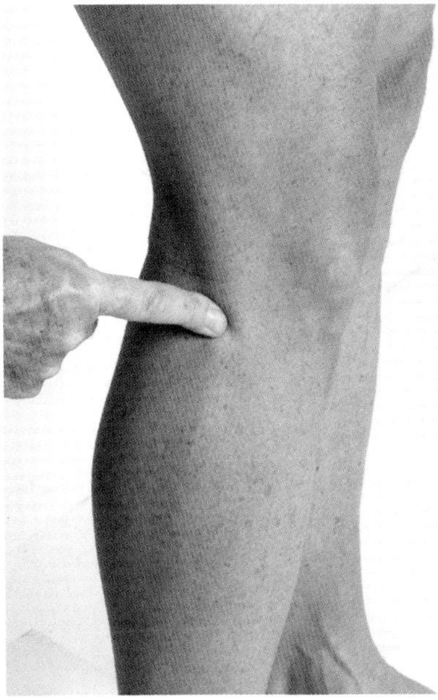

Fig. 9.7 Palpating the head of the fibula
The finger tip lies immediately above the head

## TALUS

With the subject lying prone, the knee flexed to 90° and the ankle held in dorsiflexion, the examiner's thumb can

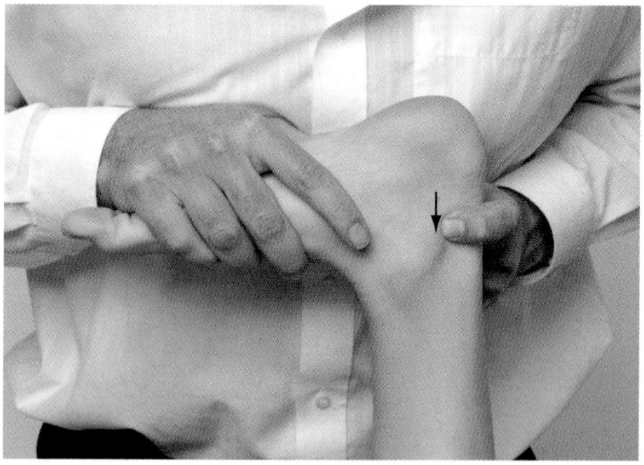

Fig. 9.8 Palpating the posterior talar tubercle
The arrow marks the underlying tubercle

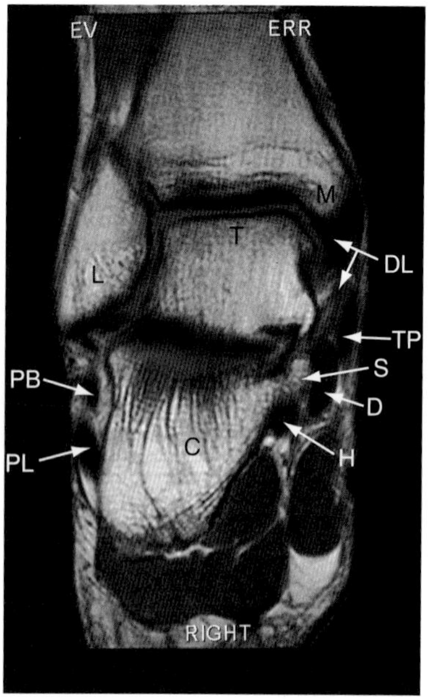


Fig. 9.9 MR coronal plane scan of an ankle
C = calcaneum, D = flexor digitorum longus tendon, DL = deltoid ligament, deep and superficial parts, H = flexor hallucis longus tendon, L = lateral malleolus, M = medial malleolus, PB = peroneus brevis, PL = peroneus longus, S = sustentaculum tali, T = dome of talus, TP = tibialis posterior

be used to palpate for a prominent **posterior talar tubercle (Steida's process)** in the depression lying anterior to the Achilles tendon, at the level of the tip of the medial malleolus (Fig. 9.8). There is considerable individual variation in the size of this tubercle and it is frequently implicated in posterior ankle impingement. Another structure that may be involved in posterior impingement, when present, is the os trigonum (a separated posterior tubercle). It can be palpated using the same method as for the posterior tubercle.

## CALCANEUM

Finally, returning to the most distal part of the posterior aspect of the leg at the heel, the subcutaneous surface of the calcaneum can be easily palpated on each side, and **immediately** adjacent to the point of attachment of the Achilles tendon.

# PALPATING THE ANKLE JOINT LINE

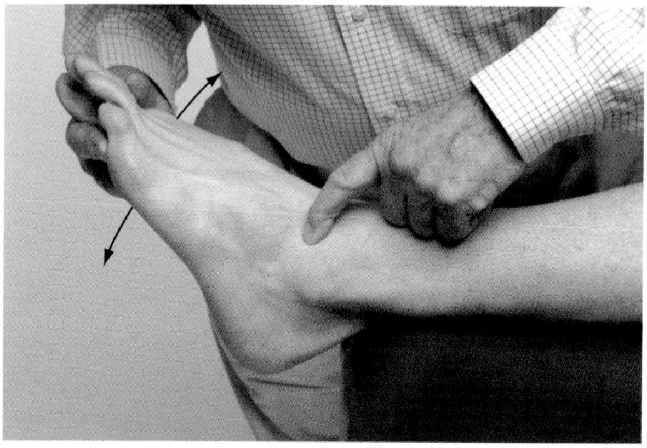

Fig. 9.10 Palpating the line of the ankle joint

The distal end of the tibia and the two malleoli form a mortise socket, into which the wedge-shaped dome of the talus closely fits. This arrangement is clearly seen on a frontal MRI scan of the ankle (Fig. 9.9).

The line of the ankle joint is not easy to define. It can be located dorsally (Fig. 9.10), although not completely. With the subject lying supine, the foot relaxed and lying at 90° to the leg, and with the examiner using deep pressure from above with the middle and index fingers, the lateral joint line can be located starting immediately in front of the lateral malleolus in the deep groove behind the soft tissues of the extensor digitorum brevis muscle. The anterior border of the lateral malleolus is first palpated and then, by moving the fingers medially, the

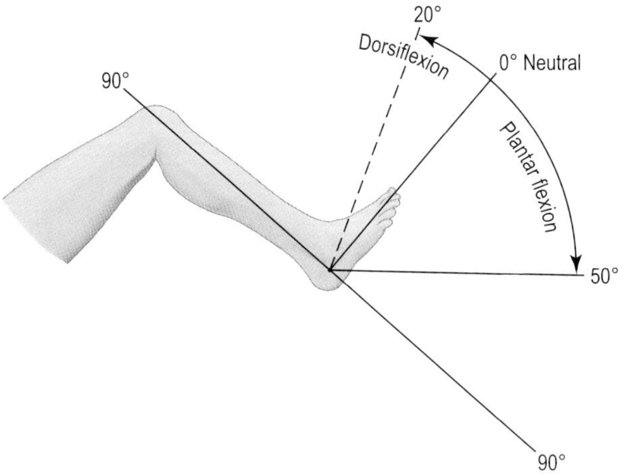


**Fig. 9.11** Range of movements at the ankle
Redrawn from *Joint motion: method of measuring and recording.* Edinburgh: E&S Livingstone, 1965 (with the permission of the American Academy of Orthopedic Surgeons, reprinted with their permission by the British Orthopaedic Association)

lower anterior margin of the tibia can be examined. Similarly, the examiner palpating medially with the tip of the index finger using firm pressure immediately in front of the malleolus, a deep groove lying at the edge of the distal surface of the tibia can be detected. The joint line is confirmed by passively dorsiflexing and plantar-flexing the foot. No other parts of the joint line can be defined due to the long tendons crossing the dorsum of the ankle. Additionally, with the subject lying supine, the feet hanging over the edge of the couch and the ankle in plantar flexion, both the **anterior border** at the **distal end of the tibia** and the **anterior superior** aspect of the **talus** can be palpated between the long tendons crossing the dorsum of the ankle. This area is a common site of anterior ankle impingement.

## RANGE OF MOVEMENTS

- Dorsiflexion
- Plantar flexion

The ankle joint is essentially a hinge joint. The range of movements is shown in Figure 9.11. The subject is seated on the edge of the examination couch, with knees flexed and legs dependent. Both active and passive movements are tested. **Dorsiflexion** ranges between **10–20°**. The opposite movement of **plantar flexion** has a wider range of **30–50°**.

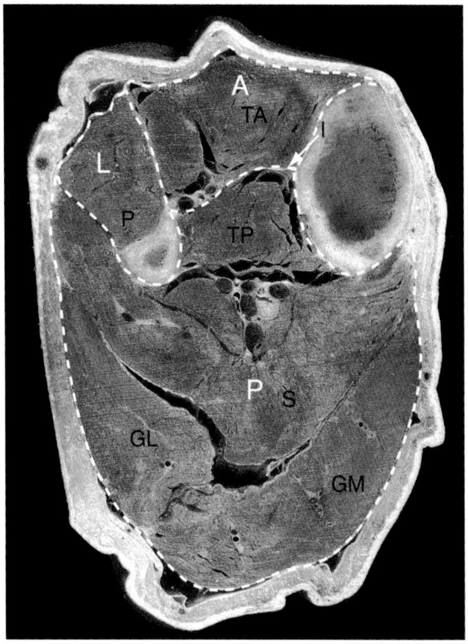


**Fig. 9.12** Prosection showing a transverse section of the leg and the muscle compartments (white dotted line)
A, L, P (large, white letters) = anterior, lateral, and posterior compartments, GL = lateral head of gastrocnemius, GM = medial head of gastrocnemius (compare with GL), I = interosseous membrane separating the large posterior compartment from the smaller anterior, P = peronei, S = soleus, TA = tibialis anterior, TP = tibialis posterior

## IDENTIFYING TENDONS AND TESTING MUSCLES

- Anterior compartment: extensor tendons
- Invertor tendons
- Lateral compartment: evertor tendons
- Posterior compartment: flexor tendons
- Gastrocnemius/soleus
- Flexor hallucis longus

Prosections showing the compartments of the leg, in addition to the muscles and tendons in the anterior compartment, are shown in Figures 9.12 and 9.13.

### ANTERIOR COMPARTMENT: EXTENSOR TENDONS

The subject sits or lies supine on the couch, with the lower limbs fully extended. The examiner places the palmar surface of the fingers of one hand across the dorsum of

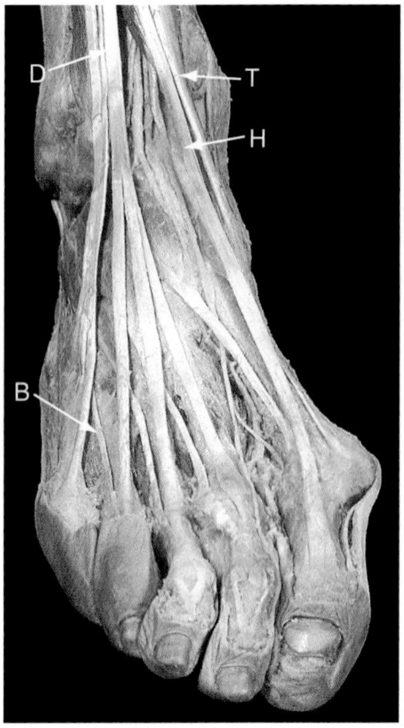


**Fig. 9.13** Prosection showing the long and short extensor tendons in the ankle and foot
B = extensor digitorum brevis, D = extensor digitorum longus (note pattern of attachment of digital slips to terminal phalanx), H = extensor hallucis longus, T = tibialis anterior (From Gosling JA, Harris PF, Whitmore I, Willan PLT. 2002 Human Anatomy, 4th edn. London: Mosby)

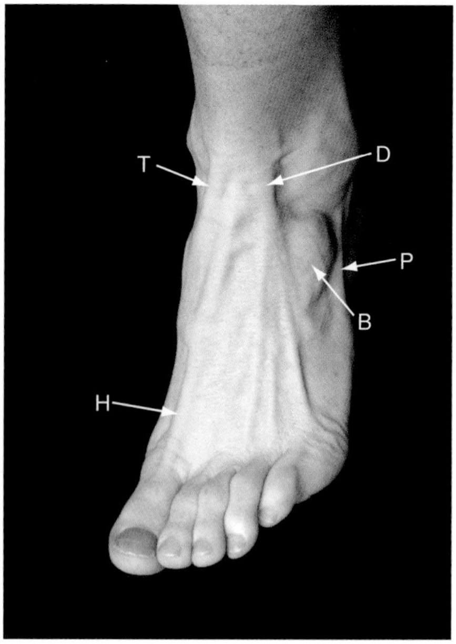


**Fig. 9.14** Long extensor tendons in the living ankle and foot
B = extensor digitorum brevis, D = extensor digitorum longus, H = extensor hallucis longus, P = peroneus longus, T = tibialis anterior

the toes, resisting attempts by the subject to extend them upward. Working from medial to lateral, the tendons of **tibialis anterior, extensor hallucis longus, extensor digitorum longus** (Fig. 9.14), and peroneus tertius (if present) become clearly defined. On the lateral side of the foot just anterior to the malleolus, a firm, visible swelling marks the belly of the extensor digitorum brevis. The long extensor tendons can be further isolated and defined by resisting extension of the great toe and individual digits.

## INVERTOR TENDONS

On the medial side of the ankle, the tendons of the invertors, **tibialis anterior and posterior,** are easily located by asking the subject to turn the foot inward and upward, the movement being resisted by the examiner grasping the forefoot across its middle (Fig. 9.15a). The tendons become prominent and are palpable just below the tip of the medial malleolus. The tibialis anterior is traced forward to its attachment on the medial border of the foot to the medial cuneiform and the adjacent base of the first metatarsal. The tibialis posterior tendon can be followed forward to the prominence of the tuberosity of the navicular, easily palpable with the index finger about 4 cm in front of the malleolus (see prosection, Fig. 9.15b).

## LATERAL COMPARTMENT: EVERTOR TENDONS

A prosection showing the evertors of the foot is provided in Figure 9.16. The tendons of **peroneus longus and brevis** can be identified immediately below the tip of the lateral malleolus (Fig. 9.17). The subject sits with the feet projecting over the end of the couch. The examiner grasps the forefoot across its middle and asks the subject to turn it outward and also to plantar-flex, these movements being resisted by the examiner. Contraction of the peronei is detected by direct palpation over the lateral side of the calf, whilst a finger tip can detect the tendons tightening immediately behind the malleoli on resisting eversion. If palpation is continued forward from below the malleolus, the prominent tendon of peroneus brevis can be traced to its bony attachment on the base of the fifth metatarsal. Additionally, the tendon of peroneus longus can be located

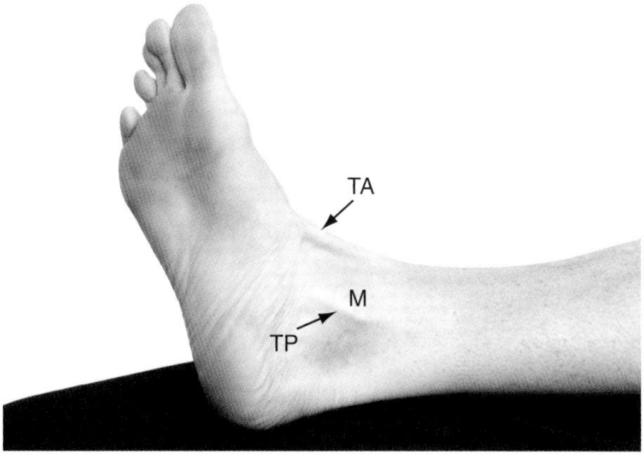


Fig. 9.15a Demonstrating the tendons of tibialis anterior and posterior and their relation to the medial malleolus
M = medial malleolus, TA = tibialis anterior, TP = tibialis posterior

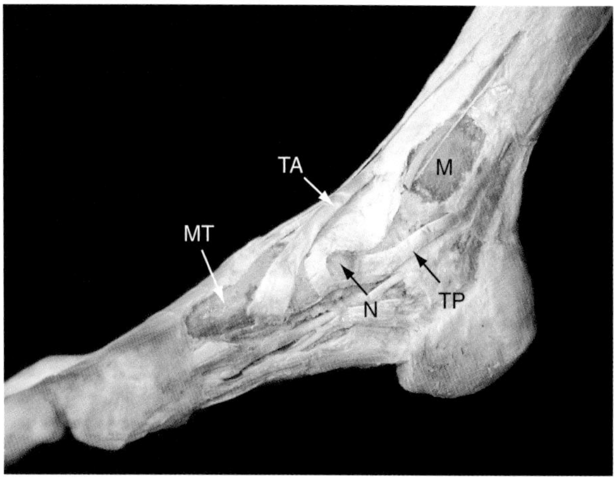


Fig. 9.15b Prosection showing the tendons of tibialis anterior and posterior
M = medial malleolus, MT = base of first metatarsal, N = navicular tuberosity, TA = tibialis anterior, TP = tibialis posterior

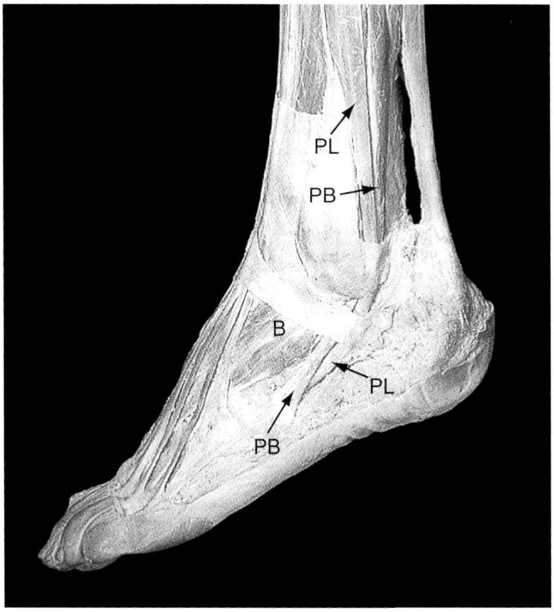


Fig. 9.16 Prosection showing the evertors of the foot in the lateral compartment of the leg and at the ankle
B = extensor digitorum brevis, PB = peroneus brevis, PL = peroneus longus (From Gosling JA, Harris PF, Whitmore I, Willan PLT. 2002 Human Anatomy, 4th edn. London: Mosby)

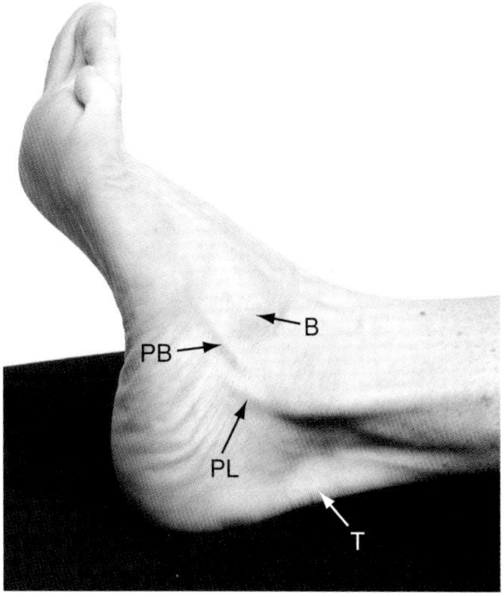


Fig. 9.17 Demonstrating the tendons of peroneus longus and brevis at the ankle
B = extensor digitorum brevis, PB = peroneus brevis, PL = peroneus longus, T = Achilles tendon

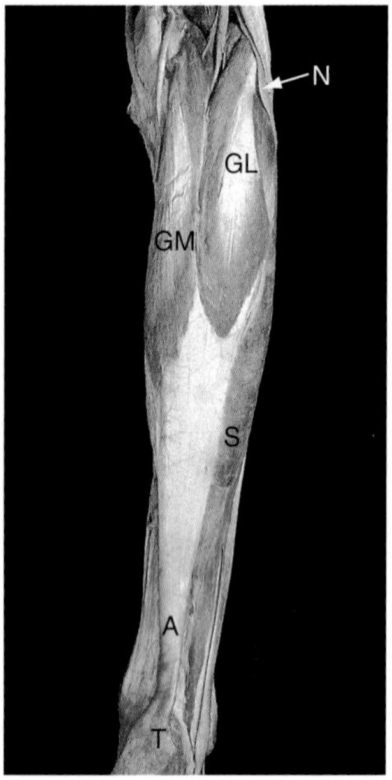


**Fig. 9.18** Prosection showing the superficial muscles in the posterior compartment of the leg
A = Achilles tendon, GL = lateral head of gastrocnemius, GM = medial head of gastrocnemius, N = common peroneal nerve crossing neck of fibula, S = soleus, T = calcaneal tuberosity (From Gosling JA, Harris PF, Whitmore I, Willan PLT. 2002 Human Anatomy, 4th edn. London: Mosby)

below the tip of the lateral malleolus below the level of the brevis tendon and passing medially and deeply in the soft tissue groove behind the base of the fifth metatarsal and beneath the lateral edge of the cuboid.

## POSTERIOR COMPARTMENT: FLEXOR TENDONS

A prosection of superficial muscles in the posterior compartment is shown in Figure 9.18. To demonstrate and test the more superficial **gastrocnemius–soleus** group, the subject stands facing away from the examiner and is instructed to rise up on tip-toe, plantar-flexing the ankle. This demonstrates the two heads of gastrocnemius, the medial being visibly the larger. Both muscle bellies are seen to attach into the more distal and flatter belly of the underlying soleus, all three of them being firmly palpable as they contract in the calf. More distally, the Achilles tendon is felt as a thick, strong band descending in the lower leg to its attachment on the back of the calcaneum (see Fig. 9.2).

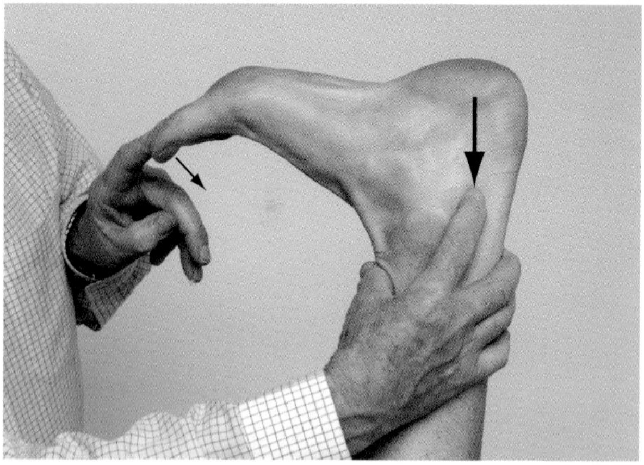

**Fig. 9.19** Palpating the tendon of flexor hallucis longus behind the medial malleolus (large arrow)

To differentiate between the actions of gastrocnemius and soleus, the subject lies face down on the couch, initially with the legs fully extended and feet hanging over the edge of the couch. The subject is then asked to plantarflex against strong resistance applied to the soles of the feet by the examiner. To distinguish the action of the soleus, the subject remains face-down but now the leg is flexed to 90° at the knee, whilst the examiner resists strong plantar flexion of the foot. This reflexes the gastrocnemius.

## FLEXOR HALLUCIS LONGUS

The deep flexors in the leg are mostly concealed by the superficial group, except in the region of the ankle, where the long tendons can be located. Deepest is flexor hallucis longus lying under the Achilles tendon. With firm, deep palpation behind the medial malleolus and forcible dorsiflexion of the hallux, the tendon can be felt to tighten (Fig. 9.19). A similar procedure whilst forcibly dorsiflexing the other toes allows detection of the extensor digitorum tendon.

# TESTING REFLEXES

- Ankle jerk

## ACHILLES (ANKLE) JERK

Cord segments and nerve roots involved are S1 and S2. The subject lies prone on the couch, with the feet projecting and dependent over the end of the couch. The examiner grasps the foot and slightly dorsiflexes it to stretch the

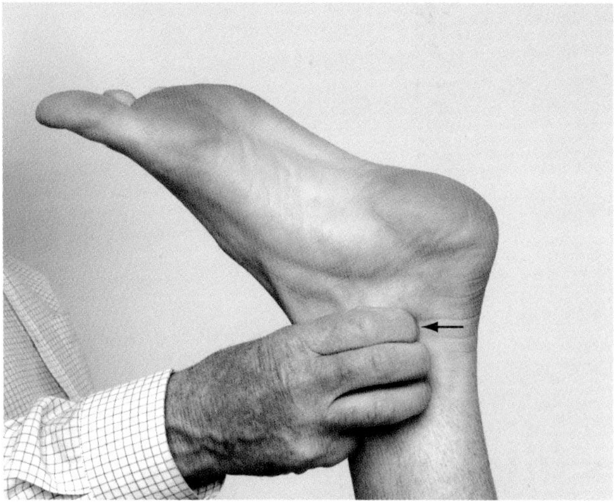

Fig. 9.20 Palpating the posterior tibial artery behind the medial malleolus (arrow)

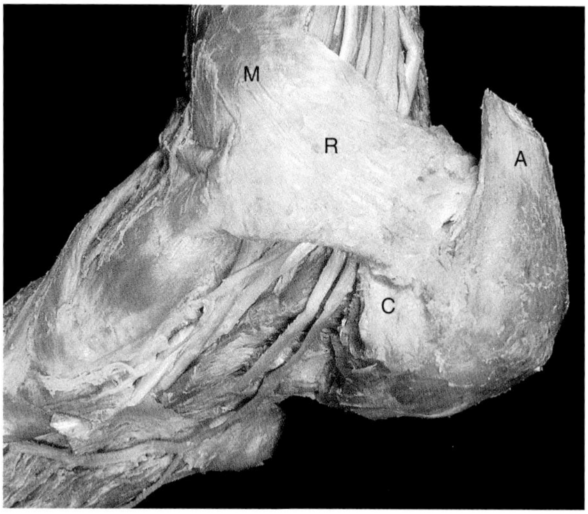


Fig. 9.21 Prosection showing the ankle flexor retinaculum and structures passing beneath it in the tarsal tunnel
A = Achilles tendon, C = calcaneum, M = medial malleolus, R = flexor retinaculum (From Gosling JA, Harris PF, Whitmore I, Willan PLT. 2002 Human Anatomy, 4th edn. London: Mosby)

Achilles tendon, which is then percussed. Alternatively, with the subject lying on one side and with the hip and knee of the uppermost limb partially flexed, the examiner grasps the foot and, whilst dorsiflexing it, percusses the Achilles tendon.

# LOCATING SOFT TISSUES

- Arteries: posterior tibial, dorsalis pedis
- Flexor retinaculum

## POSTERIOR TIBIAL ARTERY

The pulsations of this artery can be detected with the subject sitting or lying supine, and the foot relaxed and slightly plantar-flexed. The tip of the index finger is pressed firmly forward and laterally, behind the lower part of the medial malleolus (Fig. 9.20) in the soft tissue depression limited below by the firm edge of the flexor retinaculum; beneath this, the artery passes as shown in the prosection in Figure 9.21.

## DORSALIS PEDIS ARTERY

The artery is usually palpable, although not as easily as the larger posterior tibial artery. It lies lateral to the tendon of extensor hallucis longus, which serves as a landmark. Using the pads of two fingers rather than one to palpate the artery is helpful and the foot should be relaxed. Care is needed to avoid palpating too near to the line of the ankle joint, due to the presence of the thick subcutaneous inferior extensor retinaculum, which covers the artery.

## FLEXOR RETINACULUM

This lies subcutaneously and forms the roof of the tarsal tunnel, through which passes the main neurovascular bundle supplying the sole of the foot. It may be a point of entrapment. With the subject seated or lying supine, the retinaculum can be easily palpated by passively dorsiflexing and everting the foot. With the index and middle finger tips, the edge of the oblique upper border can be easily traced from the medial side of the heel upward and forward toward the malleolus (Fig. 9.22).

# SPECIAL TESTS

- Achilles tendon tears
- Ankle joint instability:
  Drawer
  Talar tilt
- Ankle impingement:
  Anterior
  Posterior

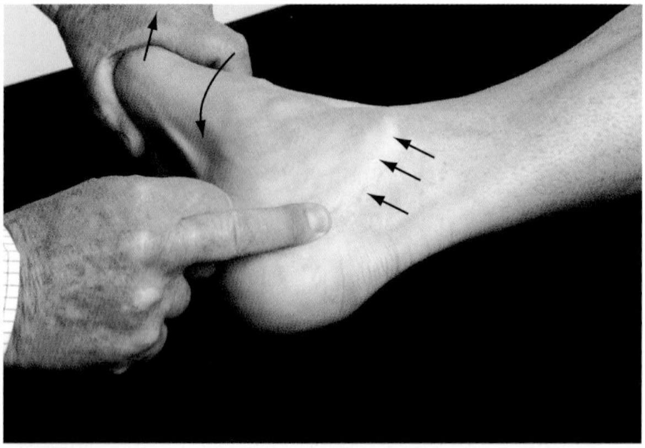

Fig. 9.22 Palpating the proximal edge of the flexor retinaculum
The skin is blanched by the underlying edge tensed by dorsiflexion and eversion of the foot

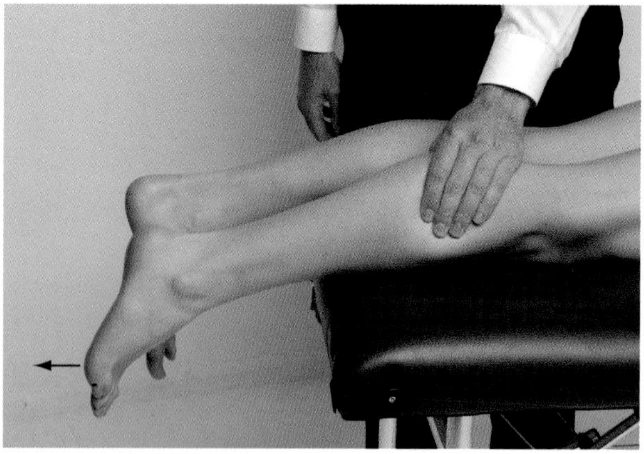

Fig. 9.23 Squeeze test for rupture of the Achilles tendon

- Syndesmosis strain:
  Tibio-fibular
  Ankle

## ACHILLES TENDON TEARS

The subject lies supine on the couch, with both feet dependent over the end of the couch.

### INSPECTION

The angle of both feet with respect to the vertical is viewed from the lateral profile and compared. Where there is tendon rupture, the foot on the injured side hangs more vertically.

### ATTEMPTED PLANTAR FLEXION

On attempting plantar flexion against resistance, an obvious depression or gap may be visible and palpable in the tendon.

### CALF SQUEEZE TEST

The examiner uses the fingers and thumb of one hand to squeeze the fleshy part of the calf comprising gastrocnemius and soleus firmly (Fig. 9.23). If the tendon is intact, the foot plantar-flexes.

## ANKLE JOINT INSTABILITY

Prosections of the ankle showing the collateral ligaments and their components from different aspects are shown in Figure 9.24.

### ANTERIOR DRAWER TEST

This is used to detect tears of the anterior talo-fibular ligament. The subject lies supine or is seated with the feet off the ground. With the subject's foot slightly (about 20°) plantar-flexed, the examiner grasps the heel in the cup of his or her own hand whilst using the other hand to stabilize the subject's leg by holding it firmly above the ankle. The examiner then attempts to pull the foot forward (Fig. 9.25). If the ligament is intact, a firm "end-feel" will be discerned after only a few millimeters of anterior translation. Pain or excessive anterior translation of the foot indicates tearing of the anterior talo-fibular ligament. This test can also be conducted with the subject sitting over the edge of a couch.

### TALAR TESTS

#### *Tilt test (inversion)*

This is used to detect injuries to the calcaneo-fibular and anterior talo-fibular ligaments, both being components of the lateral collateral ligament. The subject lies supine, with both feet over the edge of the couch. Stabilizing one leg by grasping it firmly above the ankle, the examiner uses the other hand to grip the talus and calcaneus firmly between fingers and thumb, and inverts the foot by pulling the heel inward (Fig. 9.26a).

#### *Tilt test (eversion)*

This is a stability test for the deltoid ligament. The positioning of the subject and the procedure are the same, except that the examiner grips the subject's heel and everts the foot (Fig. 9.26b).

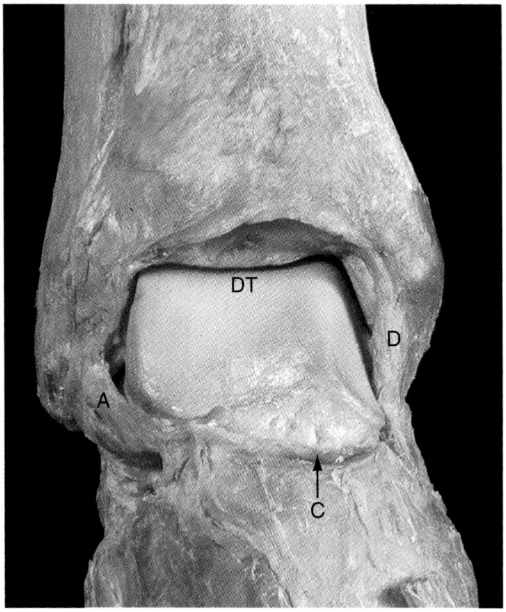


Fig. 9.24a Prosection of the ankle joint from anterior showing the anterior talo-fibular and deltoid ligaments
A = anterior talo-fibular ligament, C = capsule on neck of talus, D = deltoid ligament, DT = dome of talus (From Gosling JA, Harris PF, Whitmore I, Willan PLT. 2002 Human Anatomy, 4th edn. London: Mosby)

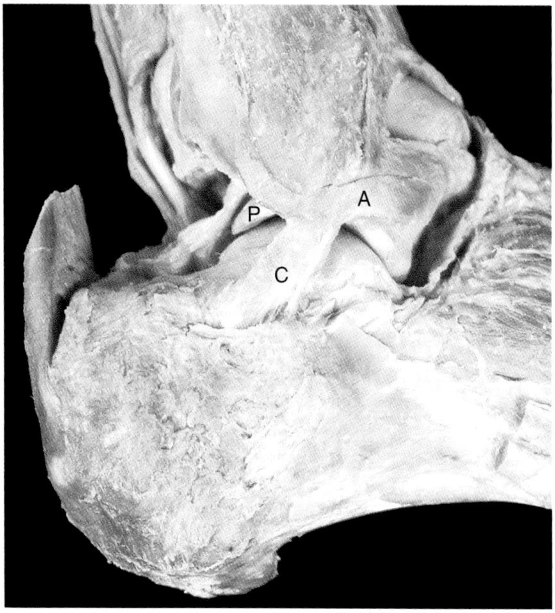


Fig. 9.24b Prosection of the ankle joint showing the components of the lateral collateral ligament
A = anterior talo-fibular, C = calcaneo-fibular, P = posterior talo-fibular (From Gosling JA, Harris PF, Whitmore I, Willan PLT. 2002 Human Anatomy, 4th edn. London: Mosby)

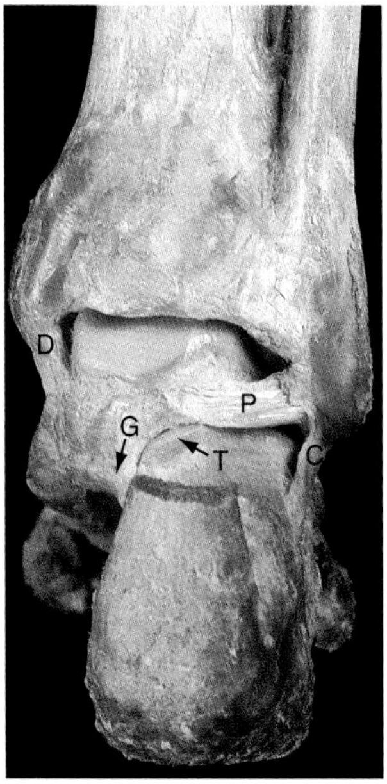


Fig. 9.24c Prosection of ankle joint from posterior showing significant structures
C = calcaneo-fibular ligament, D = deltoid ligament, G = groove for flexor hallucis longus tendon, P = posterior talo-fibular ligament, T = posterior talar tubercle (From Gosling JA, Harris PF, Whitmore I, Willan PLT. 2002 Human Anatomy, 4th edn. London: Mosby)

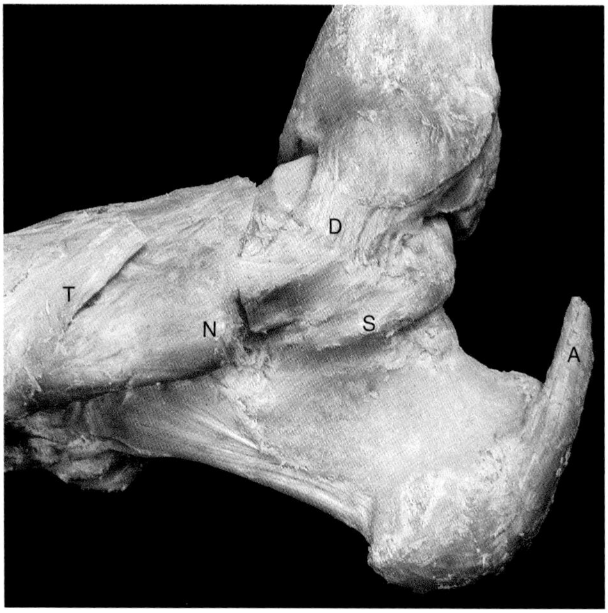


Fig. 9.24d Prosection of the ankle joint from medially, showing the collateral (deltoid) ligament
A = Achilles tendon, D = deltoid ligament, N = navicular tuberosity, S = sustentaculum tali, T = tibialis anterior tendon (From Gosling JA, Harris PF, Whitmore I, Willan PLT. 2002 Human Anatomy, 4th edn. London: Mosby)

## ANKLE IMPINGEMENT

### *Posterior impingement*

With the subject lying prone and the knee flexed 90°, the foot is gripped over the heel with one hand and over the dorsum with the other. The ankle is then passively rocked in and out of end-range plantar flexion (Fig. 9.27a). Posterior ankle pain at end-range plantar flexion may indicate posterior ankle impingement.

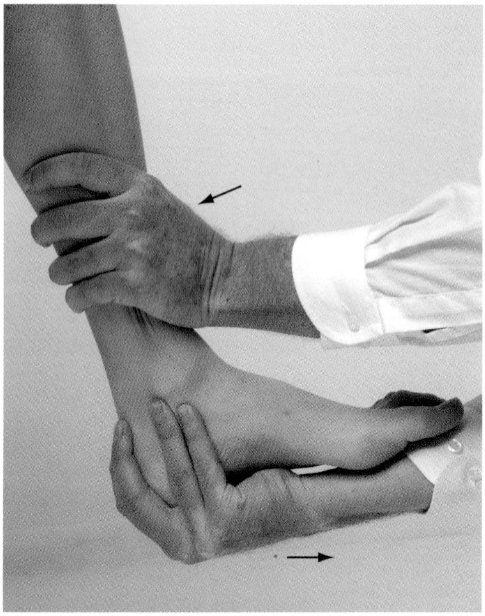

**Fig. 9.25** Drawer test for a tear of the anterior talo-fibular ligament

### *Anterior impingement*

With the subject positioned as already described, the examiner uses one hand to grip the distal leg to stabilize it, whilst the other hand is cupped over the heel with the adjacent forearm resting along the sole of the foot. The ankle is then rocked in and out of passive end-range dorsiflexion (Fig. 9.27b). Anterior ankle pain elicited at end-range dorsiflexion may indicate anterior ankle impingement.

## SYNDESMOSIS STRAIN

### WEIGHT-BEARING TIBIO-FIBULAR SYNDESMOSIS STRAIN

The subject stands on the affected limb, whilst the examiner palpates the medial and lateral malleoli with the thumb and forefinger of one hand (Fig. 9.28a). The subject then attempts to flex the knee and dorsiflex the ankle. Pain reproduced at the distal tibio-fibular joint or palpable widening of the malleoli represents a positive test. The examiner can then ask the subject to repeat this movement, whilst squeezing together the distal tibia and fibula using the palms of both hands (Fig. 9.28b). Increased dorsiflexion ROM and decreased pain confirm distal tibio-fibular joint instability.

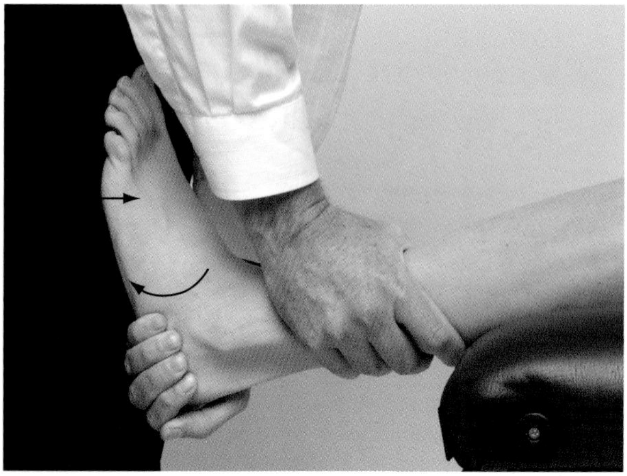

**Fig. 9.26a** Tilt test (inversion) for a tear of the calcaneo-fibular and anterior talo-fibular ligaments

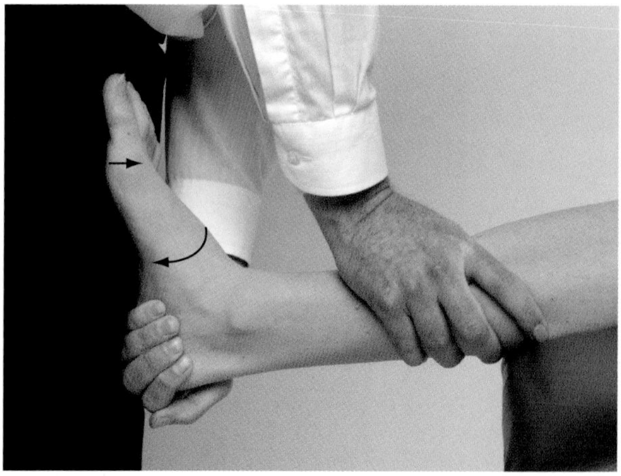

**Fig. 9.26b** Tilt test (eversion) for a tear of the deltoid ligament

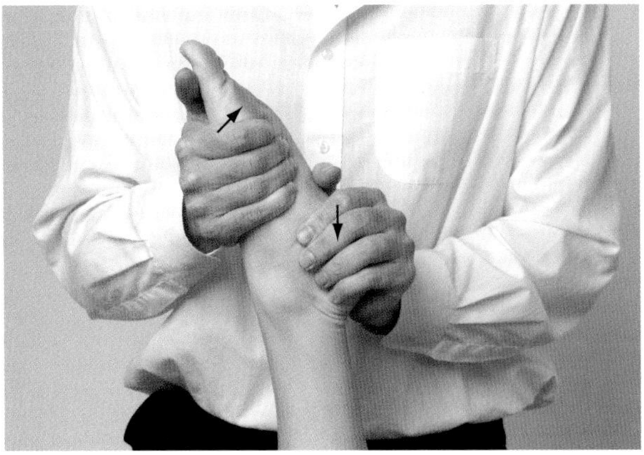

Fig. 9.27a Posterior impingement test

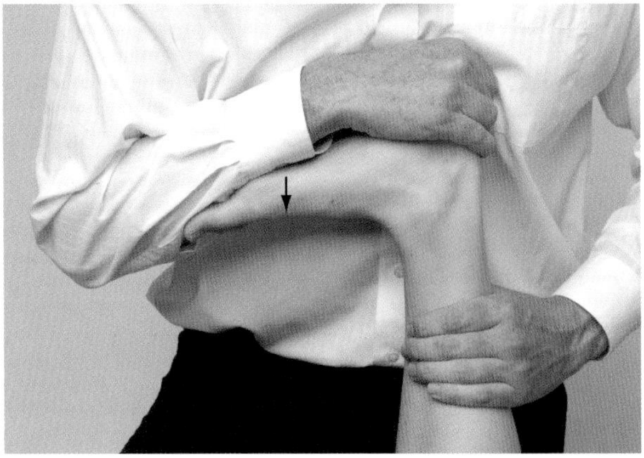

Fig. 9.27b Anterior impingement test

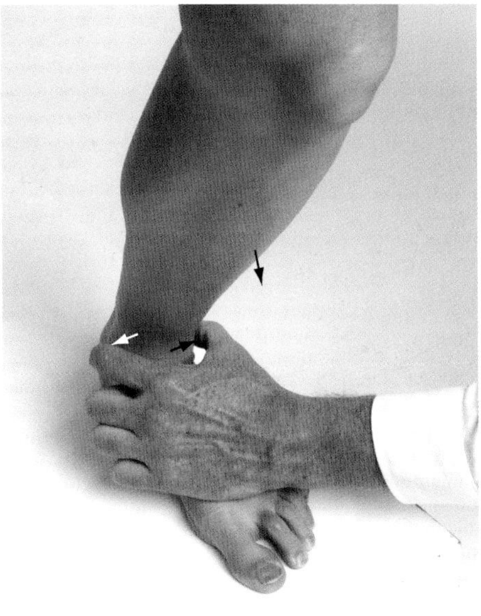

Fig. 9.28a Tibio-fibular syndesmosis strain

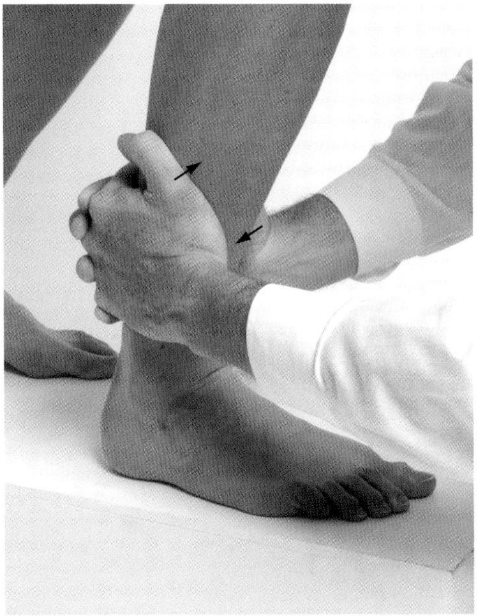

Fig. 9.28b Tibio-fibular syndesmosis strain

## NON-WEIGHT-BEARING TIBIO-FIBULAR SYNDESMOSIS STRAIN (COTTON'S TEST)

The subject sits on a chair or over the edge of the couch, with the knee at right angles and the leg dependent. The examiner firmly grips the leg just above the ankle with one hand, and using the other hand, grips the foot about its midpoint and uses it as a lever to attempt to abduct and then adduct the foot. This may evoke pain with strain or tear of the interosseous and posterior talo-fibular ligaments.

## FURTHER READING

Archbold HAP, Wilson L, Barr JB. Acute exertional compartment syndrome of the leg: consequences of a delay in diagnosis: a report of 2 cases. Clinical Journal of Sport Medicine 2004; 14: 98–100.

Giza E, Fuller C, Junge A et al. Mechanisms of foot and ankle injuries in soccer. American Journal of Sports Medicine 2003; 31:550–554.

Hopkins JT, Palmien R. Effects of ankle joint effusion on lower leg function. Clinical Journal of Sport Medicine 2004; 14:1–7.

MacDonald PB, Strange G, Hodgkinson R et al. Injuries to the peroneal nerve in professional hockey. Clinical Journal of Sport Medicine 2002; 12:39–40.

Maffulli N, Kenward MG, Testa V et al. Clinical diagnosis of Achilles tendinopathy with tendinosis. Clinical Journal of Sport Medicine 2003; 13:11–15.

Schmitt H, Lemke JM, Brocai DRC et al. Degenerative changes in the ankle in former elite high jumpers. Clinical Journal of Sport Medicine 2003;13:6–10.

Wright RW, Barile RJ, Surprenant DA et al. Ankle syndesmosis strains in National Hockey League players. American Journal of Sports Medicine 2004; 32:1941–1945.

## CASE STUDY 9 • CLINICAL PROBLEMS

**Problem 1.** *A 24-year-old male basketball player steps on an opponent's foot whilst landing from a rebound. His ankle is forcibly inverted in a plantar-flexed position. He has severe lateral ankle pain and has to be helped, without weight-bearing, from the court. Initial examination reveals antero-lateral ankle tenderness and swelling.*

a) What is the most likely diagnosis?
b) What initial orthopedic tests should be performed?
c) Name at least two other acute injuries that may have occurred with this mechanism.
d) According to the Ottawa Rules, under what circumstances is an ankle radiograph indicated for this type of injury?
e) Despite appropriate rehabilitation, this athlete continues to have lateral ankle pain 8 weeks after the injury. Name two differential or additional diagnoses that should be considered.

**Problem 2.** *Whilst pushing off from her left foot to perform a cutting maneuver, an 18-year-old female soccer player steps in a hole in the field and forcibly everts her ankle. She hears a "cracking" sound and feels pain on the inside of her ankle.*

a) What ligament is likely to have been sprained?
b) Which orthopedic test is appropriate?

**Problem 3.** *A 45-year-old male tennis player jumps to attempt a "smash" and feels a "popping" sensation and sudden sharp pain in his right lower calf. He is unable to bear weight on the right leg and needs to be carried off the court.*

a) What is the likely diagnosis?
b) What clinical tests should be used to confirm the diagnosis?
c) In what position should the ankle be immobilized?

**Problem 4.** *An 18-year-old female ballet dancer complains of posterior ankle pain when she is dancing with her foot "en pointe" (standing on one leg, supported only on the point of the hallux with the foot in extreme plantar flexion). Her physician orders an MRI scan of the ankle (Fig. 9.29).* Note: C = calcaneum; N = navicular; T = tibia; TA = talus.

a) What is the most likely diagnosis?
b) What structures might be causing the problem?
c) What is the structure labeled (*) in the MRI scan?
d) Name at least two structures that could be impinged.
e) What clinical test is used to assist in the diagnosis?

**Problem 5.** *A 22-year-old male footballer describes anterior ankle pain when running and kicking with his dominant (right) foot. He is diagnosed with having "anterior ankle impingement."*

a) What might be causing the impingement?
b) What clinical test could be used to assist the diagnosis?

**Problem 6.** *A 30-year-old male distance runner is diagnosed with "anterior compartment syndrome."*

a) What symptoms are common to this condition?
b) How is it diagnosed?
c) Which leg compartments can be affected by "chronic compartment syndrome"?

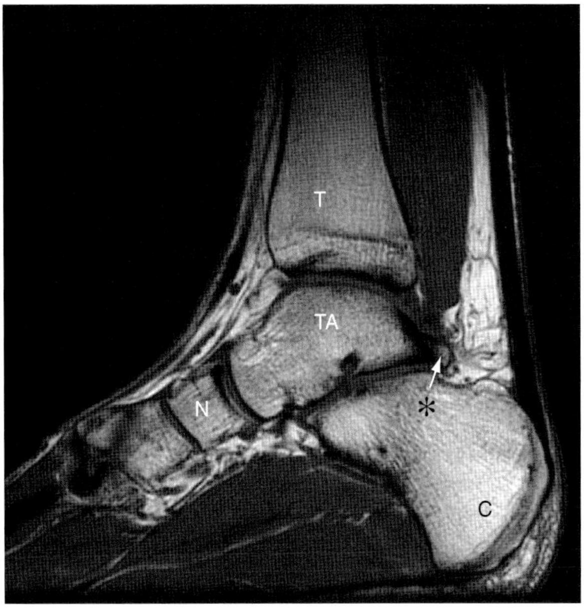


Fig. 9.29 Sagittal MRI scan of the ankle
C = calcaneum, T = tibia, TA = talus, N = navicular

CHAPTER 10

# Foot

## INTRODUCTION

The foot is the terminal segment of the lower limb. Its morphology reflects its principal functions of weight-bearing and locomotion. The bones of the forefoot, midfoot and hindfoot provide the framework for its characteristic shape. The prime function of the hindfoot is weight-bearing, as reflected by the substantial fat pad in the heel. An additional function, mainly located in the subtalar joint, is to facilitate the movements of inversion and eversion according to locomotor needs. Weight-bearing also occurs in the midfoot and forefoot, but importantly the forefoot has particular responsibility for forward thrust (propulsion) in walking, running, and jumping.

Most of the soft tissues of the foot are located in the sole. They include the plantar aponeurosis, long flexor tendons to all the toes, short intrinsic muscles, and plantar nerves and vessels. There are also well-developed deep veins, which are part of the venous pump mechanism in the lower limb.

On the dorsum of the foot, soft tissues are much less evident, comprising principally long extensor tendons to the hallux and other toes, and also the short extensor muscle and its tendons.

Tendons controlling inversion and eversion lie along the appropriate (medial or lateral) border of the foot. Superficial veins and sensory nerves lie beneath the skin.

# INSPECTION OF NORMAL CONTOURS

- Dorsal:
  Lateral border
  Medial border
- Plantar

The foot has the basic form of a modified tripod, narrow posteriorly and wider anteriorly. Its features should be examined with the subject standing, and also sitting or lying supine on a couch, the foot being viewed dorsally and from the plantar aspect.

## DORSAL ASPECT

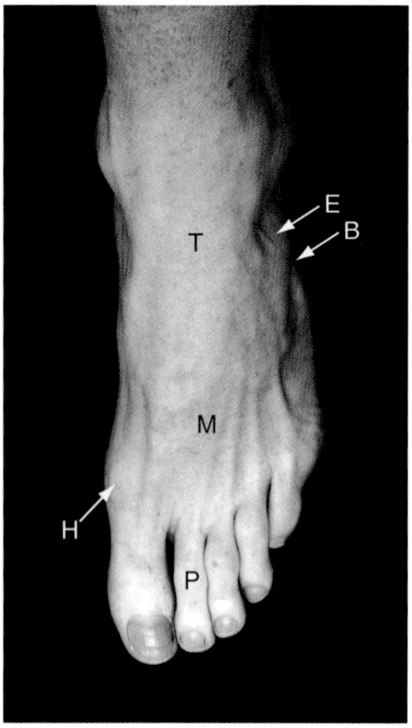


**Fig. 10.1** Dorsal view of the foot contours
Note the tapering overall profile of the toes. B = base of fifth metatarsal, E = extensor digitorum brevis, H = head of first metatarsal, P = location of phalanges, M = location of metatarsals, T = location of tarsals

From the dorsal aspect (Fig. 10.1), the hindfoot is obscured by the ankle joint. The midfoot on the medial side is elevated by the underlying medial longitudinal arch. Passing laterally, the contour slopes progressively downward to reach the outer border, which is entirely plantar-grade. Immediately in front of the lateral malleolus, but separated from it by a groove, is a fullness due to the underlying belly of the extensor digitorum brevis. Its surface color varies. In Caucasians it may appear bluish and can be confused with a bruise, particularly if there is a history of foot trauma. In the forefoot, long extensor tendons may be visible under the skin passing toward the roots of the toes. The hallux is very conspicuous and by far the most dominant toe. The digital index (length) varies, the great toe usually being the longest and the little toe the shortest. According to their comparative lengths, the profile of the toes may vary. They may taper progressively from the great toe or have a blunt spade-like form.

From the rounded contour of the heel, the **lateral border** continues forward, diverging slightly to reach the little toe. It is plantar-grade throughout its length. About its midpoint there is a slight depression marking the underlying base of the fifth metatarsal. The **medial border** passes forward from the heel, also diverging slightly. It has two characteristics. In many subjects it is elevated from the ground about its midpoint due to the medial longitudinal arch. Its other characteristic, located anteriorly, is the large prominence produced by the head of the first metatarsal at the root of the hallux.

## PLANTAR ASPECT

From the plantar aspect (Fig. 10.2a), the contours emphasize its weight-bearing role, as reflected by the characteristic thick skin and the typical footprint comprising the ball of the heel, outer part of the foot, ball of the foot (due to the underlying metatarsal heads), and pads of the digits. Medially, a depression, midfoot, marks the medial longitudinal arch. If the arch is deficient, this produces the characteristic flat foot (pes planus), widening progressively forward from the heel to the ball of the foot without the characteristic indentation of the medial longitudinal arch.

The footprint can be recorded by a simple imprint or by more quantitative methods such as a force platform (Fig. 10.2b). These records clearly demonstrate which parts bear

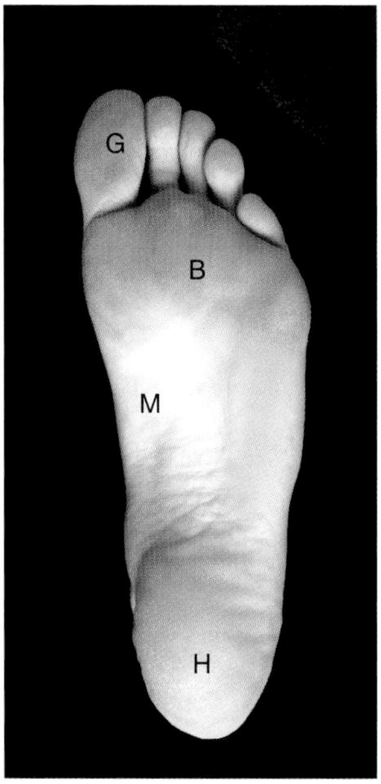


Fig. 10.2a Plantar view of the foot contours
B = ball of foot covering heads of metatarsals, G = plantar pad of hallux covering phalanges, H = heel fat pad covering calcaneum, M = medial longitudinal arch

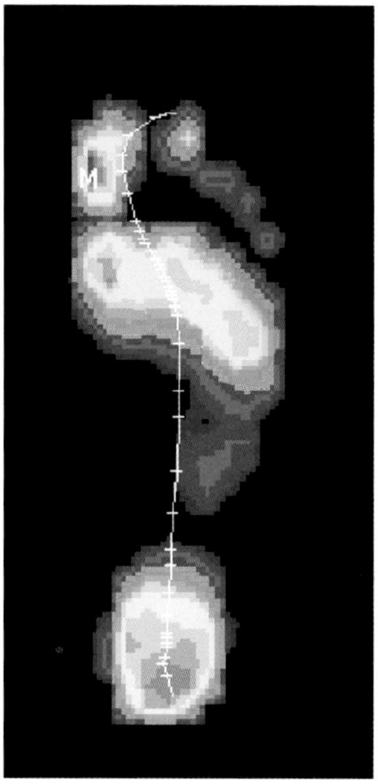


Fig. 10.2b Foot plantar pedobarograph
Note: pressure gradient highest to lowest = red, orange, yellow, green, blue

weight maximally, and particularly emphasize the role of the heads of the medial metatarsals in the ball of the foot and the great toe in propulsion. This is confirmed by the comparatively large size of the underlying skeleton in this part of the foot.

## LOCATING BONY LANDMARKS

- Calcaneum:
  Tuberosity
  Medial and lateral tubercles
  Peroneal tubercle
  Sinus tarsi
  Sustentaculum tali
- Talus:
  Head and neck
- Navicular:
  Tuberosity
- Metatarsals:
  Head
  Shaft
  Base

### CALCANEUM

Salient features of the skeleton of the foot are shown in Figure 9.4 and in the radiographs in Figure 10.3. The subject can be examined lying supine and then prone on a couch, or seated with the leg dependent. The examiner grasps and passively dorsiflexes the forefoot with one hand, and uses the pad of the thumb of the other hand to palpate deeply on the back of the calcaneum immediately below the attachment of the Achilles tendon. The upper edge of the **calcaneal tuberosity** can be clearly felt (Fig. 10.4). Continuing palpation under the heel, the examiner applies very deep pressure with the thumb through the fat pad, meeting firm resistance from the underlying **medial and lateral tubercles.** Palpating on the lateral side of the calcaneum, the examiner uses the index finger to find the bony prominence of the **peroneal tubercle** lying about 2.5 cm below the tip of the malleolus (Fig. 10.5). The region of the **sinus tarsi** can be located in the deep groove between the belly of extensor digitorum brevis, which is tensed by the subject extending the toes, and the anterior border of the lateral malleolus. The examiner uses an index finger to apply deep palpation downward and medially.

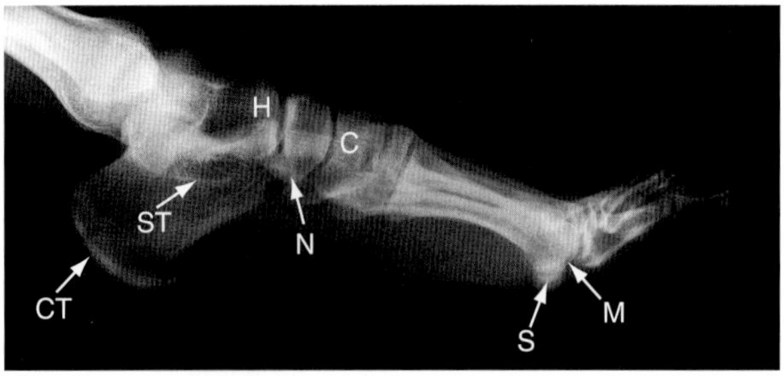


Fig. 10.3a Radiograph of the foot: medial view
C = medial cuneiform, CT = calcaneal tuberosity, H = head of talus, M = head of first metatarsal, N = navicular tuberosity, S = sesamoid, ST = sustentaculum tali

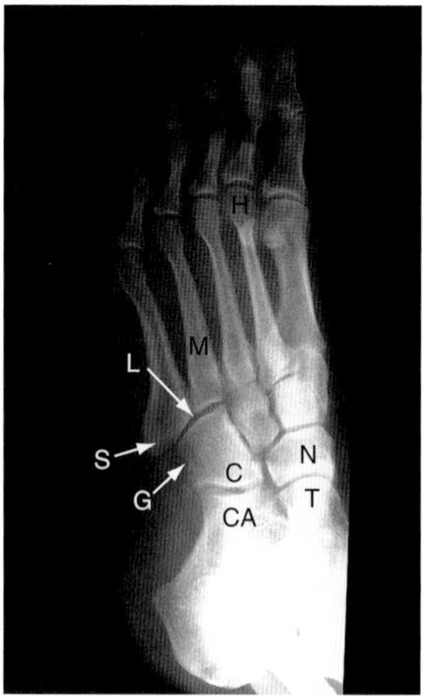


Fig. 10.3b Radiograph of the foot: dorsal view
Note: the two parts of the mid-tarsal joint, calcaneo-cuboid and talo-navicular, are clearly defined. C = cuboid, CA = calcaneum, G = groove for peroneus longus tendon, H = head of second metatarsal, L = medial part of Lisfranc's joint (tarso-metatarsal), M = fourth metatarsal shaft, N = navicular, S = styloid process, base of fifth metatarsal, T = head of talus

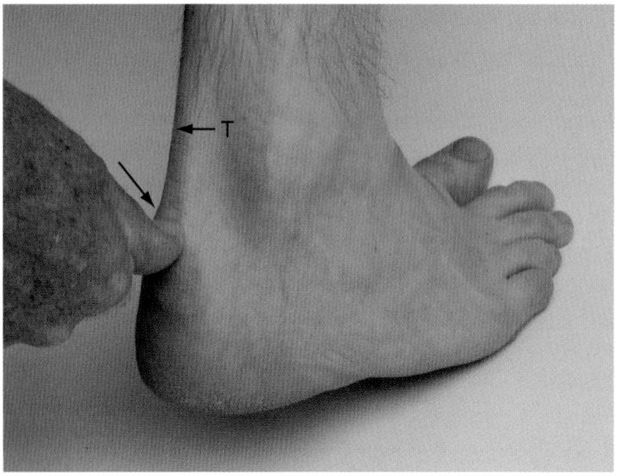


Fig. 10.4 Palpating the calcaneal tuberosity
T = Achilles tendon

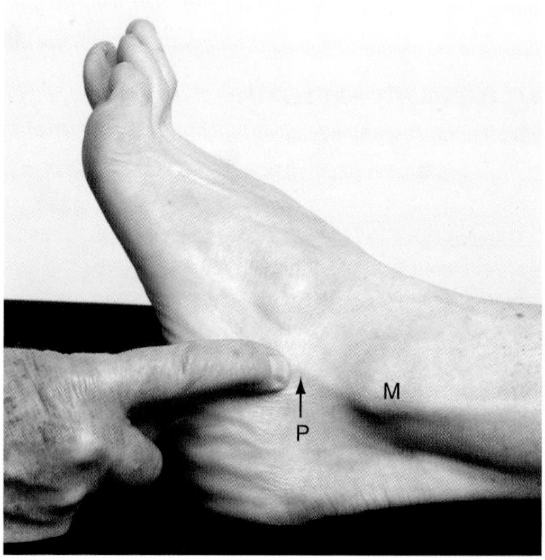


Fig. 10.5 Palpating the peroneal tubercle
M = lateral malleolus, P = peroneal tubercle immediately below tendon of peroneus brevis

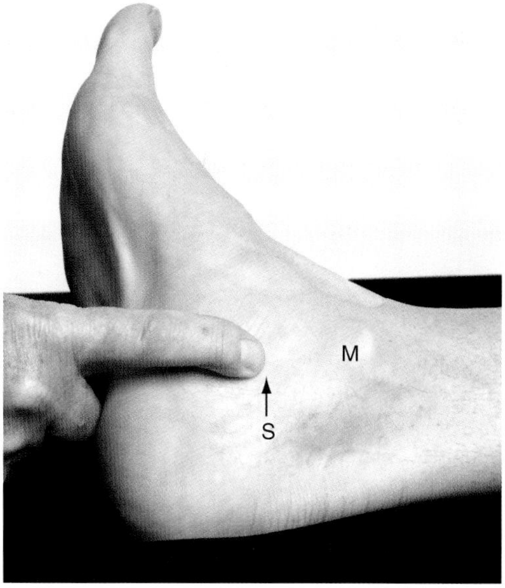


Fig. 10.6 Palpating the sustentaculum tali
M = medial malleolus, S = sustentaculum tali

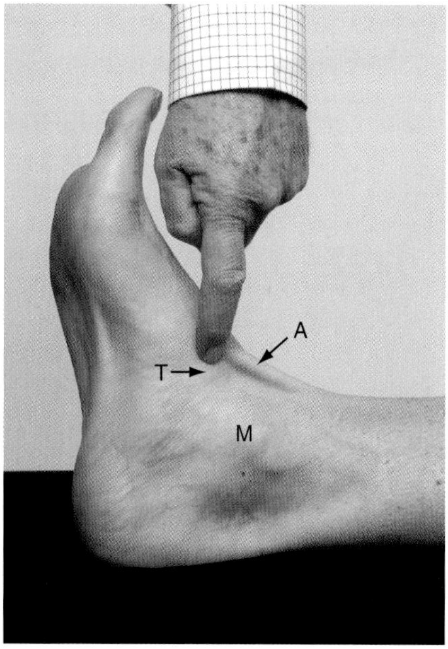


Fig. 10.7 Locating the head of talus
The head lies in the hollow between tibialis anterior and posterior tendons. A = tibialis anterior tendon, M = medial malleolus, T = head of talus

On the medial side of the heel, the **sustentaculum tali** is located by the examiner rolling a finger tip along its blunt, shelf-like eminence about 2.5 cm below the tip of the malleolus (Fig. 10.6).

## TALUS AND NAVICULAR

Continuing forward, the **head of the talus** is palpable about 2.5 cm antero-inferior to the anterior border of the malleolus. With the subject's foot inverted, the examiner rolls a finger tip over it where it lies in a depression between the tendons of tibialis anterior and posterior (Fig. 10.7). If the finger is drawn forward across the head of the talus, a groove can be felt separating it from the dorsum of the navicular. The **tuberosity of the navicular** is palpated from the dorsum of the bone. The finger is moved medially until the prominence of the tuberosity is reached (Fig. 10.8).

On the dorsum of the foot, the examiner locates the **neck of the talus** by palpating in the depression just antero-lateral to the medial malleolus and adjacent border of the tibia and lateral to the extensor hallucis longus tendon. Its location is facilitated by passive plantar flexion of the foot.

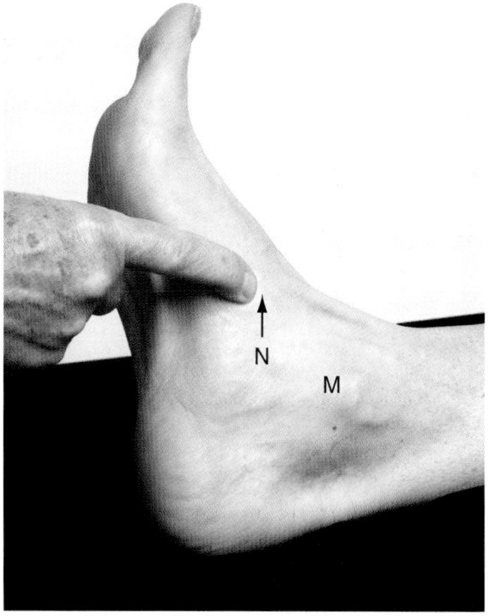


Fig. 10.8 Locating the navicular tuberosity
Tibialis posterior tendon is traced to the tuberosity
M = medial malleolus, N = navicular tuberosity

## METATARSALS

The whole of the dorsum of the **shaft of the fifth metatarsal** can be palpated from the **head** to the prominent styloid process at the **base** (Fig. 10.9). The examiner grips the subject's forefoot across the toes and, using the other hand, draws the index and middle finger tips firmly up the lateral side of the foot, starting at the little toe. Immediately proximal to the base is a groove which overlies the **cuboid.** The **heads of the first, fourth, and fifth metatarsals** are easily palpated. With the subject lying supine on the couch, foot relaxed and using the heel as a pivot on the couch the examiner locates the large head of the first metatarsal, gripping it tightly antero-posteriorly between thumb and index finger and rocking it forward and backward (Fig. 10.10a) whilst gripping the proximal phalanx firmly. Repeating this procedure on the smaller head of the fifth metatarsal provides considerable detail of its morphology. The head of the fourth metatarsal can be similarly examined but is more obscure. With the examiner applying deep pressure with the index finger on the undersurface of the head of the first metatarsal and feeling on each side of the head, the **sesamoids** can be located by their firm resistance. Their rounded shape can sometimes be defined by rolling the finger tip over them or gripping

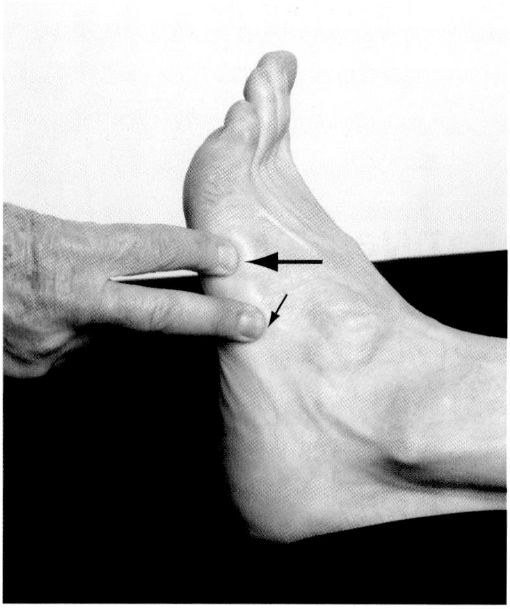

Fig. 10.9 Palpating the shaft (large arrow) and base (small arrow) of the fifth metatarsal

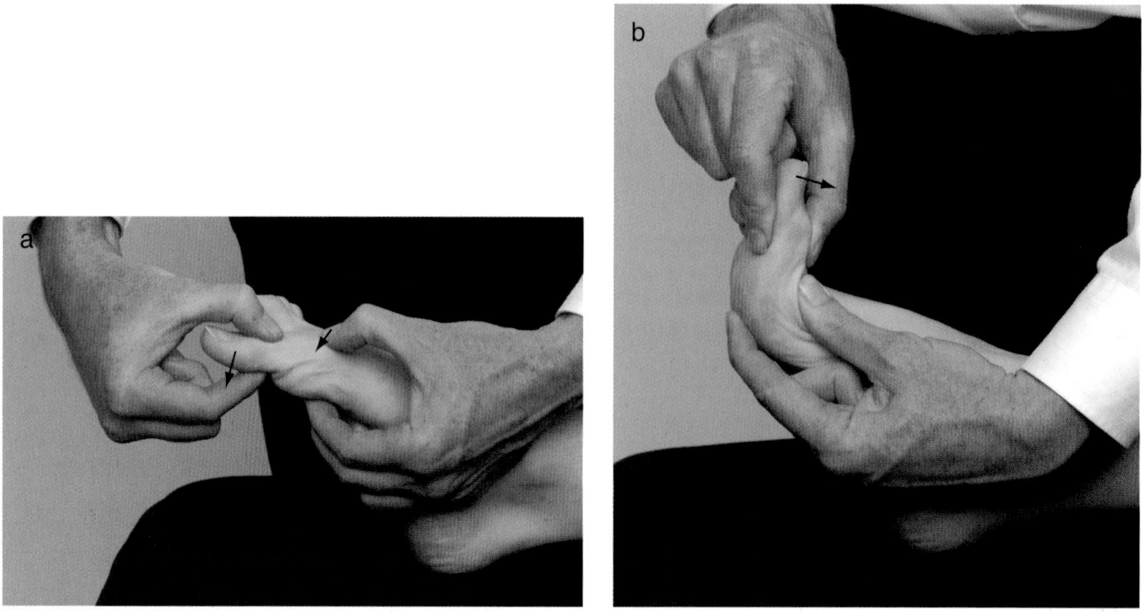


Fig. 10.10 Palpating the first metatarsal head and testing movement at the first metatarso-phalangeal joint
Note: the metatarsal is gripped firmly between the left index finger and thumb. **a** Testing plantar flexion whilst palpating the joint line with the tip of the thumb. **b** Testing dorsiflexion

between finger and thumb. The **large base of the first metatarsal** can be easily located. Starting from the head, the examiner draws the index finger firmly along the dorso-medial border of the shaft to a groove marking the joint between the base and the first cuneiform. It lies about 2.5 cm distal to the navicular tuberosity.

# LOCATING JOINT LINES

- Metatarso-phalangeal
- Metatarso-cuneiform
- Talo-navicular

Due to the close fit of the articular surfaces of the tarsals and metatarsals, very few joint lines are palpable in the foot.

## METATARSO-PHALANGEAL

The joint lines between the heads of the metatarsals and bases of the phalanges can be defined most easily in the first and fifth toes and possibly in the fourth. The subject lies supine on a couch or seated with the legs dependent. To locate the first joint, the examiner palpates deeply with the thumb over the dorsum of the metatarsal head and joint line, whilst gripping and plantar flexing and dorsi-flexing the proximal phalanx (Fig. 10.10). For the fifth joint, with the foot relaxed, the examiner grips the metatarsal head firmly over the joint line dorso-ventrally between thumb and index finger, widening the joint line by rocking the head forward and backward, whilst feeling the line with the thumb. A similar technique can be used for the fourth joint.

## METATARSO-CUNEIFORM

Only the joint between the base of the first metatarsal and first cuneiform can be located. The examiner draws the pad of the index finger firmly along the medial side of the shaft of the metatarsal toward the base until a distinct depression is reached. This marks the joint line. It may be confirmed by feeling movement here when the subject extends and flexes the great toe.

## TALO-NAVICULAR

With the foot slightly everted, this joint line is easily located by first palpating the navicular tuberosity with the tip of the index finger. The depression that indicates the joint line is palpated by drawing the finger 1 cm posteriorly, i.e. toward the medial malleolus.

# LOCATING AND TESTING TENDONS AND MUSCLES

- Long and short extensors
- Invertors and evertors
- Flexors

## LONG AND SHORT EXTENSORS

A prosection showing long and short extensor tendons of the toe is provided in Figure 9.13. The subject lies supine on the couch, with legs extended. Starting with the foot and toes in a neutral position, the subject extends the toes robustly (Fig. 10.11), if necessary assisted by the examiner, who applies downward pressure over the toes with their hand. The tendons of **extensors hallucis longus** and **digitorum longus** are clearly defined and palpable. Note that the digitorum longus tendons diverge from a common tendon easily palpable over the line of the ankle joint. Tendons to individual digits can be identified and tested by downward pressure on the digit, whilst the subject is attempting extension. The maneuver to demonstrate the long extensor tendons also causes the belly of extensor

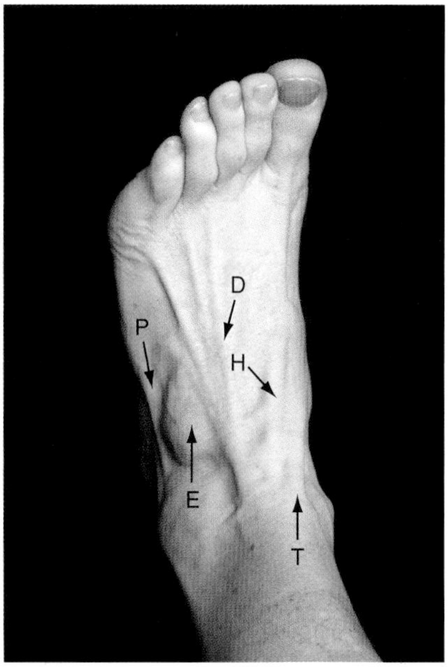


Fig. 10.11 Demonstrating the extensor tendons of the toes D = extensor digitorum longus, E = extensor digitorum brevis, H = extensor hallucis longus, P = peroneus brevis, T = tibialis anterior

digitorum brevis to contract. It appears as a tense prominence just lateral to the proximal part of the long extensor tendon to the little toe.

## INVERTORS AND EVERTORS

Prosections showing tendons that produce inversion and eversion are shown in Figures 9.15b and 9.16.

The subject is seated, with the legs dependent, and attempts full inversion of the foot whilst resisted by the examiner, who grasps the forefoot and attempts to evert it. The tendon of tibialis anterior can be easily identified and felt (see Fig. 9.15a) passing across the medial border of the foot to the base of the first metatarsal. The tibialis posterior tendon is less conspicuous. It can be palpated immediately behind and below the tip of the medial malleolus and more deeply as it passes forward to the navicular tuberosity. Identification is aided by palpating whilst the subject alternates between inversion and eversion.

Still seated, the subject attempts to evert the foot fully whilst the examiner grasps the forefoot and resists the movement. The examiner palpating with the index and middle fingers, the peroneus brevis tendon (see Fig. 9.17) can be traced forward on the lateral side of the foot immediately below the malleolus toward the base of the fifth metatarsal. The tendon of peroneus longus requires much deeper palpation. It can be felt from behind the malleolus and below the peroneal tubercle passing almost vertically to the groove behind the base of the fifth metatarsal, where it winds around the cuboid. It lies behind the peroneus brevis at the malleolus and below it in the foot. Palpation of both peroneal tendons is facilitated whilst the subject alternates between inversion and eversion.

## FLEXOR TENDONS

The long flexor tendons are shown in a prosection in Figure 10.12. Compared with the extensor tendons, those of the flexors are neither visible nor accessible for palpation due to the thickness of the skin in the sole and underlying plantar aponeurosis. However, the flexor hallucis longus tendon can be felt to tense when palpating under the sustentaculum tali whilst resisting flexion of the hallux, and that of flexor digitorum longus can be felt to tense on the side of the sustentaculum whilst resisting flexion of the toes. The action of the tendons is easily tested. Lying supine on the couch with legs extended and feet and toes in neutral position, the subject actively flexes the toes and then against resistance applied to the pads of the digits by the examiner. Individual toes can be tested separately, the tendon of flexor hallucis longus (see Fig. 9.19) being particularly powerful. The short intrinsic muscles, especially the abductors and short flexors, contribute to some of the soft tissue mass of the sole, but their actions are not readily tested.

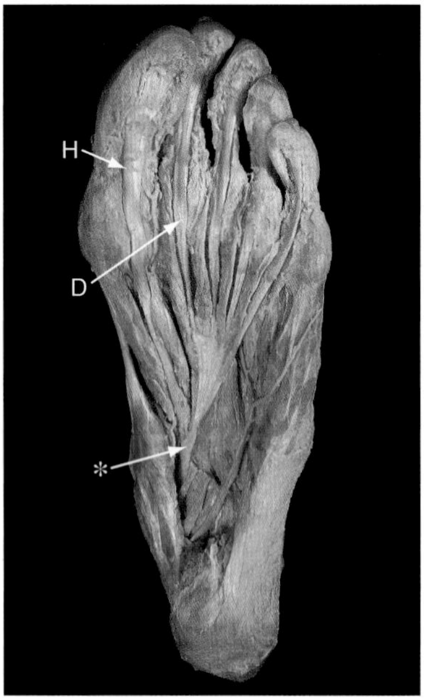


**Fig. 10.12** Prosection of the foot showing the long flexor tendons
D = flexor digitorum longus (FDL) tendon, H = flexor hallucis longus (FHL) tendon, * = tendons of FHL and FDL, which lie adjacent to the sustentaculum tali at this point (From Gosling JA, Harris PF, Whitmore I, Willan PLT. 2002 Human Anatomy, 4th edn. London: Mosby)

# LOCATING SOFT TISSUES

- Plantar aponeurosis
- Heel fat pad
- Dorsalis pedis artery

The **plantar aponeurosis** and **heel fat pad** are shown in the prosection in Figure 10.13.

## PLANTAR APONEUROSIS

With the subject lying supine on the couch, legs extended and feet in neutral position, the digital slips passing to the bases of the toes can be readily palpated. Placing the fingers of one hand firmly across the sole just proximal to

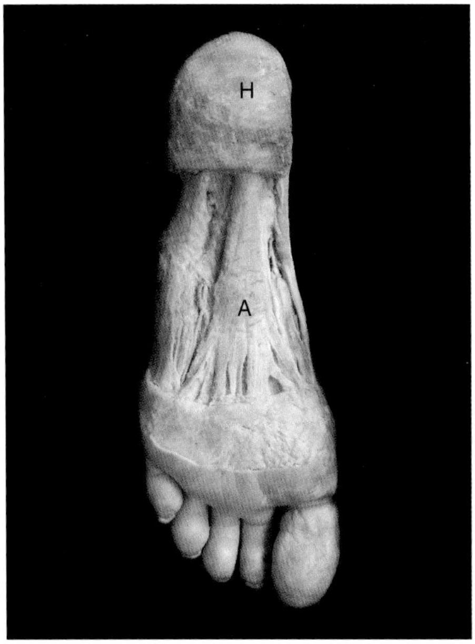


Fig. 10.13 Prosection showing the plantar aponeurosis and heel fat pad
A = plantar aponeurosis with digital slips, H = heel fat pad

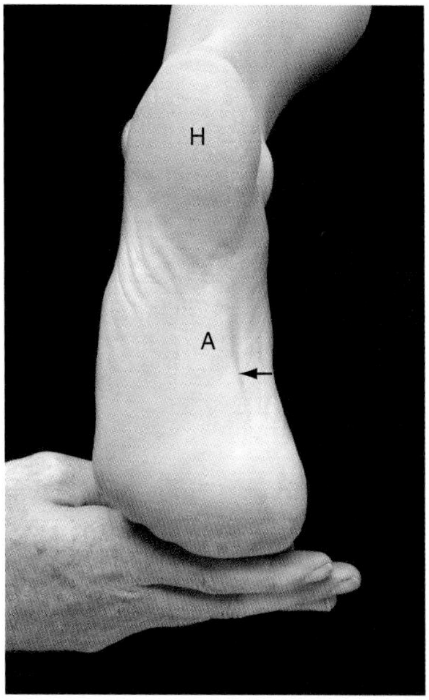


Fig. 10.14 Palpating the plantar aponeurosis in the living subject
A = plantar aponeurosis tensed by dorsiflexing the toes (medial edge indicated by the arrow), H = heel fat pad

the ball of the foot, the examiner uses the other hand to extend the toes forcibly. The aponeurosis can be seen to tense under the skin (Fig. 10.14), and the slips can be felt to tighten as the toes are extended.

## HEEL FAT PAD

The subject lies prone on the couch. The heel pad can be defined by the examiner gripping and squeezing the medial and lateral borders of the lower heel between thumb and index finger, and the thickness can be gauged by pressing firmly upward against the calcaneum with the pad of a thumb (Fig. 10.15).

## DORSALIS PEDIS ARTERY

The subject may be seated or lying on a couch. The extensor hallucis longus tendon provides a landmark for the artery, which lies lateral to it. Whilst the subject extends the great toe, the pulsations are located on the dorsum of the foot distal to the ankle, the examiner placing the pads of the index and middle fingers across the line of the artery.

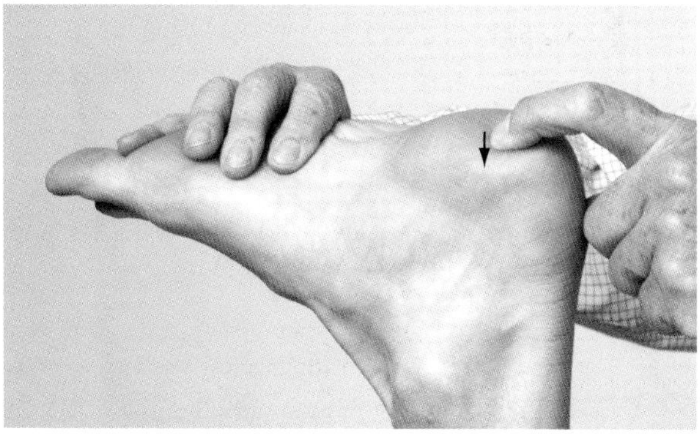

Fig. 10.15 Palpating the heel fat pad
Deep pressure impinges on the medial calcaneal tubercle

# TESTING JOINT MOVEMENTS

- Inversion and eversion
- Digital movements:
  Great toe
  Other toes

## INVERSION AND EVERSION

These movements have an oblique axis passing from the back of the calcaneum upward, forward, and medially through the head of the talus, each movement having three components. These are medial rotation, adduction, and plantar flexion with inversion, and lateral rotation, abduction, and dorsiflexion with eversion. The subject is examined sitting with the feet dependent. Active movements are tested first, followed by passive. The examiner cups a heel in one hand and, with the other, grips the more medial digits, firmly rotating the foot inward and then outward. Inversion has a greater range compared with eversion (Fig. 10.16). Two components, abduction and adduction, can be isolated and tested separately. Whilst cupping the heel in one hand, the examiner grips the toes and turns the foot horizontally, first outward (abduction, average about 10°) and then inward (adduction, average about 20°).

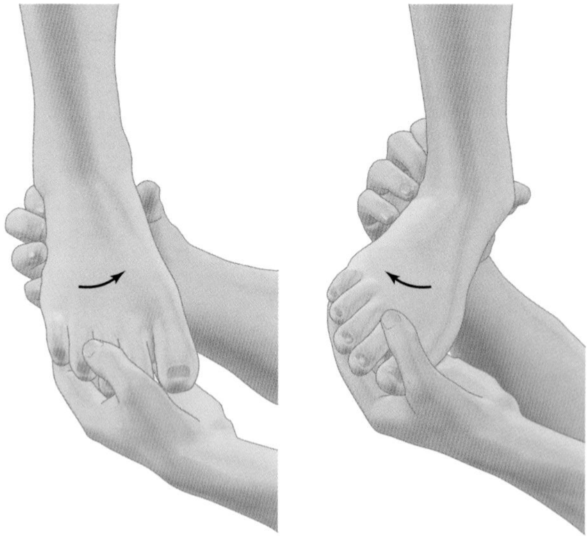

## DIGITAL MOVEMENTS

It is more practical if the examiner tests these movements passively with the subject lying supine on a couch, grasping the end of the toe between finger and thumb.

### GREAT TOE

Starting from neutral, the metatarso-phalangeal joint can be plantar flexed to about 45°; dorsiflexion is greater at 70°. At the interphalangeal joint, up to 90° flexion can be achieved.

### OTHER TOES

Greater movement occurs at the most distal joint, with 60° plantar flexion at the distal interphalangeal, and about 40° at the proximal interphalangeal and metatarso-phalangeal joints.

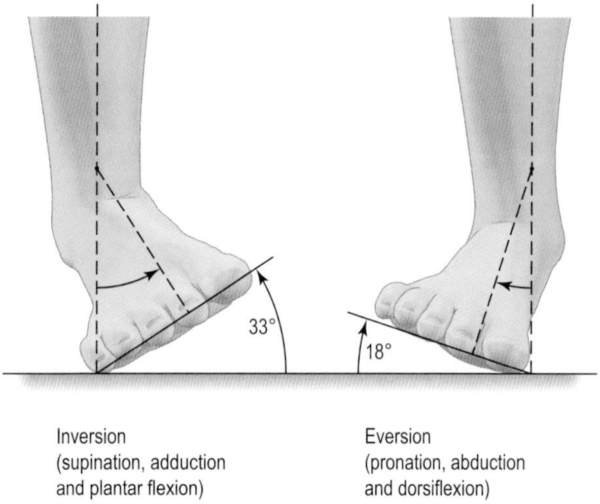


**Fig. 10.16** Diagram of the average range of movements of inversion and eversion of the foot (Redrawn from *Joint motion: method of measuring and recording.* Edinburgh: E&S Livingstone, 1965 (with the permission of the American Academy of Orthopedic Surgeons, reprinted with their permission by the British Orthopaedic Association))

# INNERVATION

- Dermatomes
- Peripheral nerves

Sensory innervation can be tested using light touch or pin-prick, with the subject lying supine on the couch and the lower limbs extended.

## DERMATOMES

The dermatomes of the lower limb involve spinal segments L1–S4 and are shown in Figure 10.17. The pattern is simple and can be easily rehearsed. A hand placed over the front of the thigh below the inguinal ligament covers L1 territory; about mid-thigh is L2; over the distal thigh, above the patella, is L3. The medial side of the leg from knee to malleolus is L4 territory; L5 extends from the lateral side of the knee distally across the front of the leg

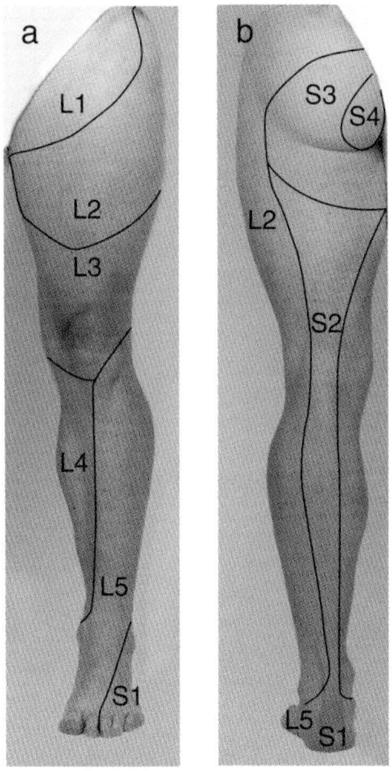


Fig. 10.17 Dermatomes of the lower limb
a Anterior surface. b Posterior surface

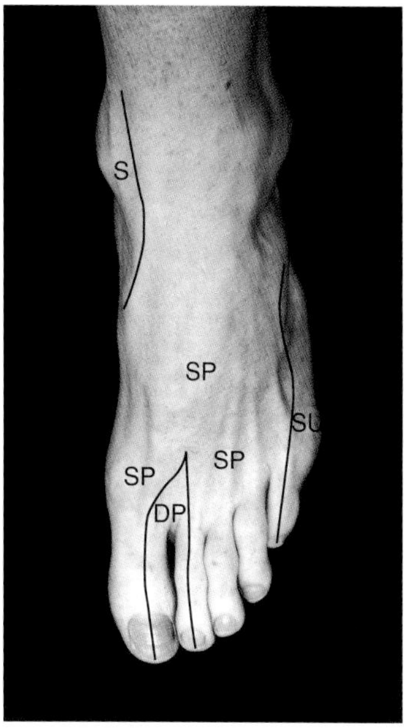


Fig. 10.18 Peripheral nerve innervation of the dorsum of the foot
DP = deep peroneal nerve, S = saphenous nerve, SP = superficial peroneal nerve, SU = sural nerve

on to the medial part of the foot. The lateral side of the foot and footprint area on the sole (the "standing" area) are S1 territory; an extensive area up the back of the leg and thigh is S2; S3 covers the buttock region (the "sitting" area); and S4 is the perineum.

## PERIPHERAL NERVES

Peripheral nerve distributions in the foot are shown in Figure 10.18. The whole of the dorsum is supplied by the superficial peroneal nerve, except for the web area between the great and second toes, which is supplied by the deep peroneal nerve. The medial border of the foot below the malleolus is supplied by the saphenous nerve, but this does not extend on to the great toe, which is supplied by the superficial peroneal nerve. The whole of the lateral border of the foot, including the little toe, is supplied by the sural nerve. On the sole of the foot, the heel region is supplied by calcaneal branches of the tibial nerve, whilst the lateral plantar nerve supplies skin of the lateral $1\frac{1}{2}$ toes and an equivalent area over the midfoot, with the medial plantar nerve supplying the medial $3\frac{1}{2}$ toes and an equivalent area over the midfoot.

# SPECIAL TESTS

- Flexor hallucis longus
- Tarsal tunnel
- Morton's neuroma
- Plantar fasciitis
- Lisfranc's joint
- Foot alignment

The subject lies supine on the couch, with legs extended and feet at 90° to the leg.

## FLEXOR HALLUCIS LONGUS TENDINOPATHY

The examiner palpates firmly over the flexor hallucis longus tendon, with the index finger about 2 cm behind the medial malleolus. The other hand grips the great toe and forcibly extends it (see Fig. 9.19). This causes pain in the presence of tendinopathy.

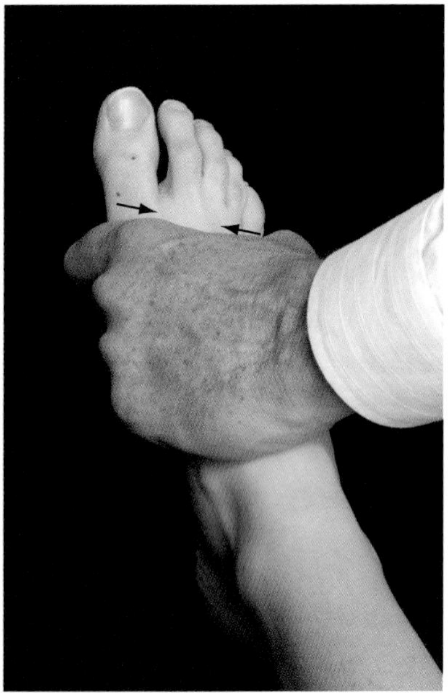

Fig. 10.19 Testing for Morton's neuroma
Compression is applied by a firm grip across the forefoot

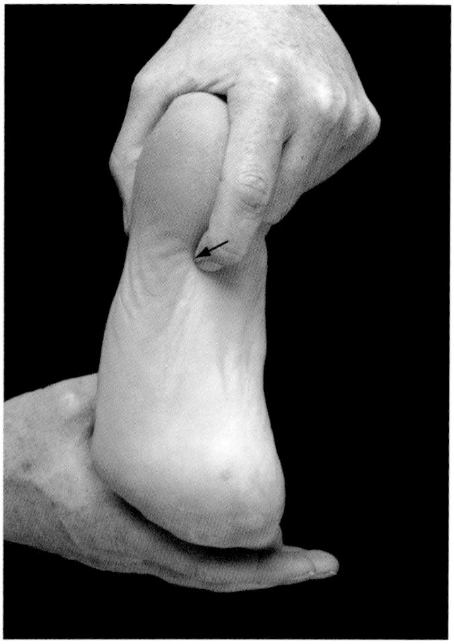

Fig. 10.20 Testing for plantar fasciitis
Deep pressure is applied close to the calcaneal attachment of the plantar aponeurosis

## TINEL'S SIGN

The tip of one finger can be used to percuss the tibial nerve as it passes inferior to the tip of the medial malleolus of the tibia. Reproduction of paresthesia (tingling, pins and needles, or anesthesia) distal to the site of percussion may be associated with tarsal tunnel syndrome. The peroneal nerve and the sural nerve may both be damaged with lateral ankle sprains, and can be tested in the same fashion by percussion: the peroneal at the neck of the fibula, and the sural where it passes behind and below the lateral malleolus.

## MORTON'S NEUROMA (METATARSALGIA)

Essentially, the test compresses the heads of the metatarsals together by applying pressure. The whole forefoot can be squeezed by a hand spanning the dorsum of the foot just behind the roots of the toes (Fig. 10.19), or the flat of one hand is firmly pressed against each border of the foot, squeezing tightly opposite the roots of the toes. Alternatively, whilst steadying the foot, the examiner uses the palmar surface of the fingers on one hand to extend the toes forcibly. This stretches the digital nerves over the deep transverse metatarsal ligaments, causing pain if a neuroma is present.

## PLANTAR FASCIITIS

With the subject lying prone, the knee flexed 90° and the feet at 90° to the leg, the examiner uses one hand to dorsiflex the toes forcibly in order to tense the plantar fascia. The thumb of the other hand is used to palpate for any tenderness of the plantar fascia; palpation should commence at its origin on the anterior calcaneus and move anteriorly along its length. In the presence of plantar fasciitis, tenderness is most commonly found just anterior to the origin (Fig. 10.20).

## STABILITY OF THE TARSO-METATARSAL (LISFRANC'S) JOINT

With the subject lying prone, the examiner stabilizes the tarsus by gripping it with the thumb over the dorsal

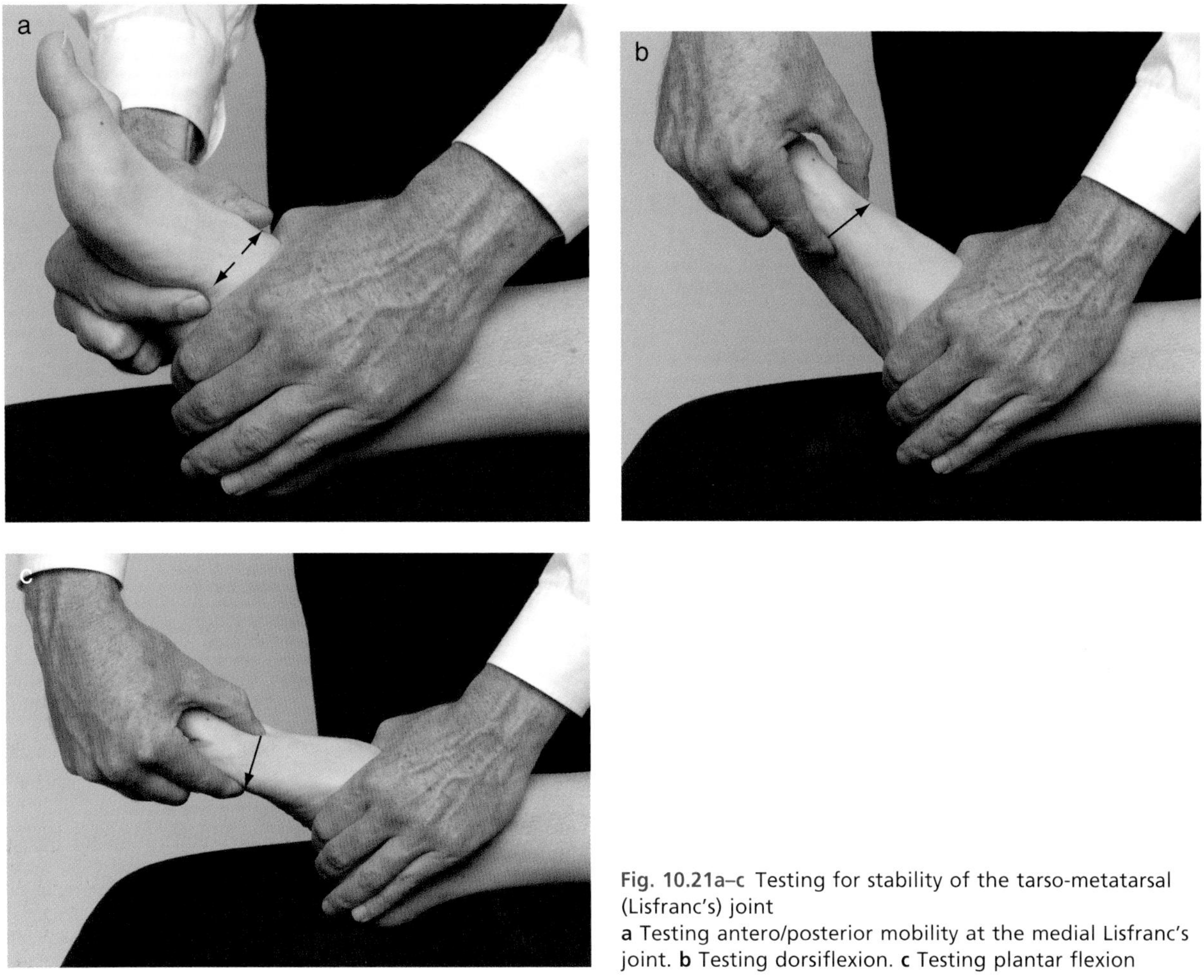


**Fig. 10.21a–c** Testing for stability of the tarso-metatarsal (Lisfranc's) joint
**a** Testing antero/posterior mobility at the medial Lisfranc's joint. **b** Testing dorsiflexion. **c** Testing plantar flexion

aspect of the distal row of tarsals and the fingers under the plantar aspect. The examiner's other hand then grips the base of the first metatarsal between thumb and forefinger, and assesses the degree of passive antero-posterior glide of this bone on the medial cuneiform (Fig. 10.21a). With the same grip, the degree of passive plantar and dorsiflexion of the joint is also assessed by moving the metatarsal on the medial cuneiform in both these directions (Fig. 10.21b and c). These tests, for laxity or stiffness, are repeated at each of the other four tarso-metatarsal joints.

## FOOT ALIGNMENT

The subject stands on a platform or couch, facing away from the examiner who observes the profiles of the feet, ankles, and Achilles tendons for asymmetry or malalignment (see Fig. 9.3).

The test is repeated following positioning of the talus in a neutral position. To do this, facing the subject, the examiner grips the talus between thumb and forefinger. The subject is then asked to invert or evert the foot actively (Fig. 10.22), stopping when the examiner can palpate both the medial and lateral talar processes. Foot alignment should also be examined with the subject standing on tip-toe.

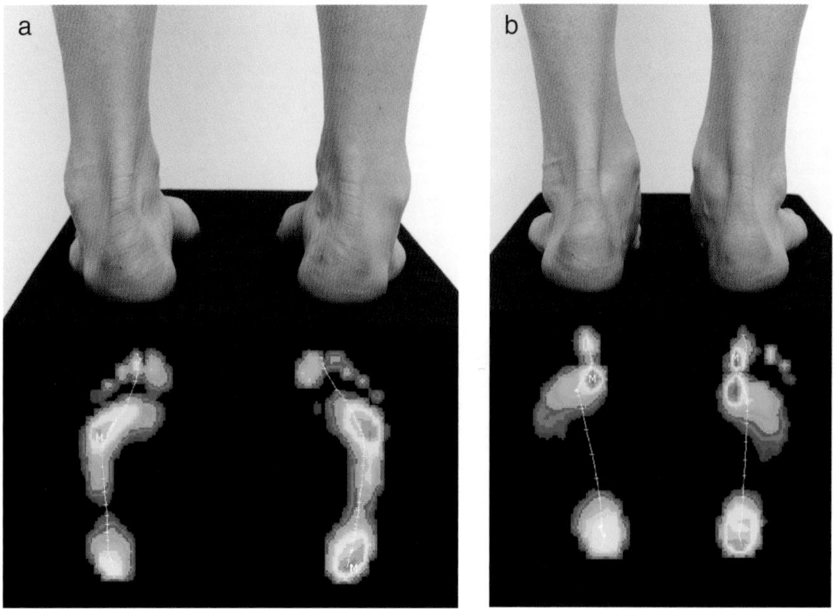


**Fig. 10.22a and b** Assessing foot and ankle alignment
**a** Ankle inversion and foot supination with matching pedobarograph. **b** Ankle eversion and foot pronation with matching pedobarograph
Note: the colors indicating different pressures are explained in Figure 10.2b

## FURTHER READING


Bradshaw C, Khan K, Brukner P. Stress fracture of the body of the talus in athletes demonstrated with computer tomography. Clinical Journal of Sport Medicine 1996; 6:48–51.

Dyck DD, Boyajian–O'Neill LA. Plantar fasciitis. Clinical Journal of Sport Medicine 2004; 14:305–309.

Fredericson M, Standage S, Chou L et al. Lateral plantar nerve entrapment in a competitive gymnast. Clinical Journal of Sport Medicine 2001; 11:111–114.

Roehrig GJ, McFarland EG, Cosgarea AJ et al. Unusual stress fracture of the fifth metatarsal in a basketball player. Clinical Journal of Sport Medicine 2001; 11:271–273.

Saxena A, Fullem B. Plantar fascia rupture in athletes. American Journal of Sports Medicine 2004; 32:662–665.

Stavinoha RR, Scott W. Osteonecrosis of the tarsal navicular in two adolescent soccer players. Clinical Journal of Sport Medicine 1998; 8:136–141.

Warren ET, Armen JH, Booher MA. Unusual cause of midfoot pain in a pole vaulter. Clinical Journal of Sport Medicine 2004; 14:360–361.

## CASE STUDY 10 • CLINICAL PROBLEMS

**Problem 1.** *A 30-year-old male 400 m hurdler has sudden sharp pain in the right medial sole of his outside (right) foot when hurdling a barrier during the first 100 m bend of a race.*

a) What are two possible diagnoses?

**Problem 2.** *A 26-year-old netball player experiences central forefoot pain whenever she runs. Her physical therapist suggests that she might have a Morton's metatarsalgia. As a precaution, an MRI scan is taken (Fig. 10.23). This reveals periostitis of the neck of the third metatarsal, with associated bone marrow edema (white arrow).*

a) What is Morton's metatarsalgia?
b) What test can be used for this condition?
c) What other symptom might also be present in this condition?
d) Given the findings in the MRI scan and the absence of paresthesia, what is the most likely diagnosis?

**Problem 3.** *A 45-year-old male tennis player complains of pain in the posterior sole of the foot when sprinting. The foot is often painful to walk on first thing in the morning.*

a) What are at least two possible causes of these symptoms?
b) How can the plantar fascia be placed under tension in order to palpate it effectively?
c) What is a possible complication of plantar fasciitis?

**Problem 4.** *A 25-year-old male field hockey player is told he has turf toe.*

a) What is turf toe and which joint needs to be examined?
b) On what type of playing surface does this condition commonly occur?

**Problem 5.** *A 17-year-old female cross-country runner complains of gradually worsening medial foot pain that now prevents her from running.*

a) Name at least two possible diagnoses.
b) Which tendon insertion should be examined and how is it located?
c) What systemic conditions that make up the so-called "female athletic triad" might also be associated with lower limb stress fracture in elite female athletes?

**Problem 6.** *A professional football (soccer) player continues to complain of lateral mid-hindfoot pain 8 weeks after a grade II lateral ankle sprain. There is no ankle joint instability or swelling, and there is full ROM.*

a) What are at least two conditions that could be causing the player's foot pain?
b) Where can the cuboid be located in the living subject?

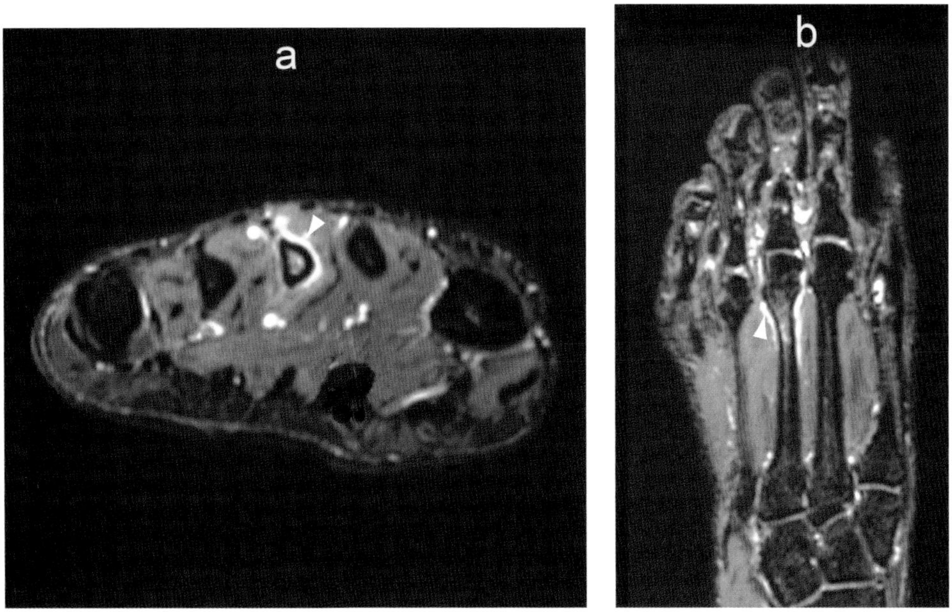


Fig. 10.23a Coronal and b axial MRI scans of a foot injury

# Answers to clinical problems

## CHAPTER 1

**Problem 1**

a) Zygoma or zygomatic arch.
b) Injury to the zygomatico-facial nerve.
c) Paralysis of the buccinator muscle.
d) Ask the patient to make sucking movements to test cranial nerve VII.

**Problem 2**

a) An orbital plate of the maxilla.
b) Blow-out fracture of orbital floor.
c) Damage to the infra-orbital nerve lying in the groove in the orbital floor.
d) Upward and outward due to disruption of the attachment of the inferior oblique muscle to the medial part of the orbital floor.

**Problem 3**

a) Maxilla; mandible and nasal bones.
b) LeFort's classification; group 1.
c) Gentle traction on the front teeth/tooth, pulling forward to detect any movement.
d) Chest radiograph.

**Problem 4**

a) Traction of the brachial plexus/cervical nerve roots.
b) Upper limb tension tests; ULTT1.
c) C6.
d) (i) Upper trapezius, scalenes, levator scapulae;
(ii) cervical facet (zygapophyseal) joints, cervical intervertebral discs, sterno-clavicular joint.

**Problem 5**

a) Masseter.
b) Elevates the mandible (closes the mouth); the subject clenches the teeth tightly whilst the examiner palpates over the muscle.
c) Parotid duct/gland; facial artery.
d) Temporo-mandibular joint. Hinging: palpation of the TMJ and observation of front tooth symmetry when the mouth is opened with the tongue resting on the roof of the mouth. Gliding: wide mouth opening with the tongue relaxed.

**Problem 6**

a) Larynx.
b) Laryngeal cartilages: thyroid (laryngeal) prominence, cricoid arch. Palpate for pain, crepitation and undue mobility, and check the groove for the median crico-thyroid ligament.
c) Laryngeal edema with potential occlusion of the airway (glottis).

## CHAPTER 2

**Problem 1**

a) Left low lumbar (L4 or L5) pars interarticularis stress fracture.
b) A left low lumbar facet joint strain; paraspinal muscle sprain; low lumbar intervertebral disc derangement; sacro-iliac joint dysfunction.
c) Stork test.
d) Magnetic resonance imaging (MRI) to identify any stress reaction (bone edema +/– stress fracture). Computed tomography (CT) might then be required to delineate the extent of the stress fracture.
e) Rest from aggravating activities for 8–12 weeks with graduated rehabilitation of trunk muscle function, followed by a graduated return to sport.

**Problem 2**

a) Mid–low thoracic wedge fracture.
b) Mid-thoracic disc herniation; disruption of the posterior spinal ligaments (e.g. posterior longitudinal); erector spinae muscle strain.
c) Female; aged over 55; dietary deficiencies.
d) Boston brace for 8–12 weeks.

**Problem 3**

a) Compression or irritation of the L5 nerve root; compromise of the sciatic or common peroneal nerve; referred pain from a central spine injury, e.g. lower lumbar disc derangement.
b) Stenosis of the lower lumbar spinal canal; herniation of a lower lumbar intervertebral disc; impingement of the sciatic nerve as it passes through or adjacent to the piriformis muscle (piriformis syndrome).
c) L5.
d) No.
e) Posterior protrusion of L4/5 intervertebral disc.

**Problem 4**

a) The sacro-iliac joint.
b) Beneath the sacral (Venus's) dimple.
c) Faber test.
d) Laxity of the lumbo-pelvic ligaments due to high levels of the hormone relaxin; stretching or disruption, and subsequent dysfunction, of muscles that stabilize the lumbo-pelvic region, e.g. the pelvic floor musculature, the transversus abdominis; strain of pelvic, lumbo-sacral and/or lumbo-pelvic ligaments during childbirth; deconditioning of the lumbo-pelvic stabilizing musculature due to a layoff from training immediately pre- and post-partum.

**Problem 5**

a) Bruising of the erector spinae muscles; fracture of a left lumbar vertebral transverse process.
b) No.
c) Trauma to the left kidney.

**Problem 6**

a) Spinal stenosis due to osteophytic ingrowth into the spinal canal.
b) No, flexion of the spine during the slump test increases the diameter of the spinal canal, relieving the nerve tension caused by spinal stenosis.
c) Surgical decompression of the spinal canal.

## CHAPTER 3

**Problem 1**

a) Costal cartilage fracture.
b) Costo-chondral subluxation; rib fracture.
c) Costal cartilage fracture.
d) Pectoralis major.
e) Costo-transverse joints, rib shaft, costo-chondral junctions.
f) Simultaneous manual compression of the anterior and posterior chest wall.

**Problem 2**

a) Anterior abdominal wall tear adjacent to the superficial inguinal ring; osteitis pubis; adductor longus tendinopathy; inguinal hernia.
b) Pain with coughing; pain with sit-ups.
c) Long and short adductor muscle test; fist squeeze test; external inguinal ring palpation.

**Problem 3**

a) Acute left rectus abdominis strain.
b) Abdominal hernia; psoas strain.
c) Forceful contraction of the muscle whilst it is in an elongated position.

**Problem 4**

a) Left internal oblique.
b) Fast bowling in cricket; tennis.
c) Intercostal muscle strain; external oblique strain; rib fracture; rib osteochondritis.

**Problem 5**

a) Transient hypertrophy of the obturator internus and externus, causing obturator nerve compression in the obturator canal.
b) Paresthesia to light touch over the medial thigh; obturator nerve conduction studies; adductor muscle weakness.
c) Slump test with hip abduction (obturator nerve bias).

## CHAPTER 4

**Problem 1**

a) Subacromial impingement syndrome.
b) Supraspinatus and infraspinatus tendon; long head of biceps tendon; shoulder joint line.
c) Neer's test; Hawkins–Kennedy test; relocation test; empty can test.

**Problem 2**

a) Shoulder capsule, anterior labrum, humeral head (Hill Sach's lesion), axillary nerve.
b) Sulcus sign; drawer test; apprehension test; full can test (deltoid muscle power test).

**Problem 3**

a) Acromio-clavicular.
b) Acromio-clavicular joint sprain.
c) Clavicular fracture; shoulder joint dislocation; fracture of the acromion process.

**Problem 4**

a) **S**uperior **L**abral **A**nterior **P**osterior.
b) Long head of biceps brachii.
c) Yergason's test and Speed's test.

**Problem 5**

a) Subscapularis.
b) Lift-off test, belly press test.

**Problem 6**

a) Supraspinatus.
b) Empty can test.
c) Hawkins–Kennedy impingement test.

## CHAPTER 5

**Problem 1**

a) Rupture of the ulnar collateral ligament of the elbow.
b) High-velocity valgus stress on the medial elbow.
c) Avulsion of one of the muscles of the common flexor origin; traction injury of the ulnar nerve.
d) Open surgical repair.

**Problem 2**

a) Extensor carpi radialis brevis.
b) Resisted middle finger extension with the elbow extended, forearm pronated and wrist in neutral.
c) Tendinosis.
d) Use a double-handed backhand; *or* alter the grip to reduce the stretch and stress on the lateral elbow structures; *or* change racket grip size; *or* use a racket that has better shock absorption.

**Problem 3**

a) Golfer's elbow.
b) Tendons of the common flexor origin; ulnar collateral ligament; ulnar nerve.
c) Varus stress on the structures of the common flexor origin.

**Problem 4**

a) Olecranon bursitis.
b) Olecranon fracture.

**Problem 5**

a) Little Leaguer's elbow.
b) Partial or complete avulsion of the medial apophysis; osteochondritis dissecans of the articular cartilage and subchondral bone of the lateral capitulum and radial head; avulsion of the posterior olecranon epiphysis; stress fracture of the proximal ulna; ulnar nerve neuritis.

**Problem 6**

a) Ulnar dislocation at the elbow.
b) Elbow fracture (ulna, radius, or humerus).
c) Rupture or occlusion of the vasculature of the cubital fossa; ulnar nerve injury; chronic elbow instability.

**Problem 7**

a) Ulnar collateral ligament stress test, UCL 90/90 stress test and the moving valgus stress test.
b) Medial epicondylitis — fist squeeze with resisted wrist flexion; ulnar neuritis — Tinel's sign.

## CHAPTER 6

**Problem 1**

a) Tear of the triangular fibro-cartilage complex (TFCC).
b) TFCC test; grip strength test.
c) Palmaris longus insertion tear; ulna-carpal joint sprain; luno-triquetral ligament strain/instability.

**Problem 2**

a) Scaphoid fracture; distal radius fracture; radio-carpal joint sprain; flexor carpi radialis avulsion.
b) Palpation of the scaphoid in the anatomical "snuff box"; the injury should continue to be managed as a scaphoid fracture until follow-up investigations exclude this condition.
c) Malunion; avascular necrosis of the proximal scaphoid.

**Problem 3**

a) Mallet finger.
b) Resisted distal phalanx dorsiflexion to test extensor digitorum muscle power.
c) Splint immobilization with the DIP joint in extension, day and night, for approximately 6–8 weeks. Larger or more complicated fractures may require internal fixation and then post-operative splinting.

**Problem 4**

a) Paresthesia (numbness, tingling, pins and needles, burning) in the median nerve sensory distribution of the hand, i.e. the radial palm, thumb, palmar index middle and radial half of the ring finger; weakness of finger flexion (especially middle and index finger)
b) Sensory testing of the median nerve distribution in the hand (sharp–blunt discrimination, light touch, hot–cold discrimination); strength testing of flexor digitorum superficialis and flexor digitorum profundus (radial digits); Phalen's test; Tinel's sign — percussion over the carpal tunnel.
c) Proximal median nerve injury (low cervical disc protrusion causing nerve root impingement, median nerve compression at the elbow (ligament of Struthers), median nerve compression by pronator quadratus); flexor digitorum superficialis or flexor digitorum profundus tenosynovitis; mid-carpal instability.

**Problem 5**

a) The ulnar nerve.
b) Guyon's canal.
c) Weakness in performing the precision grip.

**Problem 6**

a) Forced hyperextension of the PIP joint of the little finger.
b) Fracture of the proximal part of the middle phalanx with dislocation of the PIP joint.
c) The volar plate and flexor digitorum superficialis tendon.
d) Reduction under anesthetic, followed by surgical internal fixation and post-operative splinting.

## CHAPTER 7

**Problem 1**

a) Avulsion of the insertion of ilio-psoas; avulsion of the origin of rectus femoris or sartorius; tear of the proximal rectus femoris.
b) Modified Thomas test.
c) In the modified Thomas test position, the short hip flexors are tested by resisting hip flexion; the long hip flexors (rectus femoris) can be tested by simultaneously resisting hip flexion and knee extension.

**Problem 2**

a) Hamstrings.
b) Gluteus maximus: resisted hip extension with the knee straight; hamstrings: resisted hip extension with the knee flexed 90°.

**Problem 3**

a) Piriformis.
b) Find the midpoint of the line joining the dimple over the PSIS to the tip of the coccyx. Piriformis is located by drawing a second line from this midpoint to the top of the greater trochanter.
c) Direct compression from sitting on a hard boat seat for prolonged periods; lower lumbar disc protrusion on to the sciatic nerve roots; sciatic nerve compression in the posterior thigh compartment due to transient hypertrophy of the hamstrings.
d) Slump test.

**Problem 4**

a) Intramuscular hematoma of vastus lateralis.
b) Flexion, because the muscle sheath will be drawn taught compressing the muscle, thereby limiting the amount of swelling.
c) Short-term: acute compartment syndrome; long-term: heterotropic ossification.

**Problem 5**

a) Acetabular labrum.
b) Posterior abdominal wall (tear or herniation); inguinal ligament; adductor muscle origins; symphysis pubis; rectus abdominis insertion.
c) Faber test; restricted internal and/or external hip joint passive rotation; hip flexion/adduction with over-pressure

## CHAPTER 8

**Problem 1**

a) Anterior cruciate ligament rupture.
b) Lachman's test.
c) Medial collateral ligament; medial meniscus.
d) Medial collateral ligament valgus stress test; McMurray's test.

**Problem 2**

a) Patellar tendinopathy (Fig. 8.26); Sinding–Larsen–Johannsen disease (traction osteochondritis of the apex of the patella); fat pad impingement; patello-femoral pain; Osgood–Schlatter's disease.
b) Patella, especially the apex; tibial tuberosity and patellar ligament; medial and lateral fat pads.
c) Quadriceps.

**Problem 3**

a) Medial collateral ligament.
b) Medial meniscus; anterior cruciate ligament; pes anserinus tendons; knee joint capsule.
c) Wipe test. A small, slow-developing effusion indicates that there is no hemarthrosis like that associated with anterior cruciate ligament rupture.

**Problem 4**

a) Inflammation of the pre-patellar bursa.
b) Pre-patellar bursitis.

**Problem 5**

a) Patello-femoral dysfunction.
b) Patella tracking/apprehension test.

**Problem 6**

a) The lateral meniscus.
b) Lateral rotation of the tibia.
c) Meniscectomy.

**Problem 7**

a) Biceps femoris tendon and muscle; lateral head of gastrocnemius.

## CHAPTER 9

**Problem 1**

a) Anterior talo-fibular ligament +/– calcaneo-fibular ligament sprain.
b) Anterior drawer; talar tilt (ankle inversion).
c) Distal fibula fracture; talar dome fracture; peroneal tendon dislocation; peroneus brevis avulsion; tibio-fibular syndesmosis strain.
d) Inability to weight-bear on the affected limb; tenderness on palpation of the posterior aspect of either the medial or lateral malleolus; tenderness on palpation of the base of the fifth metatarsal.
e) Talar dome fracture; bifurcate ligament strain; tibio-fibular syndesmosis strain; peroneal nerve injury; sinus tarsi syndrome.

**Problem 2**

a) Deltoid ligament.
b) Talar tilt (ankle eversion).

**Problem 3**

a) Ruptured Achilles tendon.
b) Calf squeeze test; inspection of the foot angle with patient in prone lying with feet over the end of the couch; palpation for a defect of the musculo-tendinous junction of the Achilles tendon with the gastrocnemius muscle.
c) Approximately 20° plantar flexion.

**Problem 4**

a) Posterior ankle impingement.
b) A prominent posterior tubercle (Steida's process) of the talus; an os trigonum.
c) Steida's process.
d) Flexor hallucis longus tendon; capsule of posterior subtalar (talo-calcaneal) joint; posterior ankle fat pad; retrocalcaneal bursa.
e) Passive ankle plantar flexion.

**Problem 5**

a) Osteophyte(s) in the anterior subtalar joint.
b) Passive end-range dorsiflexion.

**Problem 6**

a) Pain and tightness in the antero-lateral region of the leg triggered by running and relieved by rest; numbness in the lower anterior part of the leg extending on to the dorsum of the foot and occasionally in the web between the great and second toes.
b) Intra-compartment pressure testing using manometry before, during, and after the aggravating activity.
c) Anterior compartment; deep posterior compartment; superficial posterior compartment.

## CHAPTER 10

**Problem 1**

a) Strain or rupture of the plantar fascia; sprain of a medial tarso-metatarsal (Lisfranc's) joint; adductor hallucis strain.

**Problem 2**

a) Forefoot pain caused by an interdigital nerve neuroma. Most frequently, the neuroma is formed between the distal ends of the third and fourth metatarsals.
b) Forefoot squeeze test or hyperextension of toes.
c) Paresthesia between the toes.
d) Metatarsal stress fracture.

**Problem 3**

a) Plantar fasciitis; heel fat pad inflammation; calcaneal stress fracture.
b) By holding the hallux in dorsiflexion whilst the subject is lying prone with the knee flexed to 90° and the foot and ankle held in plantar-grade.
c) Rupture of the plantar fascia.

**Problem 4**

a) Sprain of the first metatarso-phalangeal joint due to hyperextension of the hallux.
b) Artificial turf.

**Problem 5**

a) Navicular stress fracture; tarsal tunnel syndrome; tibialis anterior insertion strain.
b) Invert the foot and locate the most medial tendon crossing the front of the ankle, tracing it to its attachment to the base of the first metatarsal and adjacent medial cuneiform.
c) Amenorrhea; osteoporosis; anorexia.

**Problem 6**

a) Sinus tarsi syndrome; cuboid syndrome; peroneus brevis insertional tendinopathy or partial avulsion; peroneal nerve neuropathy.
b) In the recess on the lateral border of the foot immediately behind the base of the fifth metatarsal.

# Index

NB: page numbers in italic refer to figures; for case studies, the main page number is followed by one in brackets indicating the answer — e.g. 70 (176a)

## A



## B



## C



## D

## E



## F



## G



## H

## I



## J



## K



## L



## M

## T

## ELSEVIER DVD-ROM LICENCE AGREEMENT

## Minimum system requirements

### Windows®
Windows 2000 or higher
1.4 Ghz processor
128 MB RAM
4× DVD-ROM drive
VGA Monitor supporting 800×600 at millions of colours

### Macintosh®
Apple G4 Macintosh
Mac OS 9.1 or later
128 MB RAM
4× DVD-ROM drive
VGA Monitor supporting 800×600 at millions of colours

NB: No data is transferred to the hard disk.
The DVD-ROM is self-contained and the application runs directly from the DVD-ROM.

## Installation instructions

### Windows®
If your system does not support Autorun, navigate to your DVD drive and double click on 'Start.exe' to begin.
Alternatively, click Start, Run and type 'D:Start.exe' to begin. If D: is not your DVD drive, substitute D: with the appropriate drive letter.

### Macintosh®
If the DVD does not autorun, open the DVD icon that appears on the desktop and select 'Start' to begin.

## Using this Product
This product is designed to run with Internet Explorer 6.0 or later (PC) and Netscape 4.5 or later (Mac). Please refer to the help files on those programs for problems specific to the browser.

To use some of the functions on the DVD, the user must have the following:

a. DVD requires "Java Runtime Environment" to be installed in your system to use "Export" and "Slide Show" features. DVD automatically checks for "Java Runtime Environment" version 1.4.1 or later (PC) and MRJ 2.2.5 (Mac) if not available, it starts installing from the DVD. Please complete the installation process. Then click on the license agreement to proceed. "Java Runtime Environment" is available in the DVD Software folder. If the user manually install the software, please make sure that the user start the application by clicking the appropriate exe file.
b. Your browser needs to be Java-enabled. If the user did not enable Java when installing your browser, the user may need to download some additional files from your browser manufacturer.
c. If your system does not support Autorun, then please explore the DVD contents click on 'Start.exe' to start.

Acrobat Reader can be installed from the Software folder of the DVD.

## Viewing Images
You can view images by chapter and export images to PowerPoint or an HTML presentation. Full details are available in the Help section of the DVD-ROM.

## Frequently Asked Questions (FAQ)

### Do I need to have internet connection to run this program?
No. The program is designed to run entirely from the DVD-ROM, independent of the Internet. However the disk may contain some links to material on the Internet (website link) and to view this material you will require an Internet connection.

### When I launch the application, I get messages after N[illegible]arts. What do I do?
TCP/IP is required to run any browserbased application. TCP/IP is n[illegible]ith Windows 95, 98 and NT. To add TCP/IP in Windows 95/98/NT, go to Network in the Control Panel. Click the Add button. Click the prot[illegible]ion and click Add. Under manufacturers, select Microsoft and under Network Protrocols, select TCP/IP and click OK. Click OK again and Wi[illegible] will start to install TCP/IP. When finished you will have to restart your machine.

### What should I do if when I launch the application my ISP starts to dial out?
This application is able to run with or without a connection to the Internet. If your ISP starts to dial out, you can cancel this and the program will still run. Many ISPs will automatically dial out when a browser is launched. You may be able to turn this option off in the properties for your ISP.

### When opening the DVD-ROM in Internet Explorer on the Mac my default home page opens. What should I do?
When you run the DVD-ROM in Internet Explorer on the Mac two windows are opened — your default home page and the opening page of the DVD-ROM. Simply close the window that contains your default home page. We recommend, however, that Mac users view the DVD-ROM in Netscape.

### The export function is not working properly. What should I do?
The Export feature requires the DVD-ROM Server to run in the background. The Server application requires the "Java Runtime Environment" to be installed in the system. The Server can be started manually by selecting 'server.exe' in Windows and 'server' application in MacOS.

## Technical Support
Technical support for this product is available between 7.30 a.m. and 7.00 p.m. CST, Monday through Friday.
Before calling, be sure that your computer meets the minimum system requirements to run this software.
Inside the United States and Canada, call 1-800-692-9010.
Inside the United Kingdom, call 00-800-692-90100.
Outside North America, call +1-314-872-8370.
You may also fax your questions to +1-314-997-5080,
or contact Technical Support through e-mail: technical.support@elsevier.com.